AF773343

Atlas of Gynaecological Pathology

Current Histopathology

Consultant Editor
Professor G. Austin Gresham, TD, ScD, MD, FRC Path.
Professor of Morbid Anatomy and Histology, University of Cambridge

Volume Five

ATLAS OF GYNAECOLOGICAL PATHOLOGY

BY H. FOX and C.H. BUCKLEY
Department of Pathology
University of Manchester

MTP PRESS LIMITED · LANCASTER · ENGLAND
International Medical Publishers

Published by
MTP Press Limited
Falcon House
Cable Street
Lancaster, England

Softcover reprint of the hardcover 1st edition 1983

British Library Cataloguing in Publication Data

Fox, Harold
Atlas of gynaecological pathology.—(Current histopathology; v.5)
1. Generative organs, Female—Pathology
I. Title II. Buckley, Cathryn Hilary
III. Series
616.07 RG77

ISBN 978-94-015-7314-6 ISBN 978-94-015-7312-2 (eBook)
DOI 10.1007/978-94-015-7312-2

Typeset by Northumberland Press Limited, Gateshead.

Colour origination by Replica Photo-Litho Reproducers Limited, Stockport.

Bound by John Sherratt and Son Limited, Manchester.

Contents

	Consultant editor's note	7
	Foreword	9
1	Vulva: dermatological disorders and cysts	11
2	Vulva: inflammatory disease	15
3	Vulva: epithelial abnormalities	19
4	Vulva: neoplasms	25
5	Vagina: non-neoplastic conditions	31
6	Vagina: neoplasms	35
7	Cervix: inflammatory disease and miscellaneous non-neoplastic conditions	39
8	Cervix: epithelial abnormalities	43
9	Cervix: neoplasms	47
10	Endometrium: normal cyclical changes	51
11	Endometrium: functional disturbances	55
12	Endometrium: inflammatory disease	59
13	Endometrium: metaplasia and polypi	63
14	Endometrium: hyperplasia and intraendometrial neoplasia	67
15	Endometrium: epithelial neoplasms	71
16	Endometrium: stromal and mixed Müllerian neoplasms	77
17	Myometrium: non-neoplastic conditions and miscellaneous neoplasms	83
18	Myometrium: smooth muscle neoplasms	87
19	Fallopian tube and broad ligament: non-neoplastic conditions I	91
20	Fallopian tube and broad ligament: non-neoplastic conditions II	95
21	Fallopian tube and broad ligament: neoplasms	99
22	Ovary: normal appearances and cyclical changes	103
23	Ovary: cysts and tumour-like conditions	107
24	Ovary: miscellaneous disorders	111
25	Ovary: benign epithelial neoplasms	115
26	Ovary: epithelial neoplasms of borderline malignancy	119
27	Ovary: malignant epithelial neoplasms	123
28	Ovary: germ cell neoplasms	127
29	Ovary: sex cord stromal neoplasms	133
30	Ovary: miscellaneous neoplasms	139
31	Endometriosis and endosalpingiosis	143
32	Pregnancy	147
33	Hormone-induced changes in the female genital tract	153
34	Mechanical contraception	159
	Index	163

Current Histopathology Series

Already published in this series:

Volume 1 Atlas of Lymph Node Pathology
Volume 2 Atlas of Renal Pathology
Volume 3 Atlas of Pulmonary Pathology
Volume 4 Atlas of Liver Pathology

Other volumes currently scheduled in this series include the following titles:

Atlas of Breast Pathology

Atlas of Cytology

Atlas of Gastro-intestinal Pathology

Atlas of Joint and Connective Tissue Pathology

Atlas of Male Reproductive System Pathology

Atlas of Muscle Pathology

Atlas of Neuropathology

Atlas of Oral Pathology

Atlas of Skin Pathology

Atlas of Toxicology

Consultant Editor's Note

At the present time books on morbid anatomy and histology can be divided into two broad groups: extensive textbooks often written primarily for students and monographs on research topics.

This takes no account of the fact that the vast majority of pathologists are involved in an essentially practical field of general Diagnostic Pathology, providing an important service to their clinical colleagues. Many of these pathologists are expected to cover a broad range of disciplines and even those who remain solely within the field of histopathology usually have single and sole responsibility within the hospital for all this work. They may often have no chance for direct discussion on problem cases with colleagues in the same department. In the field of histopathology, no less than in other medical fields, there have been extensive and recent advances, not only in new histochemical techniques but also in the type of specimen provided by new surgical procedures.

There is a great need for the provision of appropriate information for this group. This need has been defined in the following terms.

(1) It should be aimed at the general clinical pathologist or histopathologist with existing practical training, but should also have value for the trainee pathologist.
(2) It should concentrate on the practical aspects of histopathology taking account of the new techniques which should be within the compass of the worker in a unit with reasonable facilities.
(3) New types of material, e.g. those derived from endoscopic biopsy should be covered fully.
(4) There should be an adequate number of illustrations on each subject to demonstrate the variation in appearance that is encountered.
(5) Colour illustrations should be used wherever they aid recognition.

The present concept stemmed from this definition but it was immediately realized that these aims could only be achieved within the compass of a series, of which this volume is one. Since histopathology is, by its very nature, systematized, the individual volumes deal with one system or where this appears more appropriate with a single organ.

This is the fifth volume of the *Current Histopathology* series. Gynaecological specimens form about one third of the work of most diagnostic histopathologists. The authors have provided a comprehensive account of the subject based upon their wide experience. The aim is to assist in the diagnostic difficulties that arise in abnormalities of the female genital tract. This volume has amply achieved that aim.

G. Austin Gresham
Cambridge

Acknowledgements

We are deeply indebted to the many colleagues who have lent us material for photography and our thanks go, therefore, to: Dr MacDonald, Manchester (Figures 1.4, 1.5, 1.6 and 1.7), Professor F. A. Langley, Manchester (Figure 31.3), Professor E. Saksela, Helsinki (Figure 9.12), Dr D. W. Buntine, Brisbane (Figures 6.3 and 9.9), Professor F. Nogales, Granada (Figure 28.5), Dr S. J. Robboy, Boston (Figure 5.8), Dr M. Wells, Leeds (Figures 18.10, 21.5, 28.8, 31.10), Dr H. J. Norris, Washington (Figure 16.1), Dr J. O. W. Beilby, London (Figure 6.1), and Dr C. D. Kooijman, Utrecht (Figures 6.9 and 24.12).

We are also most grateful to Professor Sir John Dewhurst, London, for kindly lending us Figures 6.10 and 6.11, Professor S. A. Langley, Manchester, for Figures 1.1 and 1.2, and Dr L. H. Honore, Edmonton, for Figure 4.12.

Our thanks are also due for the invaluable assistance afforded to us by the technical staff of the Department of Pathology, St Mary's Hospital, Manchester, and for the secretarial help of Mrs R. Parkinson. We are also indebted to Mrs H. Moore for typing the manuscript with speed, efficiency and skill.

Foreword

One in every three slides examined by a general diagnostic pathologist in the United Kingdom, and in most other countries, comes from a gynaecological patient. Few pathologists can hope, therefore, to escape a constant exposure to gynaecological pathology, and it is the aim of this atlas to lessen the difficulties of this diagnostic burden by acting as an illustrated guide to the histological diagnosis of female genital tract abnormalities.

Gynaecological pathology does, however, pose a number of specific problems: the range and scope of the pathological processes which may be encountered is vast, the oncological profligacy of the genital tissues is unequalled and, above all, there is, during the reproductive years of a woman's life, a constant and not uncommonly confusing morphological flux in the normal appearances of the genital tract tissues. Therefore, to illustrate not only every lesion which may occur in the gynaecological patient but also their many variants is a task which would, in itself, be beyond the compass of a relatively slim volume: to attempt further to present in pictorial form all the finer points of histological diagnosis and the frequently subtle nuances of differential diagnosis would require a massive tome. Hence, we have been forced to be highly selective in our choice of illustrations and although all may not agree with our selection, in which there are certainly a few notable lacunae, we feel that we have covered most of the lesions which are encountered with any frequency. We are, of course, also aware that many who use this volume will be well familiar with the classical, or 'textbook', appearances of most of the more common conditions and have therefore often chosen an example which, whilst being typical, is not necessarily classical.

We have deliberately chosen not to include any illustrations of gross specimens. This is partly because of our view that such illustrations are of little real value to any but the least experienced of pathologists, and partly because their inclusion would have narrowed still further our selection of histological figures.

We have tried to use illustrations of high technical excellence wherever possible, but this has not always proved possible with some of the rarer abnormalities: in such cases we have had to choose between either omitting an illustration of the lesion or illustrating a badly cut or poorly stained section. We have usually chosen to use the poor section, and we hope that our readers will forebear with us in this particular dilemma and with the imperfections of some of the illustrated sections.

Our text is clearly too brief to be anything more than synoptic but in it we have tried to concentrate on the practical difficulties which may be encountered by the pathologist; we have included a brief list of selected references for those wishing to pursue particular topics in greater depth.

H. Fox
C. H. Buckley Manchester, September 1982

Vulva: Dermatological Disorders and Cysts

1

Dermatological Disease

Psoriasis

This is a common, chronic disorder, inherited as an autosomal dominant, and characterized by the presence of well-defined, red-brown macules and plaques covered by layers of fine, silvery scales, removal of which causes punctate bleeding. In the flexural and intertriginous areas lesions often lack the silvery scales and appear shiny and red[1]. The outer surfaces of the labia majora and genito–crural folds are most commonly affected, and the distribution of the lesions is often remarkably symmetrical[2].

The histological features (Figure 1.1) include elongation and clubbing of the rete ridges, elongation and oedema of the dermal papillae, in which dilated capillaries are often apparent, relative thinning of the suprapapillary portion of the Malpighian layer, an absence of the granular layer, parakeratosis, spongiform pustules and Monroe abscesses. Monroe abscesses are the accumulation of neutrophils within the parakeratotic stratum corneum and may become sufficiently large to be clinically apparent, whilst spongiform pustules, considered to be diagnostic of psoriasis, form in the upper portion of the Malpighian layer of the suprapapillary epidermis where intercellular neutrophils lie mingled with the keratinocytes.

Lichen Planus

This is a subacute or chronic dermatosis affecting both skin and mucous membranes. The skin lesions are small, pruritic, flat-topped, violaceous papules bearing white dots or lines (Wickham's striae) which may coalesce to form plaques, whilst those on mucous membranes are white reticulate areas or plaques, which may ulcerate.

In active lesions (Figure 1.2) the histological features are those of irregular acanthosis, affecting the rete ridges and Malpighian layers, a band-like chronic inflammatory cell infiltrate at the dermo–epidermal junction associated with liquefaction degeneration of the basal layer, hyperkeratosis and an increased granular layer in the skin lesions and parakeratosis, with an absence of the granular layer and variable thinning of the epithelium, in the mucous membranes. The density of the inflammatory infiltrate, which is mainly lymphocytic, often blurs the dermo–epidermal junction and the rete ridges may acquire a saw-toothed configuration. In some cases the damage to the basal layer may lead to the formation of subepidermal bullae.

In older lesions, the basal layer of the epithelium is often absent, the inflammatory infiltrate diminishes, dermal macrophages increase in number and many of them may contain melanin derived from the damaged basal layer. The PAS positive, homogenous, eosinophilic, hyaline bodies which can be seen in the dermis and epidermis are remains of these damaged basal cells, but are not diagnostic of the disease.

Lichen Nitidus

A histologically similar but distinct condition is that of lichen nitidus. The small flesh-coloured papules remain discrete, develop parakeratosis and rarely show acanthosis. The majority of lesions (Figure 1.3) show a well circumscribed, intradermal focus of lymphocytes, epithelioid macrophages and occasional giant cells: the inflammation often extends into the covering epithelium which is thin and shows hydropic degeneration or absence of the basal layer.

Pemphigus Vulgaris

This is characterized by the presence of flaccid, easily ruptured bullae. The resultant denuded areas expand peripherally due to the progressive peripheral detachment of the epidermis.

The histological appearances are more typical in the early lesion. Progressive intercellular oedema and disappearance of the intercellular bridges lead to loss of cellular cohesion (acantholysis), and subsequently to the formation of intraepithelial bullae (Figure 1.4) in which clusters and individual cells float. The basal layer of the epithelium remaining attached to the dermal papillae produces a picture likened to a 'row of tombstones'. From the floor of the bullae, papillae, covered by basal cells, protrude into the lumen forming so-called villi; epithelium also grows down into the dermis between the villi. In older lesions, the epithelium in the base of the bullae may, due to regeneration, become multilayered. Antibodies to the intercellular substance of the squamous epithelium can be demonstrated by indirect immunofluorescence[3].

In some patients the denuded skin heals with verrucous vegetations which may be studded by pustules. This is pemphigus vegetans. In the early stages the picture is the same as that of pemphigus vulgaris, but villus formation and the downward growth of epithelium is more marked producing acanthosis and papillomatosis and there are intraepidermal eosinophilic abscesses.

Darier's Disease (*Keratosis Follicularis*)

This is inherited as an autosomal dominant and is characterized by a slowly progressive eruption of hyperkeratotic or crusted papules showing a follicular distribution. The lesions may, by coalescence, form

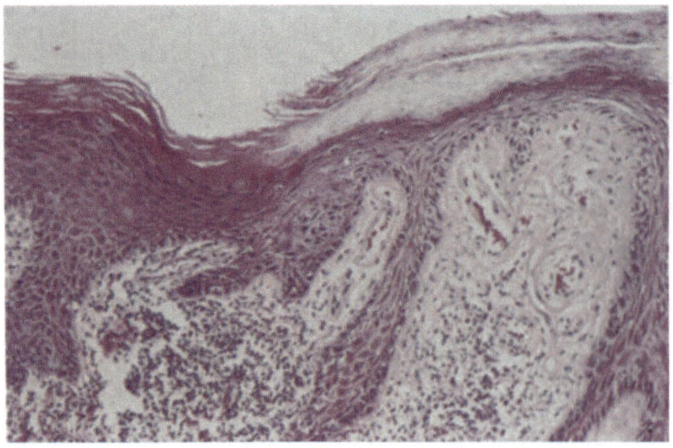

Figure 1.1 Vulva: psoriasis. This field is from the margin of a psoriatic plaque: on the right it shows the characteristic parakeratosis, elongation and clubbing of the rete ridges, thinning of the suprapapillary epidermis and congestion of the capillaries in the papillary dermis. More normal squamous epithelium is present to the left. The dermis is chronically inflamed. H & E × 250

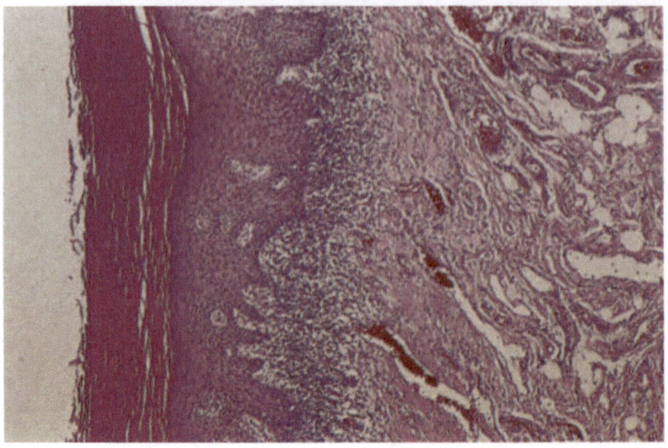

Figure 1.2 Vulva: lichen planus. There is a dense chronic inflammatory cell infiltrate at the dermo–epidermal junction and focal liquefaction degeneration of the basal epithelial layer. The rete ridges are irregular and many are spiky. There is pronounced hyperkeratosis and the dermis is congested. H & E × 100

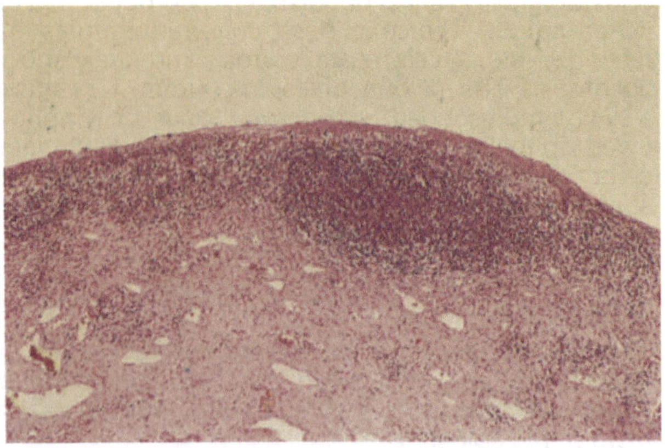

Figure 1.3 Vulva: lichen nitidus. This small papule is covered by thin squamous epithelium which shows hydropic degeneration of the basal layer. In the dermis there is a well demarcated collection of chronic inflammatory cells and there is also a scattering of lymphocytes in the dermis and epidermis. H & E × 40

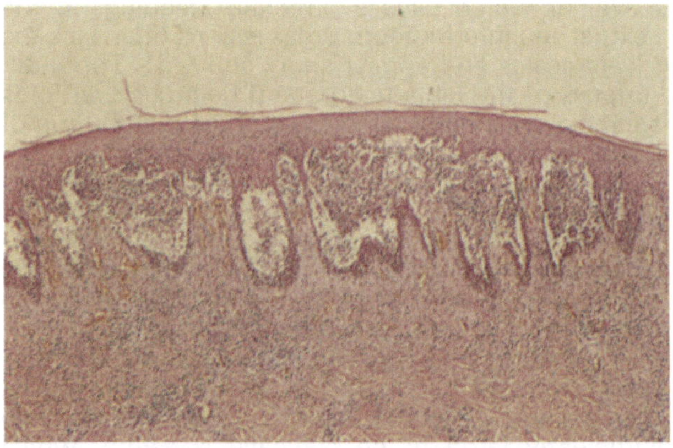

Figure 1.4 Vulva: pemphigus vulgaris. Suprabasal, intra-epithelial bullae containing acantholytic, rounded squamous cells are characteristic of pemphigus. The base of the bulla is formed by a layer of basal cells and there is a minimal dermal inflammation. H & E × 40

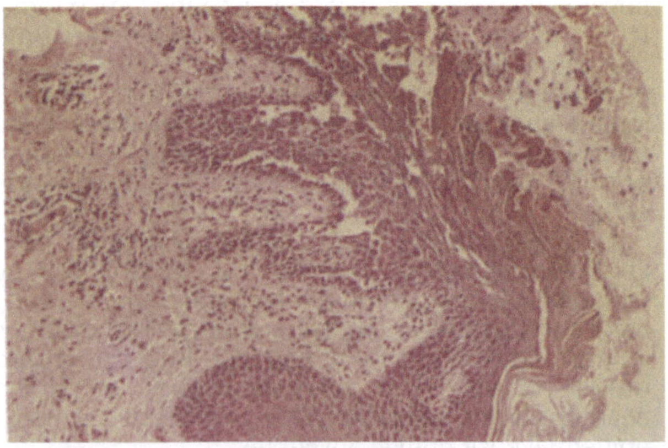

Figure 1.5 Vulva: familial benign pemphigus (Hailey–Hailey disease). An early suprabasal bulla. Dermal papillae, covered by basal cells (villi), protrude into the bulla which contains acantholytic squames. The roof of the bulla, to the right, is formed by hyperkeratotic, focally parakeratotic squamous epithelium. The dermis is focally inflamed. H & E × 100

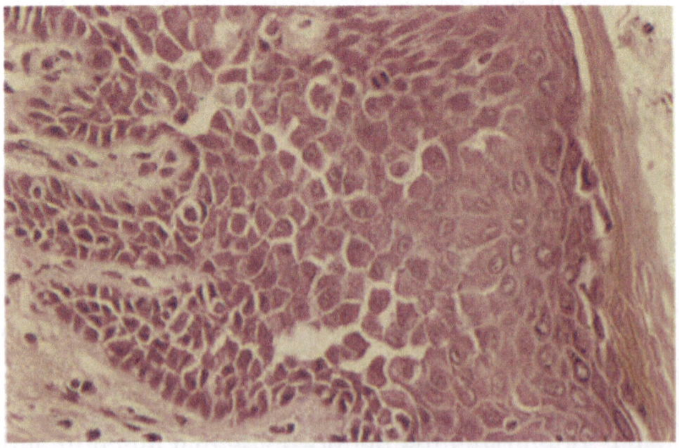

Figure 1.6 Vulva: familial benign pemphigus (Hailey–Hailey disease). An early lesion showing the so-called 'dilapidated brick wall' appearance which results from loosening of the intercellular bridges and incomplete acantholysis. H & E × 250

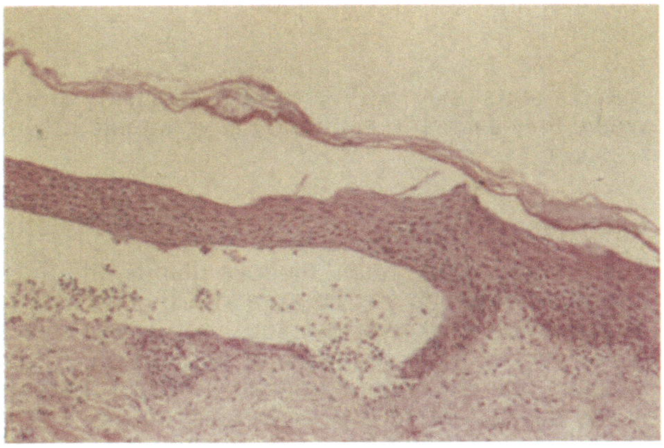

Figure 1.7 Vulva: benign mucosal pemphigoid (cicatricial pemphigoid). A subepidermal bulla of benign mucosal pemphigoid is becoming intra-epidermal as a tongue of squamous epithelium grows along the base of the bulla from its margin. There is little or no dermal inflammation. H & E × 100.

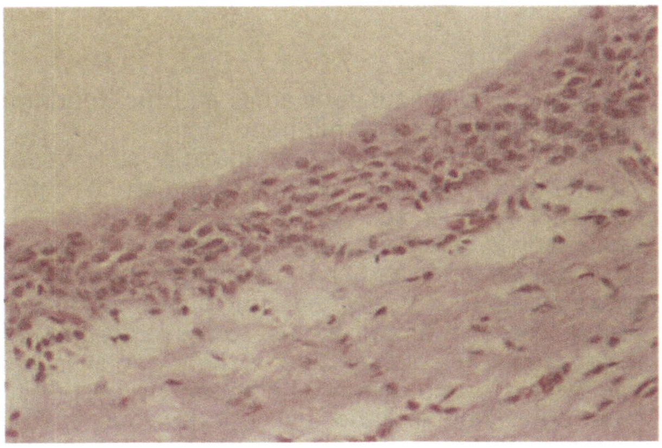

Figure 1.8 Vulva: sebaceous cyst (pilar cyst). The cyst is lined by stratified epithelium which shows no evidence of a granular layer or keratinization. The cells of the surface layer are round, their cytoplasm is eosinophilic and their nuclei round and centrally placed. The appearances are consistent with a pilar cyst, an uncommon vulval lesion. H & E × 250

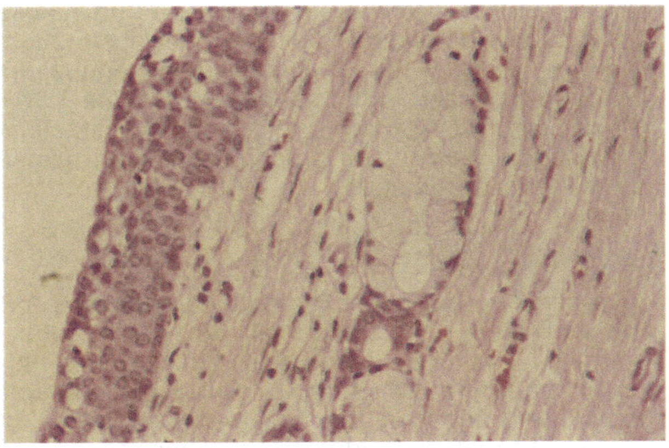

Figure 1.9 Vulva: Bartholin's duct cyst. The cyst lining (to the left) is formed by columnar epithelium undergoing squamous metaplasia: the fibrous wall contains glandular acini lined by tall mucus-secreting cells with clear cytoplasm, basal nuclei and well-defined cell margins. There is no inflammation. H & E × 250

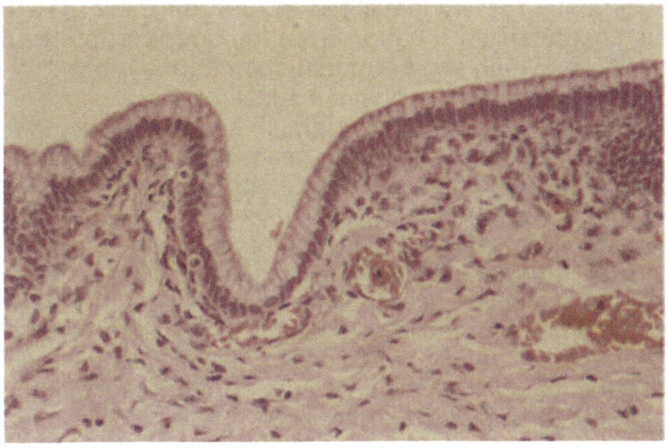

Figure 1.10 Vulva: mucinous cyst. The cyst is lined by a single layer of tall mucus-secreting cells with pale eosinophilic cytoplasm and basal nuclei. The wall is fibrovascular. H & E × 100

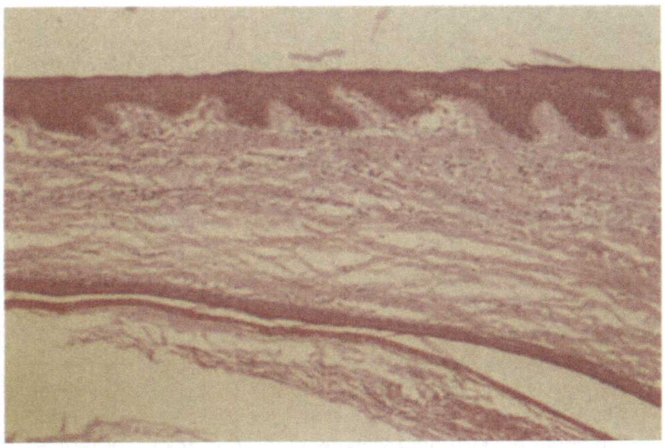

Figure 1.11 Vulva: epidermal cyst. The field shows skin in which there is a cyst lined by stratified squamous epithelium and containing laminated keratin. H & E × 40

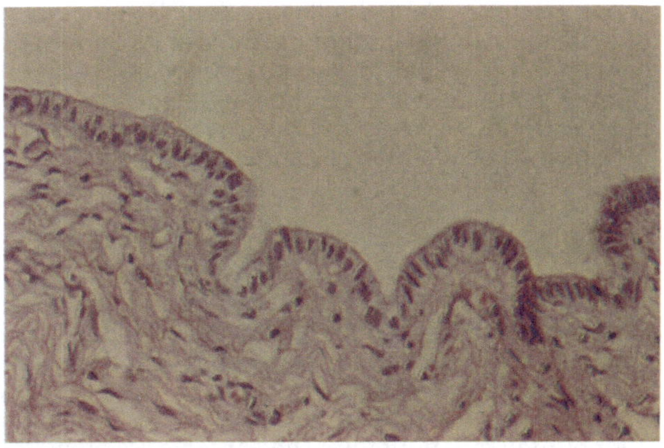

Figure 1.12 Vulva: Gartner's duct cyst. The cyst is lined by a single layer of cubo–columnar cells with pale eosinophilic cytoplasm. H & E × 250

verrucous or papillomatous areas and the condition tends to present in late childhood.

The histological features are those of supra-basal acantholysis leading to the development of intra-epithelial clefts or lacunae into which villi, similar to those seen in pemphigus, protrude. There is acanthosis, hyperkeratosis and chronic inflammation, whilst dyskeratosis is indicated by individual cell keratinization, corps ronds and 'grains'. Corps ronds are seen in the upper Malpighian and in the granular layers, and have a round, central, homogenous basophilic mass consisting of either pyknotic nucleus or dyskeratotic material, or both, surrounded by a clear halo: they are characteristic but not pathognomonic of Darier's disease. 'Grains' resemble large parakeratotic cells: their nuclei are elongated or grain-like and their cytoplasm homogenous, dyskeratotic and basophilic or, less commonly, eosinophilic.

Familial Benign Pemphigus (Hailey–Hailey Disease)

This is also a dominantly inherited disorder, although no family history is elicited in one third of cases. It is characterized by a localized, recurrent eruption of vesicles which show a predeliction for the intertriginous areas and first appear in adolescence.

The early lesions show small, suprabasal lacunae which are similar to those seen in Darier's disease, but in the established lesion acantholysis affects large sections of the Malpighian layer (Figure 1.5) and larger vesicles and bullae form into which 'villi' protrude. Groups and single epithelial cells lie in the bullae but where acantholysis is incomplete, the loose attachments of the intercellular bridges give a 'dilapidated brick wall' appearance (Figure 1.6). Occasional epithelial cells have the features of corps ronds and 'grains' (see Darier's disease).

Benign Mucosal Pemphigoid (Cicatricial Pemphigoid)

In contrast to the preceding disorders, the bullae of benign mucosal pemphigoid (cicatricial pemphigoid) are tense, subepidermal, and after rupture show no tendency to increase in size. Those which heal without scarring are associated with only mild dermal inflammation, whilst those in the rare areas of scarring show extensive dermal inflammation. Regeneration of epithelium in the floor of the bulla at its periphery, converts the bulla to an intraepithelial position (Figure 1.7) but it can be differentiated from pemphigus, Darier's disease and Hailey–Hailey disease by the absence of acantholysis and dyskeratosis.

Vulval Cysts

Sebaceous Cysts

Blockage of a sebaceous gland duct of the vulva results in the formation of a sebaceous cyst. The cysts develop in the hair-bearing areas or on the labia minora, they are mobile, attached to the skin and surmounted by a punctum. The contents are greasy or pultaceous, yellow-white material, and the cysts are lined by squamous epithelium showing sebaceous differentiation (Figure 1.8). Infection of the cysts is common, and if destruction of the lining occurs the contents may spill into the adjacent stroma where they elicit a foreign body type granulomatous reaction.

Bartholin's Duct Cyst

The vulva contains many mucous glands, the most important of which are the paired Bartholin's glands at the introitus. A cyst develops in the Bartholin's gland duct as a consequence of obstruction. A firm swelling, varying in size from 1 to 10 cm presents in the postero-lateral part of the labium major; it is lined by transitional epithelium showing foci of squamous metaplasia and mucus-secreting acini are usually present in the wall (Figure 1.9). The contents are clear, colourless, mucoid fluid. Infection of these cysts is common (see Bartholin's gland abscess).

Mucinous Cysts

These cysts which were at one time thought to arise from Müllerian (paramesonephric) duct remnants, almost certainly arise from the lesser, un-named vulval mucinous glands following duct obstruction. They are lined by tall, mucus-secreting epithelium similar to that seen in the endocervix (Figure 1.10). The rare serous cysts of the vulva, lined by epithelium of tubal type, similarly develop from small un-named intravulval serous glands.

Epidermoid Cysts

Epidermoid cysts are lined by stratified squamous epithelium (Figure 1.11) and contain greasy grey-white, laminated keratinous debris. They develop from epithelial inclusions which occur following obstetric trauma or surgery or remain at sites of fusion of epidermal structures during embryogenesis.

Cysts of the Canal of Nuck

These develop from the peritoneal remnants which persist along the path of the round ligament as it passes through the inguinal canal into the labium major. Such cysts occur most commonly in the upper part of the labium major, are lined by a single layer of flattened epithelium and contain clear, serous fluid.

Cysts of Gartner's Duct (Mesonephric or Wolffian Duct)

These lie in the lateral part of the vulva. They are lined by a single layer of shallow, columnar or cuboidal epithelium (Figure 1.12), have a thin fibromuscular wall and contain colourless clear, serous fluid.

References

1. Ridley, C. M. (1975). *The Vulva*. (London, Philadelphia: Saunders).
2. Friedrich, E. G. Jr. and Wilkinson, E. J. (1982). The Vulva. In Blaustein, A. (ed.). *Pathology of the Female Genital Tract*, 2nd edn., pp. 13–58 (New York: Springer-Verlag)
3. Lever, W. F. and Schaumberg-Lever, G. (1975). *Histopathology of the Skin*. (Philadelphia and Toronto: Lippincott)

Vulva: Inflammatory Disease 2

Non-specific Infections

The relatively common, non-specific superficial infections of the vulva, which are predisposed to by local warmth, moisture and repeated micro-organismal contamination, are indistinguishable from such infections occurring in skin elsewhere in the body.

Specific Infections

Herpes Simplex Infection

This disease, usually due to herpes simplex virus II and less commonly to type I, is acquired by sexual contact and presents clinically as a painful, sharply marginated, recurrent ulcerative vulvitis; lesions in the urethra, bladder and cervix usually coexist. One of several groups of intraepithelial vesicles form as the result of acantholysis caused by balloon and reticular degeneration. Balloon degeneration occurs mainly at the bases of the vesicles and frequently extends through the full thickness of the epithelium so that the vesicle becomes subepidermal; the epidermal appendages may also be affected. This cellular change is specific for viral vesicles and is characterized by uniform, eosinophilic cytoplasmic swelling, intranuclear viral inclusions, occasional multinucleation and loss of intercellular bridges. Reticular degeneration is recognized mainly in the upper parts of the vesicles and at their margins, and is not specific for viral infections: intracellular oedema leads to cellular rupture, and coalescence of neighbouring cells creates a multilocular vesicle which gradually becomes unilocular as cell membranes disappear. The underlying dermis is usually inflamed and in severe reactions there may be a vasculitis.

Molluscum Contagiosum

The lesions of this disease are discrete, asymptomatic or mildly pruritic, umbilicated, smooth-surfaced, waxy or pearly, skin-coloured nodules or papules. They may be single or multiple and, when mature, cheesy-like material can be expressed from their centres. They are caused by a DNA pox virus, transmitted by sexual contact, and involution is spontaneous though frequently slow. The specific histological findings are of a nest of well-demarcated, pear-shaped lobules of acanthotic squamous epithelium (Figure 2.1). The epithelial cells of the lower Malpighian layer contain small, ovoid, eosinophilic intracytoplasmic viral inclusions (molluscum bodies) and as the cells approach the surface, these inclusions increase in size and, at the level of the granular layer, become basophilic (Figure 2.2). Ultimately they attain a diameter of 35 μm, compress the nucleus to a fine crescent at the periphery of the cell[1] and are shed from the central crater or umbilicus. The surrounding dermis is rarely inflamed, but if the lesion ruptures into the dermis there is a severe inflammatory reaction which may include foreign body giant cells.

Lymphogranuloma Venereum

This is a sexually transmitted disease caused by a *Chlamydia*. The primary lesion is a papule or painless ulcer near the urethra on the vulva, or in the vagina, which develops within a few days of exposure and heals rapidly. This is followed, in about 30% of cases, by a suppurative, painful inguinal lymphadenopathy which drains through multiple sinuses[2]. Vaginal and posterior perineal lesions are followed by a perirectal lymphadenopathy. The third stage of the disease is characterized by chronic lymphoedema and post-inflammatory scarring. The histology of the initial papule is non-specific, and whilst the stellate abscesses seen in the lymph nodes are characteristic of lymphogranuloma they are not specific for this disease; initially, clusters of epithelioid cells, interspersed with occasional giant cells, form throughout the node and as these increase in size, their centres undergo necrosis and become filled with neutrophil polymorphs and macrophages whilst fibrous tissue, infiltrated by plasma cells, forms at their margins. The epithelioid cells around the abscesses form a palisade and ultimately the abscesses coalesce. In the late stages the nodes show focal acellular necrosis and numerous plasma cells.

Granuloma Inguinale

This is a venereal disease due to infection by *Calymmatobacterium granulomatis*. Primary lesions occur on the labia minora and mons pubis as painful papules or ulcers filled with exuberant granulation tissue which bleeds easily. In the early stages of the disease, the lesions expand by direct peripheral infiltration but later spread occurs via the lymphatics. The central ulcer base is composed of non-specific granulation tissue containing histiocytes and plasma cells with occasional small abscesses composed of neutrophil polymorphs (Figure 2.3), but very few lymphocytes. Many of the histiocytes contain the intracytoplasmic bacterial inclusions or Donovan bodies which are difficult to see in a haematoxylin and eosin stained section but are more easily demonstrated by Giemsa or silver stains where they appear as encapsulated, bipolar bodies 1–2 μm long. The squamous epithelium at the ulcer margins frequently shows pseudoepitheliomatous hyperplasia (Figure 2.4).

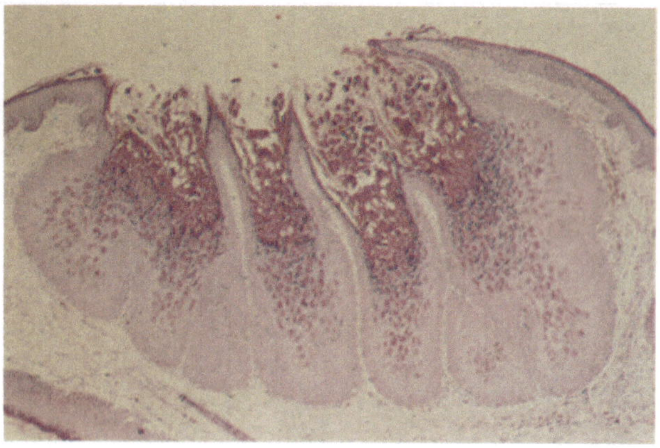

Figure 2.1 Vulva: molluscum contagiosum. A typical lesion formed by lobules of hyperplastic, acanthotic squamous epithelium each of which opens into the central crater on the convexity of the nodule. It is from this central umbilication that the molluscum bodies can be expressed as a curd-like material. H & E × 40

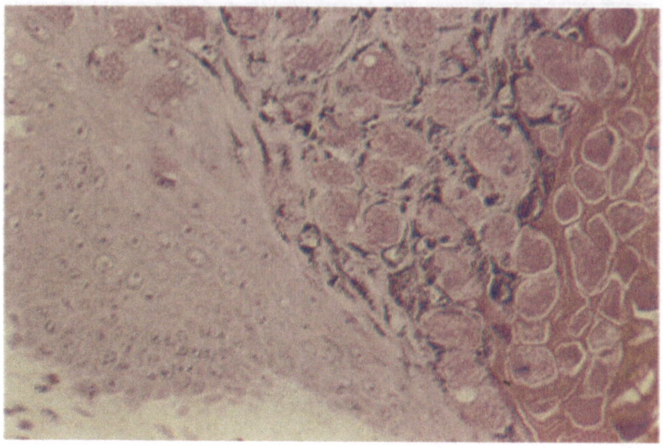

Figure 2.2 Vulva: molluscum contagiosum. This high power detail from a lobule shows the normal basal and lower Malpighian layers of the squamous epithelium to the lower left and the granular, intracytoplasmic, eosinophilic viral inclusions, 'molluscum bodies' to the right. Note that the inclusions are most numerous in the stratum granulosum where they are intermingled with the dark purple staining keratohyaline granules, and in the stratum corneum where they are surrounded by keratin. H & E × 250

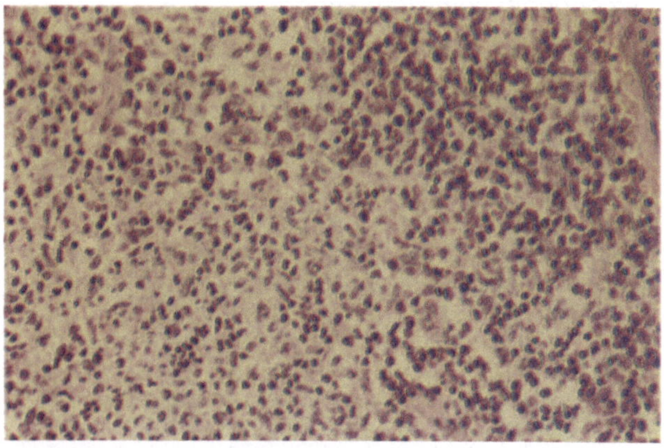

Figure 2.3 Vulva: granuloma inguinale. Non-specific granulation tissue from the base of a vulval ulcer. The inflammatory cell infiltrate consists predominantly of plasma cells and histiocytes but in the centre of the field can be seen a collection of polymorphonuclear leukocytes forming a micro-abscess at the advancing margin of the lesion. H & E × 250

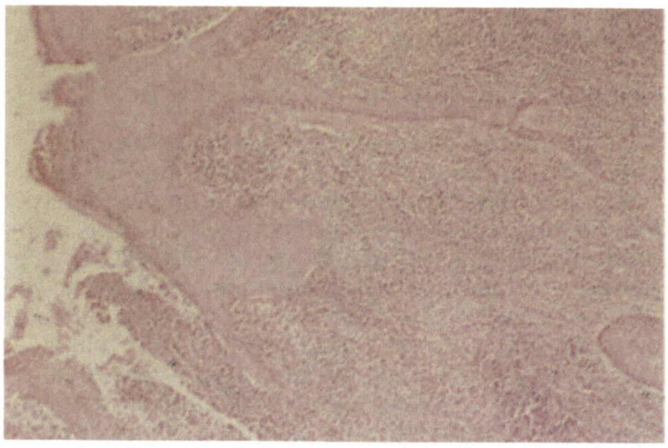

Figure 2.4 Vulva: granuloma inguinale. The squamous epithelium at the margin of an ulcer (to the left) shows acanthosis and elongation of the rete ridges, but no cytological atypia. There is a dense, non-specific, inflammatory cell infiltrate in the dermis and at the lower margin of the section the exuberant granulation tissue in the ulcer base can be seen. H & E × 40

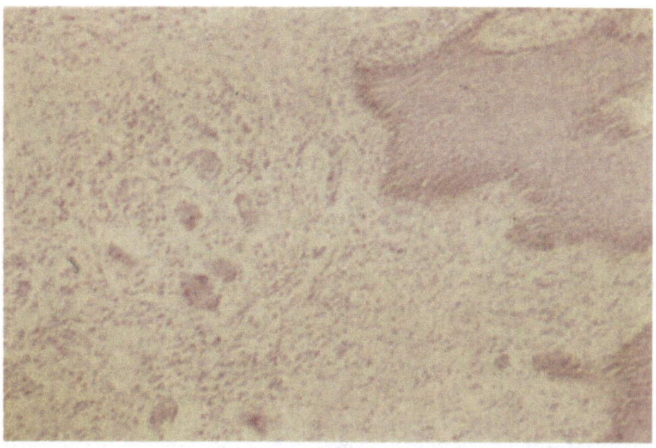

Figure 2.5 Vulva: schistosomiasis. Schistosomal ova in the vulval dermis. A focal, active, non-specific chronic inflammatory cell infiltrate can be seen and there is granulation tissue formation. Note the heavily pigmented basal layer of the covering epithelium, to the right. The patient was Egyptian. H & E × 100

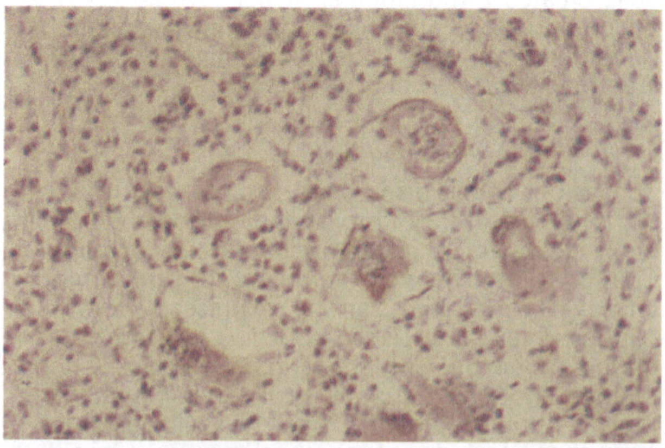

Figure 2.6 Vulva: schistosomiasis. The ova are surrounded by granulation and fibrous tissue and the inflammatory cell infiltrate contains lymphocytes, eosinophils and an occasional plasma cell. In long standing cases, the ova may become calcified. H & E × 250

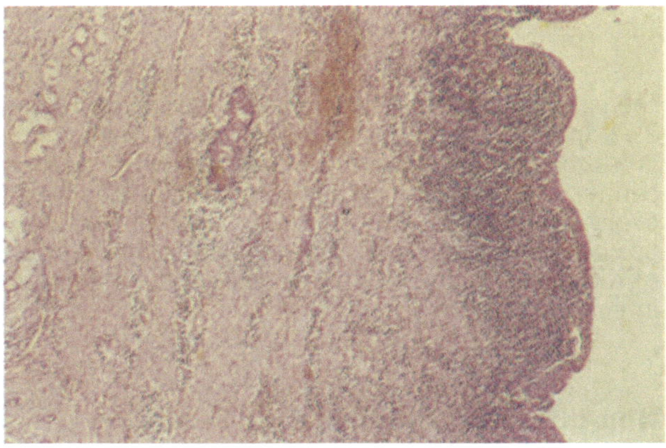

Figure 2.7 Vulva: Bartholin's gland abscess. To the right can be seen part of the wall of a dilated duct: its epithelium shows squamous metaplasia and sloughing with focal ulceration. Immediately deep to the epithelium is a dense band of chronic inflammatory cells consisting predominantly of lymphocytes and plasma cells. Within the fibrous wall of the abscess (to the left) there are foci of lymphocytes and residual glandular acini can be seen, these being formed by tall pale, mucus-secreting, epithelial cells. H & E × 40

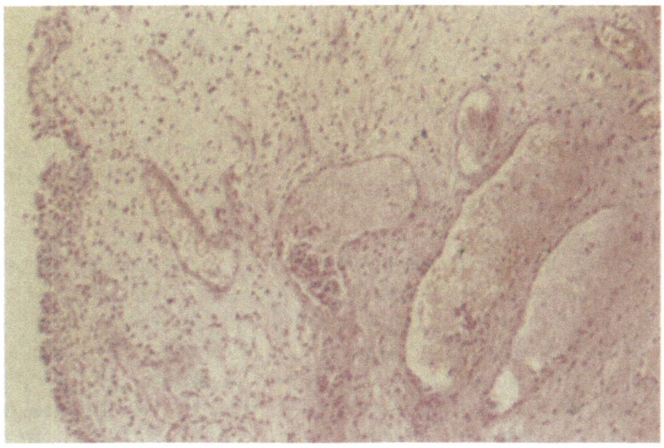

Figure 2.8 Vulva: urethral caruncle. This oedematous and intensely congested caruncle was removed from a 72-year-old woman who complained of bleeding. The stroma is composed of young, extremely oedematous fibroblastic granulation tissue and the covering epithelium (to the left) is transitional in type. Note that inflammation is minimal. H & E × 100

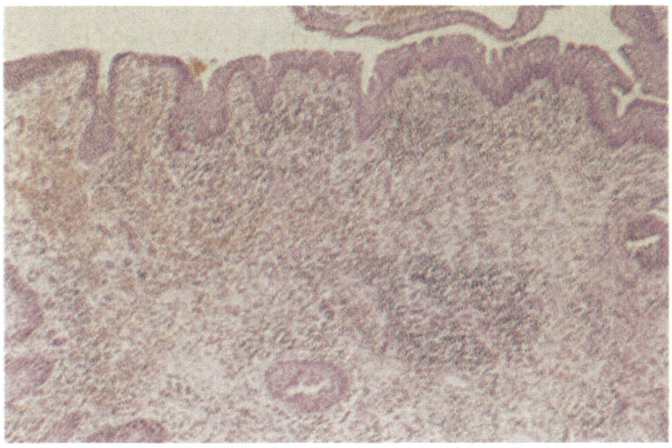

Figure 2.9 Vulva: urethral caruncle. In this caruncle the stroma is more densely fibrous although younger granulation tissue can be seen to the left. It is heavily infiltrated by a chronic inflammatory cell infiltrate which is predominantly lymphocytic. The covering epithelium is of transitional type above and is squamous in nature at the left margin. H & E × 100

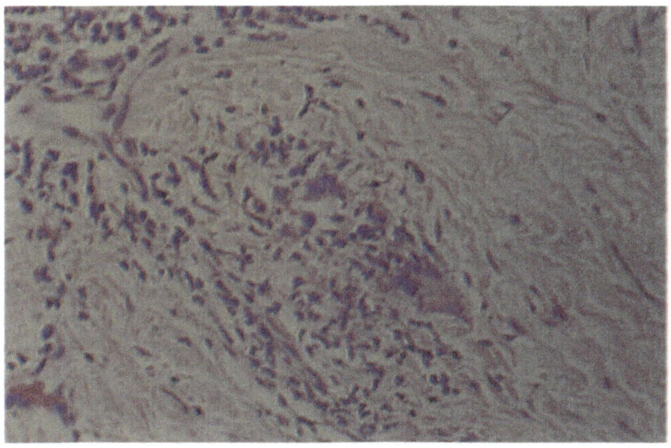

Figure 2.10 Vulva: Crohn's disease. This vulval biopsy was taken from a site adjacent to an ulcer and the plasmocytic infiltrate in the ulcer wall is just visible in the upper left corner. The centre of the field is occupied by a small, rather ill-formed, granuloma in which epithelioid cells, lymphocytes and two macrophage giant cells can be identified. This picture is fairly typical of vulval Crohn's disease. H & E × 250

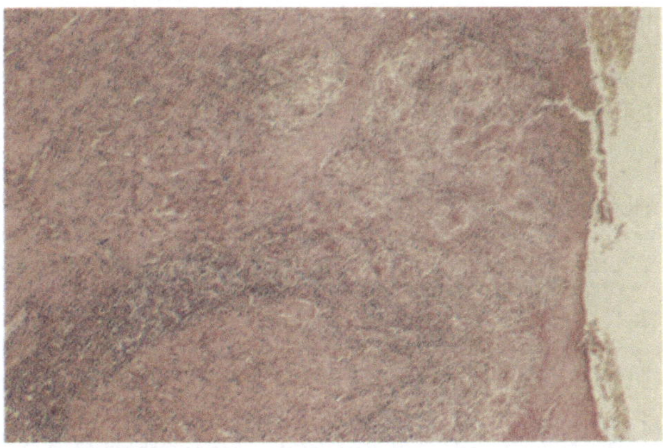

Figure 2.11 Vulva: Behcet's disease. The section shows the base and margin of an ulcer. To the upper right, the ulcer base is covered by non-specific, fibrinous exudate containing polymorphonuclear leukocytes and to the lower right, the mildly acanthotic epithelium at the ulcer margin can be seen. The ulcer base is formed by non-specific granulation tissue heavily infiltrated by lymphocytes and containing large numbers of thick-walled blood vessels which are showing an endarteritis. H & E × 40

Syphilis

The primary lesion of this disease, the chancre, occurs within 3 weeks at the site of innoculation with *Treponema pallidum*. It is a firm, indurated, red-brown nodule or plaque with surface erosion or, occasionally, painless, punched out ulceration; it becomes painful if secondary infection occurs. The chancre, which is usually single, is found on the labia or at the introitus: healing occurs within 3–6 weeks and the lesion may pass unobserved. The most striking histological feature is a dermal infiltrate of lymphocytes and plasma cells. The dermal capillaries show endothelial proliferation and the inflammatory infiltrate may extend into their walls. The covering epidermis shows acanthosis at the margins of the lesion, and becomes progressively thinner towards the centre of the chancre where it may be entirely lost or oedematous and heavily infiltrated by inflammatory cells. Silver stains, e.g. Levaditi's stain, will reveal spirochaetes around the dermal capillaries but they are hard to distinguish from the reticulin fibres and a fluorescent stain on frozen tissue is preferred. A painless, rubbery lymphadenopathy develops 4–5 weeks after the chancre, and microscopic examination shows chronic inflammation including plasma cells, numerous spirochaetes and, on occasions, non-caseating sarcoid-like granulomata.

Secondary lesions develop in the untreated patient 6 weeks to 6 months after initial infection, and usually present as a generalized, red-brown maculopapular rash involving skin and mucous membranes. The macules rarely contain spirochaetes and their histological picture is not diagnostic; the superficial dermal capillaries show endothelial swelling and there is an infiltrate of lymphocytes and plasma cells. In contrast, the papular lesions team with spirochaetes and in the ano–genital area may be large, moist and verrucous, the so-called condylomata lata: their histological appearances are specific, for the capillaries of both superficial and deep dermis show endothelial swelling and proliferation with a perivascular infiltrate in which plasma cells are conspicuous. In the superficial dermis there is also a diffuse inflammatory infiltrate which may include epithelioid granulomata and occasional giant cells. In condylomata lata additional features are seen in the epidermis. These are acanthosis, intra- and intercellular oedema and migration of polymorphs. Tertiary syphilitic lesions rarely affect the vulva.

Schistosomiasis

Involvement of the vulva is relatively common in those areas of the world where the disease is endemic. Infection is usually due to *S. haematobium* (Figures 2.5 and 2.6).

Infection of Bartholin's Gland

This may be due to *Neisseria gonorrhoea, staphylococcus* or *enterobacilli*. Initially there is an acute adenitis characterized by a periacinar neutrophil polymorph infiltrate, and neutrophil polymorphs are also seen in the lumen of a somewhat dilated duct (Figure 2.7). Infection can subside at this stage but may progress to suppuration and abscess formation: healing can result in residual fibrosis whilst there may be an evolution into a persistent chronic adenitis. Repeated episodes of inflammation may ultimately lead to a cyst of the duct which in turn increases susceptibility to infection.

Non-infectious Inflammatory Processes

Urethral Caruncle

This presents as a sessile or polypoidal, red nodule at the urethral meatus in the elderly patient; it may be asymptomatic but more frequently causes dysuria, or, because it is friable, bleeding. It is formed of highly vascular, young, myxomatous, fibroblastic granulation tissue (Figure 2.8) and the overlying epithelium, which may be ulcerated, is of transitional or squamous type (Figure 2.9); the lesion is usually infiltrated by lymphocytes, which are more numerous following ulceration. At times the vascular channels attain a large size and resemble haemorrhoids. Aetiologically, the lesion may be a localized mucosal prolapse or non-specific, inflammatory granulation tissue.

Crohn's Disease

In occasional patients with perianal Crohn's disease there is also vulval oedema and deep, fissuring vulval ulceration which is often secondarily infected[3]. Histologically, the fissures are lined by non-specific granulation tissue but the surrounding dermis contains the more typical non-caseating tuberculoid granulomata (Figure 2.10).

Behcet's Syndrome

This term refers to the triad of oral and genital ulceration with uveitus. The vulval ulcers may be histologically non-specific with necrotic material and neutrophil polymorphs at the surface and round cells more deeply and, under such circumstances, diagnosis must depend largely on the associated systemic features. In some cases, however, an obliterating endarteritis or necrotizing arteritis is seen in the ulcer base (Figure 2.11), this latter being regarded as pathognomonic by some authors[4].

References

1. Lever, W. F. and Schaumburg-Lever, G. (1975). *Histopathology of the Skin*. (Philadelphia and Toronto: J.B. Lippincott)
2. Fox, H. and Buckley, C. H. (1982). *Pathology for Gynaecologists*. (London: Edward Arnold)
3. Ridley, C. M. (1975). *The Vulva*. (London, Philadelphia and Toronto: W. B. Saunders)
4. Friedrich, E. G. and Wilkinson, E. J. (1982). The Vulva. In Blaustein, A. (ed.) *Pathology of the Female Genital Tract*. 2nd edn., pp. 13–58. (New York, Heidelberg, Berlin: Springer-Verlag)

Vulva: Epithelial Abnormalities 3

Vulval Dystrophies

The vulval dystrophies are a group of conditions characterized by disordered growth, and sometimes maturation, of the vulval squamous epithelium: their aetiology is unknown though recently an association between vulval dystrophy and achlorhydria has been demonstrated whilst papilloma virus has been identified in a few cases. A rationalized and simplified classification and nomenclature of vulval dystrophies[1] has replaced an earlier system which was based almost entirely on the naked eye appearance of the lesions, but which subsequently acquired a pathological connotation which was confusing, unsatisfactory and, at times, misleading. Thus terms such as kraurosis, leukoplakia and neurodermatitis are no longer acceptable as pathological diagnoses, and the vulval dystrophies are classified as hyperplastic dystrophy, with or without cellular atypia, lichen sclerosus and mixed dystrophy.

Hyperplastic Dystrophy

This diagnostic category encompasses those conditions previously classed as neurodermatitis, lichen simplex chronicus, hypertrophic (or early) leukoplakia and hypertrophic vulvitis: it accounts for about 50% of all vulval dystrophies. Patients with this condition are usually less than 50 years old and complain of vulval pruritis or soreness. The vulval skin has a variegated appearance with well demarcated or ill-defined, thickened white areas of hyperkeratosis alternating with reddish, non-keratinized areas. The lesions occur most commonly on the clitoral prepuce, the labia majora, the interlabial sulci, the lateral surface of the labia minora and the posterior commissure.

Histologically (Figure 3.1), there is hyperkeratosis and irregular thickening of the Malphigian layer of the epidermis with elongation, widening and variable fusion of the rete ridges. The individual squamous cells have regular nuclei with finely dispersed chromatin, intercellular bridges are clearly seen and, in the hyperkeratotic areas, a thickened granular layer is seen. The dermal papillae may be oedematous and there is often a plasmalymphocytic infiltration of the papillary and reticular dermis.

Lichen Sclerosus

The suffix *'et atrophicus'* was previously added to this condition but has been abandoned since the demonstration that the vulval epithelium showing this abnormality is metabolically highly active: included with the diagnosis of lichen sclerosus are conditions previously diagnosed as kraurosis or atrophic leukoplakia. Extravulval lesions are often present and may, indeed, occur in the absence of vulval involvement. Lichen sclerosus is of unknown aetiology but occurs at all ages, and whilst sometimes asymptomatic can cause pruritus and soreness: dyspareunia is, because of tissue shrinkage, common and the disease tends to progress in an insidious, but relentless, manner.

The affected areas show low, irregular, flat-topped or depressed white maculo-papules which may coalesce to form well defined plaques: in newly involved areas the lesions may be oedematous or bullous, these changes being seen particularly in children. In longstanding cases the skin may be parchment-like, the labia minora atrophic and the normal vulval contours obliterated.

Histologically (Figure 3.2), the affected skin has a shallow squamous epithelium, sometimes only 2 or 3 cell layers thick, with hyperkeratosis and follicular plugging. Loss of rete ridges may be partial or complete whilst hydropic degeneration of the basal layer may lead to subepidermal bullae (Figure 3.3) and pigmentary incontinence. The superficial dermis is oedematous and hyalinized with loss of elastic fibres: in the deeper layers of the dermis there is a dense band of non-specific chronic inflammatory cells.

Mixed Dystrophy

In about a third of cases of lichen sclerosus areas of hyperplastic dystrophy are also present, this being a mixed dystrophy (Figure 3.4). The hyperplastic areas may be typical or hyperplastic epithelium may overlie dermis showing the characteristic features of lichen sclerosus. There is no evidence that the hyperplastic areas eventually become atrophic, and indeed the two components of a mixed dystrophy each behave as would be expected had they occurred in isolation.

Dystrophy with Cellular Atypia: Vulval Intraepithelial Neoplasia

Controversy and doubt exist over the malignant potential of the vulval dystrophies[2]. About 5–10% of women with a dystrophy will eventually develop an invasive squamous cell carcinoma, whilst 5% of patients presenting with symptoms due to a dystrophy already have a carcinoma; conversely, dystrophic epithelium is found adjacent to the tumour in nearly 50% of patients presenting with a squamous cell carcinoma[3]. It is clear, however, that a dystrophy in which there is no cellular atypia carries no increased risk of malignancy, that between 10 and 25% of dystrophies with severe atypia will progress to a carcinoma, and that cellular atypia occurs only in hyper-

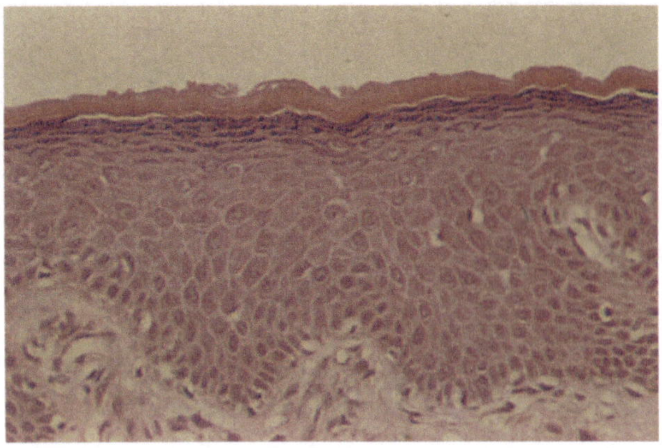

Figure 3.1 Vulva: hyperplastic dystrophy. In this biopsy from an elderly woman, the epithelium is only mildly hyperplastic but there is a prominent stratum granulosum and mild hyperkeratosis. There is no cytological atypia or dermal inflammation. The degree of epithelial hyperplasia often varies within a single sample and areas of mild hyperplasia such as this may be underdiagnosed. H & E × 250

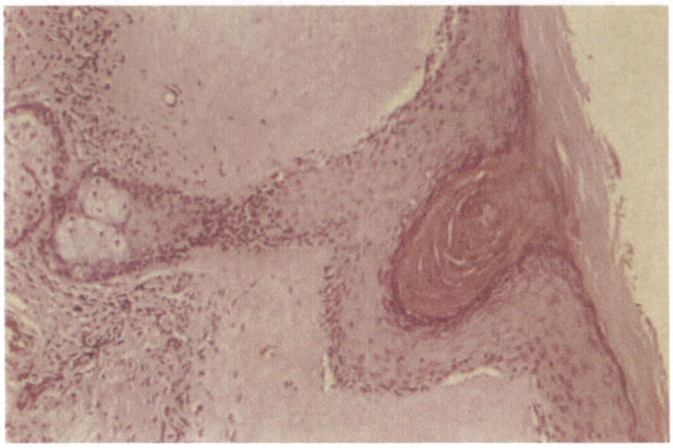

Figure 3.2 Vulva: lichen sclerosus. The epidermis, to the right, is atrophic, has no rete ridges and is markedly hyperkeratotic. The sebaceous gland traversing the field contains a keratin plug. A dense band of chronic inflammatory cells lies deep to the hyalinized papillary and superficial reticular dermis. H & E × 100

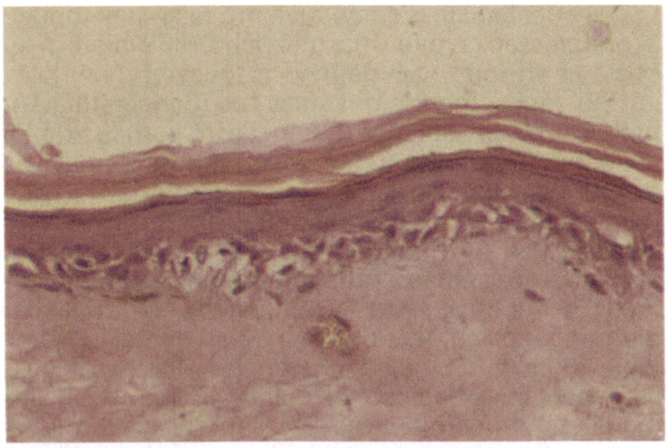

Figure 3.3 Vulva: lichen sclerosus. In this example the squamous epithelium is extremely atrophic, being only two or three cells thick, although the stratum granulosum and stratum corneum are conspicuous. There is hydropic degeneration of the basal layer and melanin pigment lies within macrophages in the hyalinized dermis to the left of the field. H & E × 250

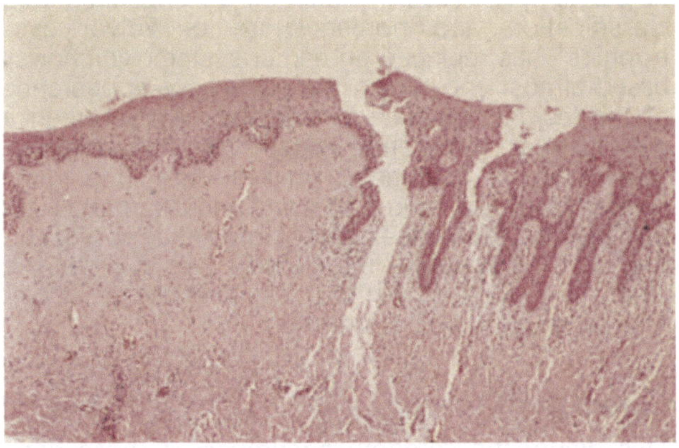

Figure 3.4 Vulva: mixed dystrophy. The squamous epithelium to the left of the field shows no significant abnormality but the underlying dermis shows the hyalinization characteristic of lichen sclerosus: by contrast the squamous epithelium to the right of the field shows hyperplastic dystrophy with cellular atypia and the dermis is chronically inflammed. This is only one of the possible combinations of epithelial abnormality seen in a mixed dystrophy. H & E × 40

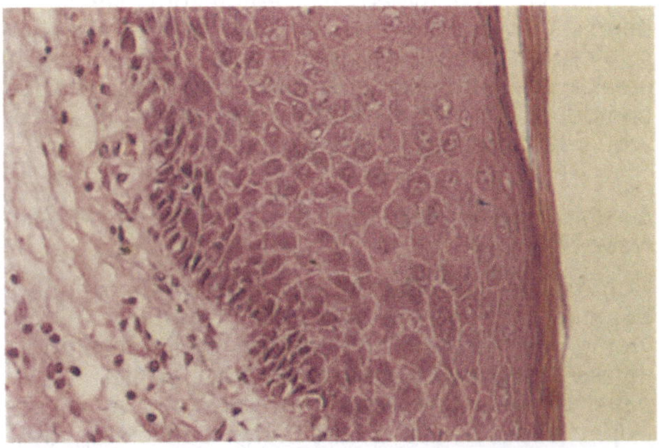

Figure 3.5 Vulva: dystrophy with atypia. Vulval intraepithelial neoplasia grade I (VIN I). The squamous epithelium in this example shows an abnormality of epithelial maturation, multinucleate cells being present. H & E × 250

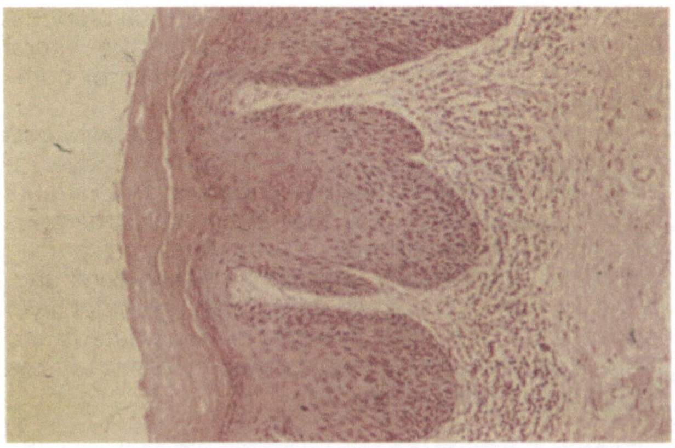

Figure 3.6 Vulva: dystrophy with atypia. Vulval intraepithelial neoplasia grade II (VIN II). The squamous epithelium shows acanthosis together with marked hyperkeratosis, and there is a band of lymphocytes in the dermis immediately deep to the epithelium. The epithelium shows abnormalities of stratification with basal and parabasal cells extending into the lower half of the Malpighian layer and abnormalities of cellular maturation as shown by the epithelial pleomorphism and multinucleation. H & E × 100

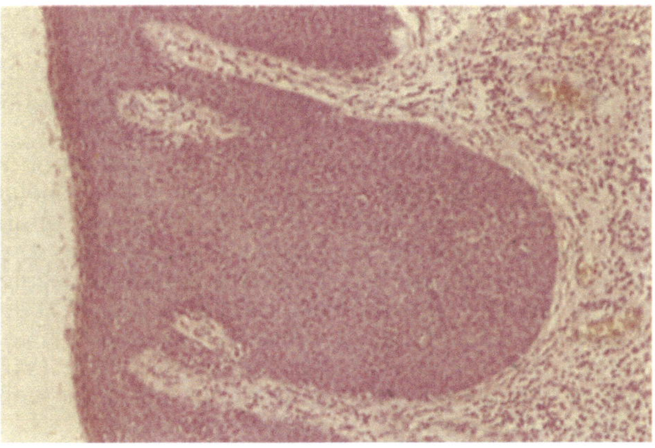

Figure 3.7 Vulva: dystrophy with atypia. Vulval intraepithelial neoplasia grade III (VIN III). This is an example of VIN III (squamous carcinoma *in situ*) in which the full thickness of the acanthotic, hyperplastic epithelium is occupied by fairly uniform regular cells of basal or parabasal type with high nucleo–cytoplasmic ratios; there is parakeratosis. The dermis shows a uniform lymphocytic infiltrate and this was limited to the dermis beneath the epithelium showing the greatest atypia. H & E × 100

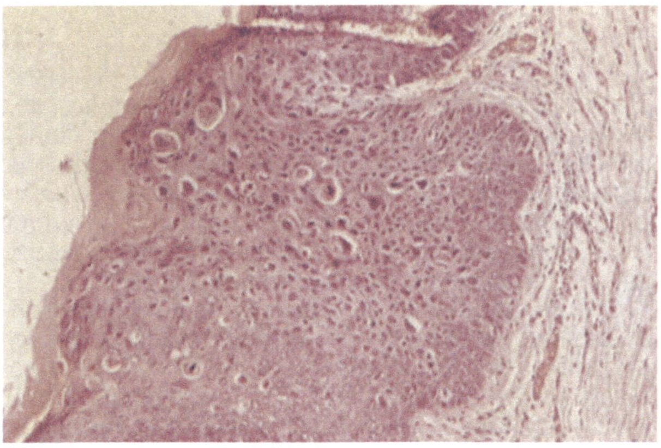

Figure 3.8 Vulva: dystrophy with atypia. Vulval intraepithelial neoplasia grade III (VIN III). The squamous epithelium in this field shows hyperplasia with acanthosis and is hyperkeratotic. There is a severe abnormality of cellular maturation characterized by individual cell keratinization with nuclear pyknosis and cytoplasmic eosinophilia, corps ronds, cellular pleomorphism and clear perinuclear vacuoles (koilocytosis). This form of VIN is thought to be of viral aetiology. H & E × 100

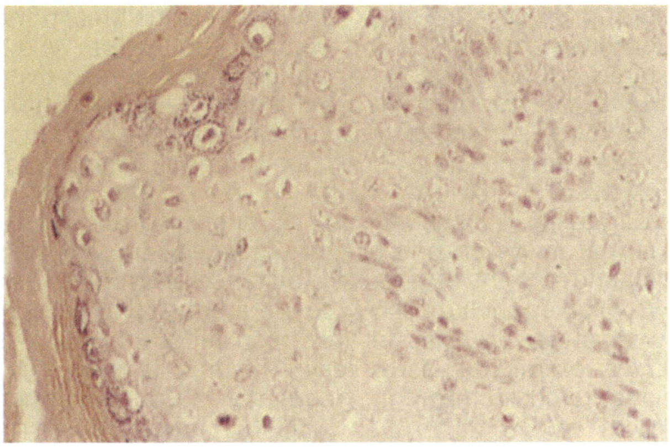

Figure 3.9 Vulva: flat condyloma acuminatum. The epidermis shows minimal nuclear enlargement and epithelial multinucleation. Individual cells show dense eosinophilic, premature cytoplasmic keratinization and there is perinuclear vacuolation (koilocytosis). H & E × 250

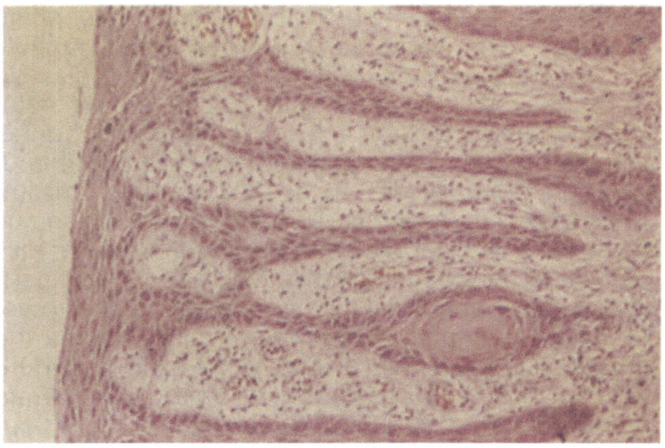

Figure 3.10 Vulva: hyperplastic dystrophy. In this field there is extreme elongation of the rete ridges with parakeratosis and cellular atypia. In one rete ridge there is a well-formed squamous epithelial pearl similar to that seen in squamous carcinoma (Figure 4.3); the dermis is mildly inflamed. Similar epithelial pearls may also be seen in dystrophic epithelium showing little or no other evidence of cellular atypia. H & E × 100

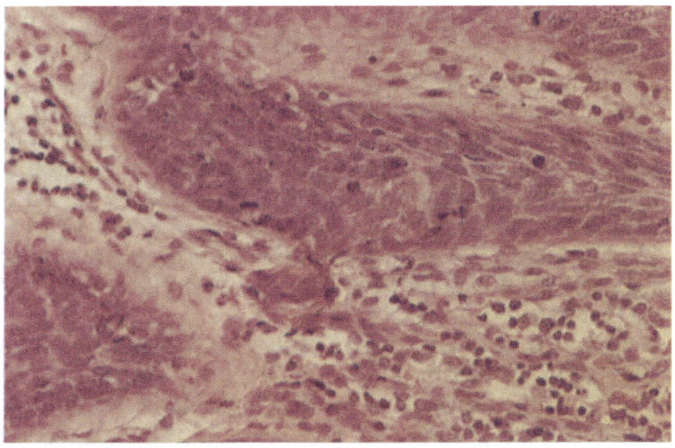

Figure 3.11 Vulva: microinvasive squamous carcinoma. This is the rete ridge from a hyperplastic dystrophy showing cytological atypia. Along the lower margin of the ridge there is focal, premature cytoplasmic maturation as shown by more copious cytoplasm staining eosinophilically in contrast to the adjacent basophilic cells. A tongue of these atypical cells breaches the basement membrane and penetrates the stroma. The site of such microinvasion is marked by premature cytoplasmic maturation, cellular enlargement and a focal dermal plasmo–lymphocytic infiltrate. H & E × 250

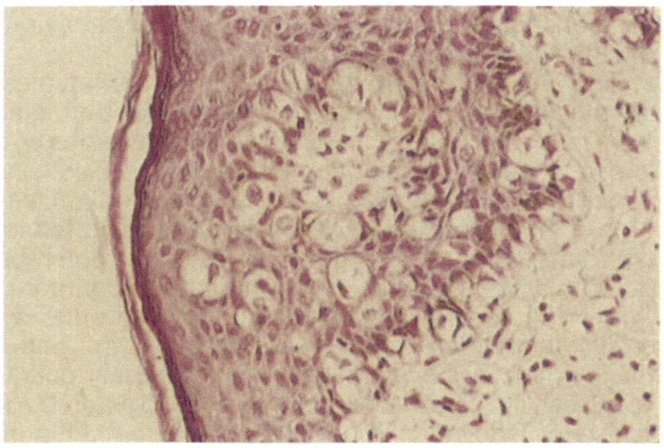

Figure 3.12 Vulva: Paget's disease. The basal layers of this intrinsically normal squamous epithelium are infiltrated by large cells with clear cytoplasm and central round or ovoid nuclei. Clusters of similar cells also lie higher in the Malpighian layer. Mucin stains demonstrate intracytoplasmic mucus and help to distinguish the cells from those of malignant melanoma to which they may bear a close resemblance. H & E × 250

plastic dystrophy and in the hyperplastic areas of a mixed dystrophy. Atypia is never seen in lichen sclerosus; reported examples of this condition that have apparently progressed to an invasive neoplasm probably being cases of mixed dystrophy, in which the hyperplastic component was either overlooked or subsequently obliterated by the neoplasm.

Cellular atypia may also develop in flat vulval condylomata or in the adjacent epithelium and is, in such circumstances, often associated with cervical neoplasia. Whether, however, cellular atypia can arise in previously fully normal vulval squamous epithelium is a debatable point to which there is, as yet, no answer.

Areas of atypical epithelium may appear flat or warty: reddening with an atypical vascular pattern often indicates the site of the most marked cytological abnormalities.

Histologically, atypia may be recognized by disturbances of normal epithelial stratification and abnormalities of cellular maturation. Two basic patterns are seen, one in which cells of basal or parabasal type with a high nucleo–cytoplasmic ratio and basophilic cytoplasm extend into the upper layers of the epidermis, and a second in which premature cytoplasmic maturation of individual cells occurs in the deep layers of the epithelium. In both forms mitotic figures are seen higher in the epithelium than normal and, in severe cases, these may be of abnormal or bizarre form: other atypical cellular features include multinucleation, nuclear pleomorphism with irregular dispersion of chromatin, parakeratosis and koilocytosis. When these abnormalities are limited to the lower third of the epithelium and are of minor degree the condition is usually described as mild atypia (Figure 3.5), extension into the middle third is moderate atypia (Figure 3.6) whilst involvement of more than two thirds of the epithelial thickness is classed as a severe atypia: involvement of the full thickness of the epithelium (Figure 3.7) is regarded as carcinoma *in situ*[1]. There is an increasing tendency to use the terms vulval intraepithelial neoplasia (VIN) grades I, II and III to correspond, respectively, with mild atypia, moderate atypia and severe atypia/carcinoma *in situ*, but this terminology is less well established than is that for the corresponding cervical lesions, largely because of the greater uncertainty about the interrelationships between, and the biological behaviour of, the various grades of vulval atypia.

The individual histological features in an atypical epithelium vary from patient to patient and from area to area in individual patients, but in general terms two types of vulval carcinoma *in situ* (VIN III) are encountered, these often being multifocal. Multinucleation and the presence of mitotic figures, often of abnormal form, above the basal layers are common to both types but in the most frequently encountered form (Figure 3.7) a parakeratotic layer overlies an epithelium which is otherwise occupied throughout its full thickness by immature, atypical basal or parabasal cells (a picture previously described as 'erythroplasia of Queyrat'). The less common form (Figure 3.8) of carcinoma *in situ* (VIN III) is that in which premature individual cell keratinization, corps ronds, giant cells and pleomorphism, together with a variable degree of hyperkeratosis, are the predominant features: this latter form (sometimes called 'Bowen's disease' or 'Bowenoid atypia') is virtually identical to the pattern seen if cellular atypia develops in a flat condyloma (Figure 3.9), and it is possible that all such cases originate in warty epithelium and are of viral aetiology[4].

Rarely, the disturbance in epithelial maturation is principally indicated by the presence of epithelial pearls in the rete ridges (Figure 3.10), a feature thought to indicate a prognosis worse than that which would be predicted from the degree of cellular atypia alone[5,6]; it should be noted, however, that the prognosis for all types of vulvar cellular atypia is uncertain, for it is known that carcinoma *in situ* (VIN III) in this site can regress and does not commonly appear to progress to an invasive neoplasm.

Microinvasive Squamous Cell Carcinoma (Figure 3.11)

This term has been introduced in an attempt to define a group of early or minimally invasive carcinomata which can be treated conservatively. Agreed criteria for the diagnosis of vulval microinvasive carcinoma have not been established, but these tumours appear to fall into one or other of two groups[7]. In the first group, small, spray-like confluent lesions breach the basement membrane and arise from epithelium which rarely shows evidence of intraepithelial atypia. Even when the depth of invasion is less than 5 mm from the lower surface of the epithelium from which they have arisen, 10% of such tumours will have metastasized to regional lymph nodes at the time of diagnosis. The second, and apparently distinct, type is that in which one or more isolated cords of cells extend into the stroma, to a distance of 2 mm or less, from an epithelium showing intraepithelial neoplasia: metastases have so far not been reported with this type of microinvasive lesion, which is being encountered increasingly frequently in young women with carcinoma *in situ* (VIN III) having arisen in association with condylomata. Any evidence of vascular invasion, no matter how small the lesion is, negates a diagnosis of microinvasive vulval carcinoma.

Paget's Disease

Vulval Paget's disease is rare and occurs most commonly after the menopause. It presents as poorly demarcated, erythematous, eczematoid, often multifocal, lesions, subsequent histological examination shows large, round or oval cells with palely basophilic or neutrophilic cytoplasm lying singly or in nests in the epidermis, clusters of cells being seen predominantly in the basal layers (Figure 3.12). These cells stain positively with PAS (after diastase), Alcian blue, and Gomori's aldehyde fuchsin, whilst staining variably with Masson–Fontana, and giving a negative DOPA reaction, characteristics which differentiate them from the cells of a malignant melanoma or of a Bowenoid type of atypia.

In up to 50% of cases there is intraepithelial or invasive neoplasia in the adjacent cutaneous adnexae, and it appears that the Paget cells are adenocarcinomatous cells which have migrated into the epidermis. However, in other cases there is no associated neoplasm, and it is thought that under these circumstances the Paget cells have developed *in situ* from undifferentiated or uncommitted cells in the germinative zone and represent therefore a type of primary intraepithelial neoplasia. On very rare occasions invasion of the dermis by Paget cells has been recorded, but this is exceptional and most cases pursue an indolent but progressive course. The prognosis is poor for those patients with invasive adnexal tumours at the time of diagnosis, but is better in those with no extraepidermal neoplasia; the histological extent of the disease often extends, however, beyond the margins of the clinically visible lesion and this, together with the *in situ* development of the neoplasia, probably explains the high incidence of recurrence after local excision.

References

1. International Society for the Study of Vulvar Disease. (1976). New nomenclature for vulvar disease. Report of the Committee on Terminology. *Obstet. Gynecol.*, **47**, 122–124
2. Buscema, J., Woodruff, J. D., Parmley, T. H. and Genadry, R. (1980). Carcinoma *in situ* of the vulva. *Obstet. Gynecol.*, **55**, 225–230
3. Buscema, J., Stein, J. and Woodruff, J. D. (1980). The significance of the histologic alterations adjacent to invasive vulvar carcinoma. *Am. J. Obstet. Gynecol.*, **137**, 902–909
4. Stein, D. S. (1980). Transmissible venereal neoplasia: a case report. *Am. J. Obstet. Gynecol.*, **137**, 864–865
5. Buscema, J. and Woodruff, J. D. (1980). Progressive histobiologic alterations in the development of vulvar cancer. *Am. J. Obstet. Gynecol.*, **138**, 146–150
6. Zacur, H., Genadry, R. and Woodruff, J. D. (1980). The patient-at-risk for development of vulvar cancer. *Gynecol. Oncol.*, **9**, 199–208
7. Barnes, A. E., Crissman, J. D., Schellhas, H. F. and Azoury, R. S. (1980). Microinvasive carcinoma of the vulva: a clinicopathologic evaluation. *Obstet. Gynecol.*, **56**, 234–238

Vulva: Neoplasms

4

Tumours of the vulva are not common but are, as are all skin neoplasms, extremely varied[1].

Benign Epithelial Tumours

Basal Cell Papilloma (Seborrhoeic Keratosis)

This is common, occurs mainly after middle age and appears as a velvety, granular or verrucous, exophytic pigmented plaque. Histologically (Figure 4.1), it is composed of sheets and cords of variably pigmented, small, uniform basaloid cells with relatively large nuclei: horny invaginations which appear as keratin lined cysts and true horn cysts may be present; irritation may result in the formation of keratinized squamous cells in sheets or whorls. The adjacent papillary dermis is usually inflamed.

Condylomata Acuminata.

These are sexually transmitted, papilloma virus-induced neoplasms; they occur on the vulva, perineum and perianal area in young women, are frequently multiple and may be papillary or verrucous, pedunculated or sessile (Figure 4.2). Histologically, hyperkeratotic or parakeratotic squamous epithelium showing koilocytosis, epithelial multinucleation and individual cell keratinization is supported by fine, fibrovascular papillary cores. Condylomata may be associated with, or followed by, vulval intraepithelial neoplasia.

Keratoacanthoma

This usually appears in the older patient on the hair-bearing skin of the vulva as a solitary, firm, dome-shaped nodule with a central keratin-filled crater. It usually reaches its maximum size of 1–2 cm in a few weeks, involuting spontaneously within a few months and healing with a small depressed scar. The general morphology is typical: a central epithelial invagination is filled with keratin and irregular strands of squamous epithelium extend down into the dermis and up into the crater, the underlying dermis is inflamed. In the immature lesion, the infiltrating epithelial strands show individual cell keratinization, cells of atypical appearance and mitoses, whilst in the mature lesion keratinization is more extensive, mitoses are fewer and atypical cells rare. As the lesion resolves, dermal inflammation decreases, the epithelium shows more widespread keratinization and the crater gradually flattens and disappears.

Malignant Epithelial Tumours

Squamous Carcinoma

This is the most common malignant neoplasm of the vulva comprising 4% of all malignant disease of the genital tract and 90% of malignant vulval tumours. The majority of patients with this neoplasm are more than 50 years old, less than 6% are premenopausal and almost one third are nulliparous.

Squamous carcinoma may follow long term irritation or granulomatous inflammation of the vulva and in about 50% of cases there is histological evidence of an associated vulval dystrophy. The association of this neoplasm with sexually transmitted diseases and with multicentric carcinoma in the lower genital tract (between 6 and 15% of patients have synchronous or asynchronous cervical neoplasia) suggests the possibility of a venereally transmitted carcinogen, perhaps a virus.

Almost three quarters of the tumours arise from the labia and most of the remainder arise equally from the posterior commissure and the clitoris[2]. Approximately equal proportions appear indurated, ulcerated or exophytic. In 2–3% of patients there is more than one invasive focus and in 25–30%, multicentric intraepithelial neoplasia is also present.

Histologically, 90–95% of these neoplasms are well well-differentiated, consisting of irregular masses of epithelial cells showing intercellular bridges and minimal cytological atypia and, with progressive keratinization towards the centres of the masses, the familial epithelial pearls (Figure 4.3). Other cellular strands consist of partially keratinized cells. A dermal inflammatory infiltrate is common.

In the less common poorly differentiated tumour the cell masses are less clearly demarcated from the surrounding stroma, show focal or individual cell keratinization, lack intercellular bridges and show greater cellular atypia and more frequent, often atypical mitoses. Occasionally, particularly following irradiation, a spindled cell form occurs[1]. The dermal inflammatory infiltrate is often scanty.

There is no correlation between the histological grade of the tumour and the clinical stage at presentation, although the well-differentiated tumours do appear to run a more indolent course. The 5 year survival is directly related to the clinical stage and the extent of lymph node involvement, and ranges from 90% for stage I disease with no metastases to less than 25% in stage II and IV disease with bilateral inguinal or pelvic node metastases.

Verrucous Carcinoma

This is a distinct, but rare, neoplasm which usually occurs in the elderly. It mimics the condyloma acuminatum both clinically and histologically, and forms a condylomatous mass with acanthotic epithelium supported by fine fibrovascular, papillary cores. The diagnosis may be missed because of the extraordinarily good cellular differentiation (Figure 4.4), absence of epithelial pearls and rarity of mitoses. Cellular atypia is rare, but occasionally occurs at the bases of the rete ridges, and individual cell keratinization is seen. The bland histological appearances are in sharp contrast to the locally aggressive nature of the neoplasm, which has a marked tendency to recur and requires extensive local resection: it does not, however, metastasize. Radiotherapy appears to enhance its aggressiveness.

Malignant Melanoma

Only 2–9% of vulval cancer is of this type, which occurs in a generally older age group than does squamous carcinoma.

There are two main patterns of growth, the superficial spreading, formed by large cells with large nuclei and nucleoli and finely granular cytoplasm, and the nodular, with epithelioid or spindle-like cells (Figure 4.5); both have irregular margins and show variable pigmentation. The former grows by lateral spread in the epidermis with later dermal invasion, whilst the latter invades the dermis deeply *ab initio* without a horizontal growth phase.

Melanomata are staged by, and the prognosis is directly related to, the depth of invasion[3], the nodular lesions thus having the worse prognosis. Tumours limited to the epidermis (Level I) are extremely rare and their potential for metastasis is uncertain. Extension of the tumour for less than 1 mm from the granular layer, invading but not filling the papillary dermis, is Level II for which 100% survival is expected after adequate treatment. Tumour filling and expanding the papillary dermis with spread to the border of the reticular dermis (1–2 mm) is Level III and with extension into the reticular dermis (more than 2 mm), Level IV, a 40% survival rate is expected. Once tumour has penetrated the subcutaneous fat (Level V), a 20% survival is the most that can be hoped for.

Basal Cell Carcinoma

These are rare in the vulva, and tend to develop in the elderly. Most occur on the labia and histologically they resemble basal cell carcinoma elsewhere in the body. The individual tumour cell has a large oval or elongated darkly staining nucleus, poorly defined cytoplasm and cell margins and lacks intercellular bridges on light microscopy. They are arranged in a variety of patterns, solid (Figure 4.6) and cystic masses, fine trabeculae and small scattered groups, the cells at the periphery of the cell masses typically form a palisade; the adjacent stroma shows immature fibrous tissue which often appears mucinous. Local excision is usually curative but the tendency of the tumour to have a superficial peripheral component which is not clinically apparent emphasizes the necessity for wide excision.

Urethral Tumours

Neoplasms at this site are uncommon; those developing in the distal urethra are usually squamous, but may be transitional, whilst those in the upper urethra are more commonly transitional: very exceptionally a urethral adenocarcinoma may arise from the paraurethral glands.

Tumours of the Skin Appendages

Papillary Hidradenoma

This is an exclusively vulval, benign neoplasm of apocrine sweat gland origin. Generally an asymptomatic nodule arises from the labia majora, the interlabial sulcus or the lateral surface of the labia minora. Occasionally the covering epithelium becomes ulcerated, tumour protrudes and bleeding may occur.

Histologically (Figure 4.7), the tumour comprises a complex of tubules and glands lined by a single or, typically, a double layer of epithelium, the outer layer being myoepithelium. The absence of cellular atypia and the infrequency of mitoses distinguish this neoplasm from adenocarcinoma to which it bears a superficial resemblance.

Rare Sweat Gland Tumours

Clear cell hidradenoma and syringoma, benign neoplasms arising from the epithelial matrices in the eccrine sweat gland primordia and eccrine ducts respectively occur only in the vulva, whilst sweat gland carcinoma of acintic cell origin (Figure 4.8) are unusual and usually associated with Paget's disease. Ductal carcinoma, morphologically similar to that of breast carcinoma, and not associated with Paget's disease has been reported[4].

Adenosquamous carcinoma[5] of the vulva arising from the mucin secreting cells of the skin appendages is a rare and highly aggressive neoplasm with a very poor prognosis. Histologically, it comprises areas of poorly differentiated squamous carcinoma and glandular or adenoid spaces lined by cuboidal cells with basophilic granular cytoplasm.

Connective Tissue Neoplasms

Small benign connective tissue tumours such as leiomyomata or neurofibromata can develop in the vulva but show no predeliction for the site.

Angiokeratoma

This tumour has a predeliction for the vulva, it occurs in the child-bearing years, forms a purple sessile nodule and consists of dilated, endothelial-lined channels in the papillary and reticular dermis (Figure 4.9); the overlying squamous epithelium is hyperkeratotic and extremely acanthotic, rete ridges extending deeply to separate the vascular channels. The adjacent dermis is often mildly inflamed.

Granular Cell Tumour (Granular Cell Myoblastoma)

In the vulva this forms an ill-defined, grey or yellow-grey, subcutaneous nodule[6]. Histologically (Figure 4.10) it is composed of large polyhedral cells with indistinct cell margins, granular, eosinophilic cytoplasm and round vesicular nuclei. Bands of fibrous tissue create a lobular pattern. The covering epithelium is often hyperplastic (or pseudoepitheliomatous) and may be mistaken for carcinoma. The lack of a capsule and the infiltrating margins of this benign neoplasm necessitates wide excision to prevent recurrence, whilst very occasionally malignant forms occur.

Sarcomata

Vulval sarcomata are rare, accounting for only 1–3% of malignant vulval neoplasms. They may be of any type but most commonly are leiomyomata[7].

Metastatic Tumours

The possibility of metastatic tumour should always be considered when presented with a vulval tumour of unusual appearance. Most commonly the primary site lies in the cervix but the endometrium, kidney, urethra, breast, lung and lymphoma must all be considered.

The vulva is a particularly important site of metastasis of choriocarcinoma, (Figure 4.11) but it is essential to differentiate between the villus-containing deposits which occur in invasive mole and true choriocarcinoma metastases which show a typical biphasic pattern and lack villi.

Bartholin's Gland Tumours

Adenoma of Bartholin's Gland

This is an unusual neoplasm which is probably related to age and inflammation[8]. It is a well-defined nodule composed of branching and closely packed alveoli lined by mucigenic epithelium (Figure 4.12).

Carcinoma of Bartholin's Gland

These rare neoplasms present as a painless nodule in middle aged women[9].

Histologically 50% are adenocarcinomata, 30% squamous and the others adenoid cystic, transitional or indeterminate. The prognosis is poor, this usually being attributable to the extensive lymphatic drainage, the deep seated nature of the tumour and the tendency to delay treatment whilst regarding swellings of Bartholin's gland as inflammatory.

References

1. Lever, W. F. and Schaumburg-Lever, G. (1975). *Histopathology of the Skin.* (Philadelphia and Toronto: Lippincott)
2. Japaze, H., Garcia-Bunuel, R. and Woodruff, J. D. (1977). Primary vulvar neoplasia: a review of *in situ* and invasive carcinoma 1935–1972. *Obstet. Gynecol.*, **49**, 404–411
3. Chung, A. F., Woodruff, J. M. and Lewis, J. L. (1975). Malignant melanomas of the vulva. *Obstet. Gynecol.*, **45**, 638–646
4. Rich, P. M., Okagaki, T., Clark, B. and Prem, K. A. (1981). Adenocarcinoma of the sweat gland of the vulva. *Cancer*, **47**, 1352–1357
5. Underwood, J. W., Adcock, L. L. and Okagaki, T. (1978). Adenosquamous carcinoma of skin appendages (adenoid squamous cell carcinoma, pseudoglandular squamous cell carcinoma, adenoacanthoma of sweat gland of Lever) of the vulva. *Cancer*, **42**, 1851–1858
6. Lieb, S. M., Gallousis, S. and Freedman, H. (1979). Granular cell myoblastoma of the vulva. *Gynecol. Oncol.*, **8**, 12–20
7. Davos, I. and Abell, M. R. (1976). Soft tissue sarcomas of the vulva. *Gynecol. Oncol.*, **4**, 70–86
8. Honore, L. H. and O'Hara, K. E. (1978). Adenoma of the Bartholin's gland: report of three cases. *Eur. J. Obstet., Gynecol. Reprod. Biol.*, **8**, 335–340
9. Wahlström, T., Vesterinen, E., and Saksela, E. (1978). Primary carcinoma of Bartholin's glands: a morphological and clinical study of six cases including a transitional cell carcinoma. *Gynecol. Oncol.*, **6**, 354–362

Figures 4.1–4.12 will be found overleaf.

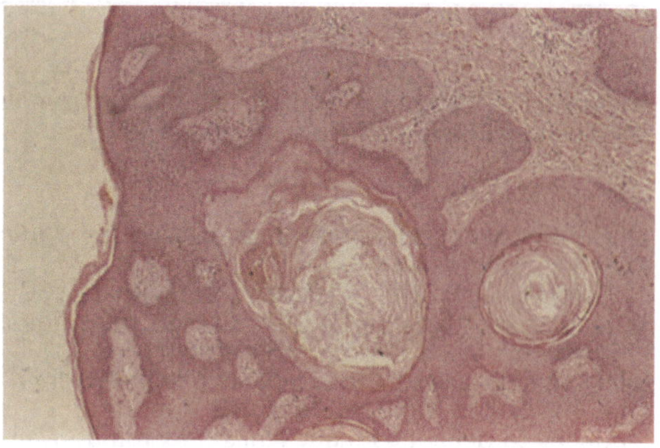

Figure 4.1 Vulva: basal cell papilloma. The lesion is composed of sheets and bands of uniform, focally pigmented, basaloid squamous cells around the margins of which there is a sharply defined regular layer of basal cells. The surface epithelium (to the left) is hyperkeratotic and the cellular islands contain invaginations and cysts in which there is laminated keratin. The fibrous stroma is chronically inflamed. H & E x 40

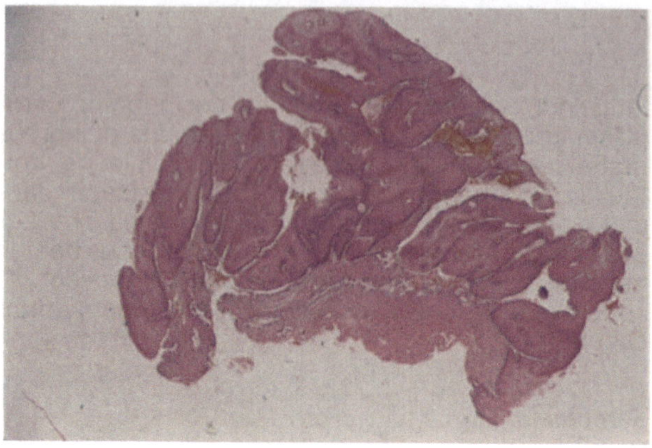

Figure 4.2 Vulva: condyloma acuminatum. This complete papillary condyloma acuminatum, removed from a patient receiving immunosuppressives after renal transplantation, is formed by fibro-vascular cores covered by acanthotic squamous epithelium. Flat condylomata similar to those seen in the cervix (Figure 8.8) also occur on the vulva. The cytological characteristics of both forms of condyloma are similar. H & E x 40

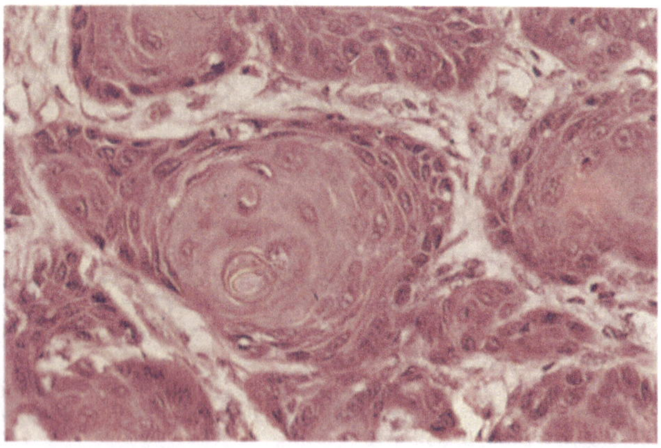

Figure 4.3 Vulva: squamous carcinoma. The sharply demarcated, infiltrating islands of well differentiated squamous carcinoma are composed of cells showing progressive cytoplasmic maturation (keratinization) towards the centres of the islands with the formation of epithelial pearls. The individual cells show only a little pleomorphism, have well-formed intercellular bridges and an occasional nucleolus; mitoses are rare. H & E x 250

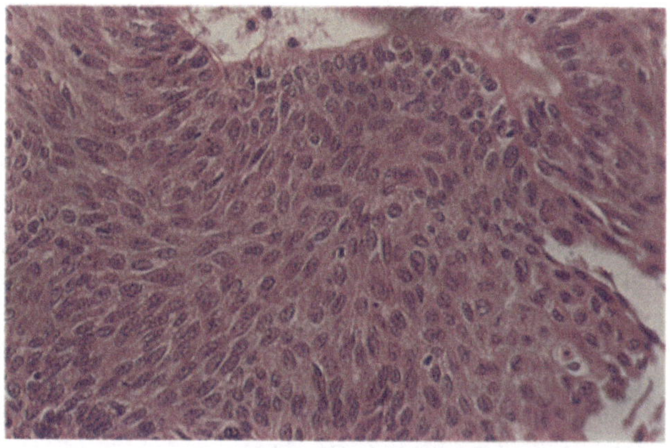

Figure 4.4 Vulva: verrucous carcinoma. The tumour is composed of well differentiated squamous cells showing remarkably little pleomorphism and only occasional multinucleation or individual cell keratinization, features which emphasize its similarity to a papillary condyloma acuminatum. H & E x 250

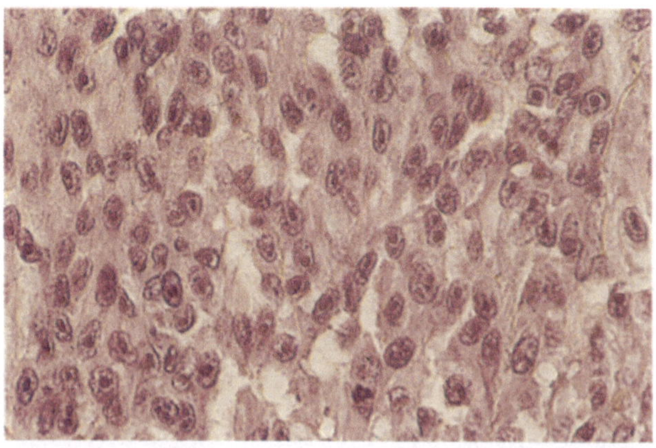

FigureFigure 4.5 Vulva: malignant melanoma. The epithelioid cells of this nodular melanoma are large, have a high nucleo–cytoplasmic ratio and prominent eosinophilic nucleoli. This example was virtually amelanotic. H & E x 400

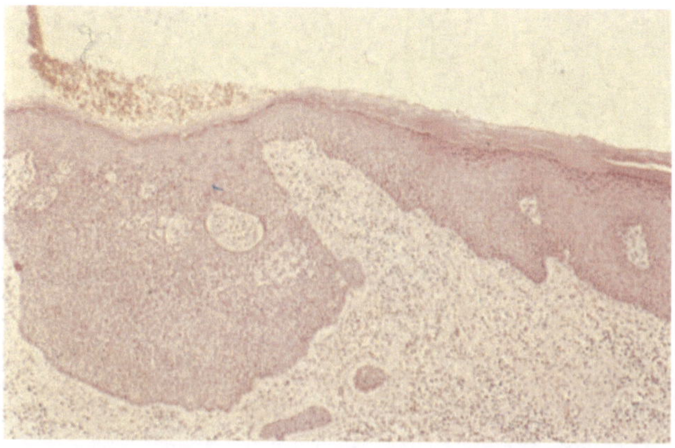

Figure 4.6 Vulva: basal cell carcinoma. One of the foci of a solid, basal cell carcinoma showing its origin from the squamous epithelium. The peripheral cellular palisade is visible even at this magnification. H & E x 40

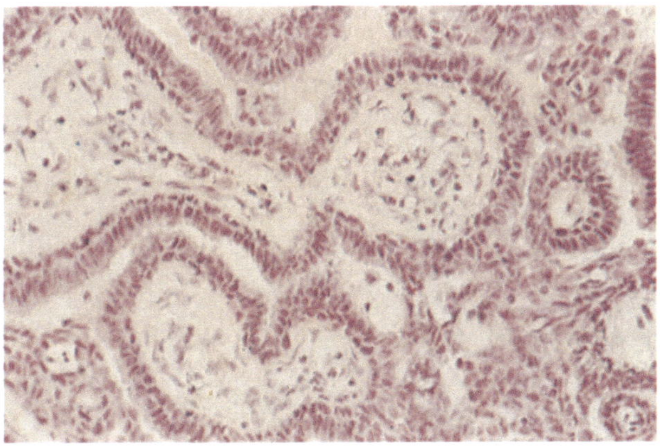

Figure 4.7 Vulva: papillary hidradenoma. The glands are lined and the papillae are covered by a double layer of epithelium. The deeper layer is formed by small, regular myoepithelial cells with ill-defined cytoplasm and darkly staining flattened nuclei lying parallel to the basement membrane. The outer columnar cells have larger vesicular nuclei whose long axes lie at right angles to the basement membrane, and their cytoplasm is well-defined though pale. There is a fine fibrous stroma. H & E × 250

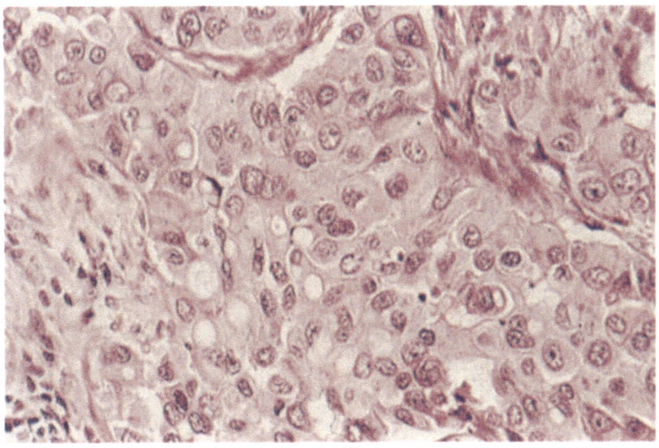

Figure 4.8 Vulva: adnexal carcinoma. This sweat gland tumour was associated with Paget's disease of the vulva (Figure 3.12). It is composed of large cells with well-defined cellular margins, pale eosinophilic cytoplasm and rather pleomorphic nuclei with irregularly dispersed chromatin and prominent nucleoli. H & E × 250

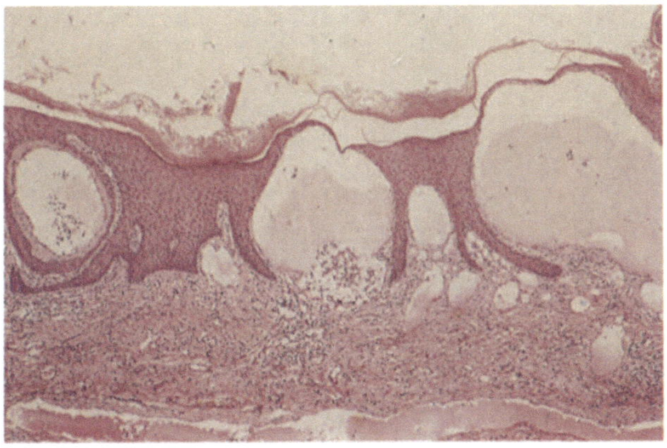

Figure 4.9 Vulva: angiokeratoma. The rete ridges of the epidermis are elongated and enclose thin-walled vascular channels. The epithelium is mildly hyperkeratotic and the dermis is chronically inflamed. H & E × 40

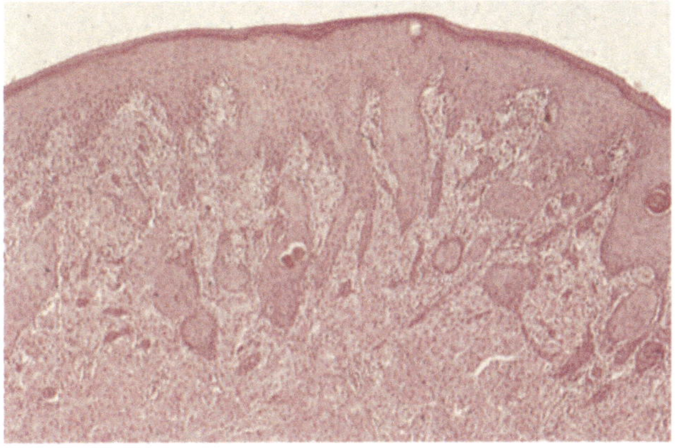

Figure 4.10 Vulva: granular cell tumour. The tumour cells are large, have round vesicular nuclei and granular eosinophilic cytoplasm. They infiltrate and pack the dermis and subcutaneous tissue. The covering epidermis shows a striking degree of pseudoepitheliomatous hyperplasia and elongated rete ridges, some with well formed 'epithelial pearls', appear to penetrate deeply into the dermis. The absence of cellular atypia and/or mitoses and the presence of the characteristic granular cells distinguishes the condition from infiltrating squamous carcinoma. H & E × 40

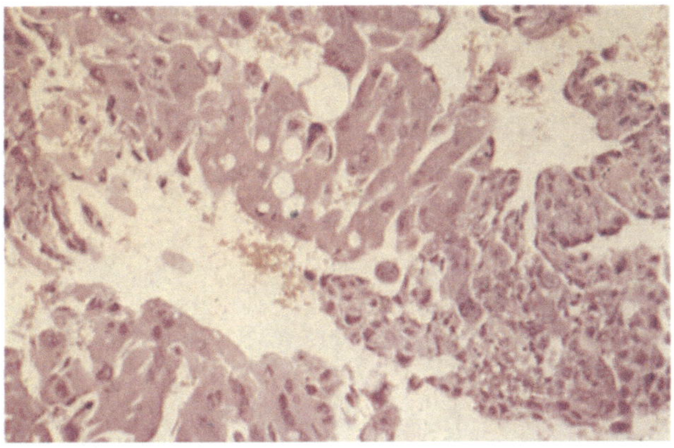

Figure 4.11 Vulva: metastatic choriocarcinoma. This vulval nodule contains areas of multinucleate syncytiotrophoblast with dense eosinophilic cytoplasm to the upper left and cytotrophoblast with its paler cytoplasm to the lower right. No villi were present in the lesion thus distinguishing it from an invasive mole. H & E × 100

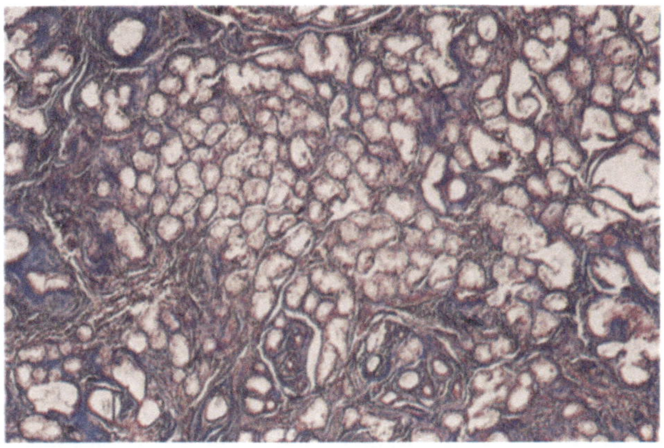

Figure 4.12 Vulva: Bartholin's gland adenoma. The field shows the closely packed glandular acini and relative paucity of stroma and ducts which characterize this neoplasm. Masson Trichrome × 40

Vagina: Non-Neoplastic Conditions

5

Inflammatory Disease

Non-infective Vaginitis

Many instances of vaginitis are of a non-infective nature and result from trauma, surgery, foreign bodies, irradiation, chemical irritants, ill-fitting pessaries or prolapse (Figure 5.1). In most such cases the histological appearances are quite non-specific but post-irradiation vaginitis is characterized by a plasma cell infiltrate, obliterative endarteritis, atypia of stromal fibroblasts and hyalinization of stromal collagen.

When plasma oestrogen levels are low, i.e. in the pre-menarchal and post-menopausal years and during lactation, the vaginal epithelium becomes thin and an atrophic vaginitis may develop: contrary to general belief, however, this is a rare condition and probably non-infective in nature[1]. Histological examination in such cases shows a thin epithelium, which is occasionally focally ulcerated, and a sub-epithelial lymphoplasmacytic infiltrate. A particular form of atrophic vaginitis is the very rare 'desquamative inflammatory' vaginitis which exactly mimics, both clinically and histologically, an atrophic vaginitis but in which plasma oestrogen levels are normal: this condition, currently of unknown pathogenesis, does not respond, as does an atrophic vaginitis, to oestrogen therapy.

Infective Vaginitis

About a third of vaginal infections are classed as 'non-specific': it is, however, now firmly established that this condition is due to infection with the sexually transmitted organism *Gardnerella vaginalis*, probably in association with anaerobic bacteria. Infections of this type are characterized by a malodorous, thin, greyish, vaginal discharge but are not accompanied by any tissue damage or inflammatory reaction[2].

N. gonorrhoeae can cause slight oedema and congestion of the vagina in adult women but is incapable of producing a true vaginitis, the thick squamous epithelium being resistant to the organism[3]. In children, however, the thinner mucosa is permeable to *N. gonorrhoeae* which is able to evoke a chronic vaginitis characterized by stromal oedema and congestion associated with a chronic inflammatory cell infiltrate.

Fungal infection of the vagina, usually due to *Candida albicans*, is common and usually associated with a vulvitis: *Candida albicans* is frequently present as part of the normal flora of the vagina and, in many cases, it is far from clear why it should assume a pathogenetic role. *Candida vaginitis* is characterized by a 'cottage cheese' discharge and white patches, which can be easily removed, on the vaginal mucosa: histological examination reveals fungal hyphae, a polymorphonuclear leukocytic exudate on the surface and a chronic inflammatory cell infiltrate of the underlying stroma.

Trichomonal vaginitis (Figure 5.2), is caused by the flagellate protozoan *Trichomonas vaginalis*, is common during the reproductive years and is usually, though not invariably, sexually transmitted. In the acute stage the mucosa is reddened and granular: oedema, congestion and a lymphocytic infiltration of the stroma, which may extend into the epithelium to form pseudo-abscesses, are the typical histological features. Following an acute episode the infection may pass into a chronic phase with persistence of the inflammatory process in the vagina, albeit in a somewhat damped down fashion: other patients become asymptomatic carriers, the protozoan continuing to inhabit the vagina but not eliciting any inflammatory reaction.

A herpetic vaginitis is present in most cases of herpes infection of the vulva, but is often overshadowed by the vulval lesions and hence overlooked. The histological features are similar to those seen in the vulva but occasionally there may be extensive ulceration.

Tampon-associated Vaginal Ulceration

Vaginal ulceration associated with tampon usage is uncommon, has been reported principally from the United States and tends to occur in women who change tampons unduly frequently[4]. The ulcers usually develop in the fornices and have rolled or irregular margins with a granular base. Histologically, the floor of the ulcer is formed of non-specific granulation tissue in which fibres may be embedded: biopsy of the ulcer edge shows regenerating epithelium which can be mistaken for squamous carcinoma.

Cysts

Vaginal cysts are uncommon, the type most frequently encountered being the mesonephric (or Gartner's duct) cyst (Figure 5.3) which, although typically arising in the anterolateral wall of the vagina, can also develop in the midline: although usually small these cysts may attain a size sufficient to present at the vulva. Histologically, the cysts are lined by an epithelium of cuboidal or low columnar cells and contain smooth muscle in their wall. Occasionally, multiple cysts of this type form a chain along the vaginal wall.

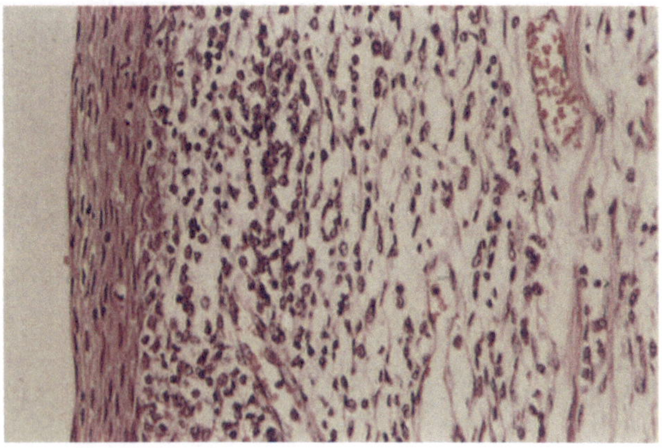

Figure 5.1 Vagina: non-specific inflammation. The vaginal epithelium (to the left) is rather atrophic and not glycogenated. In the stroma there is an inflammatory infiltrate of lymphocytes and plasma cells. The biopsy is from a patient with recurrent vaginitis. H & E × 250

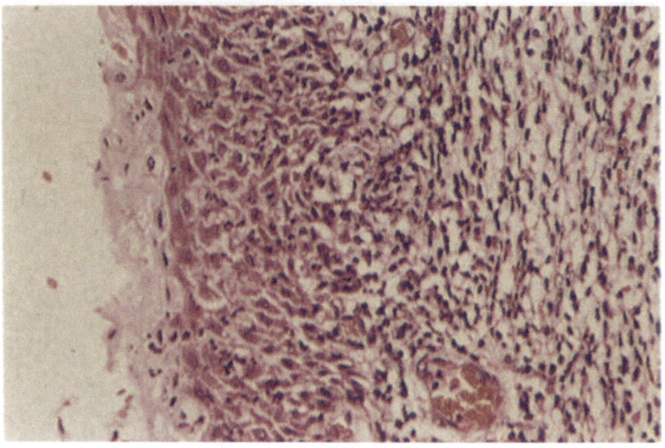

Figure 5.2 Vagina: Trichomonal vaginitis. The vaginal epithelium (to the left) is oedematous, infiltrated by lymphocytes and occasional polymorphonuclear leukocytes and there is sloughing of the superficial layers. The stroma is infiltrated by lymphocytes and plasma cells and the capillaries are dilated and congested. H & E × 250

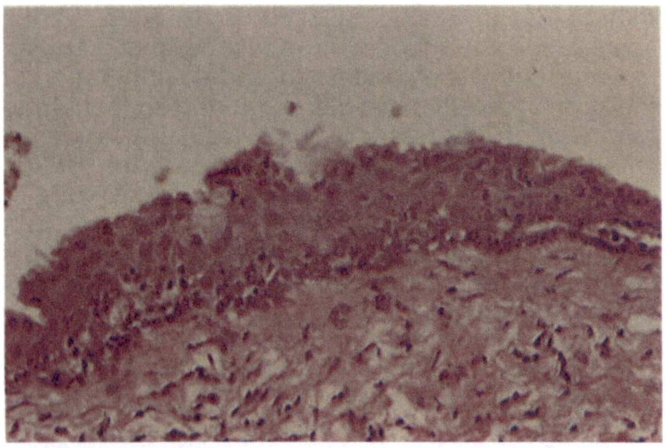

Figure 5.3 Vagina: Gartner's duct cyst. This is the wall of a series of cysts from the anterolateral vaginal wall. It is lined by cubo–columnar epithelium which is undergoing squamous metaplasia. Residual columnar cells are visible as an incomplete layer covering immature squamous epithelium. H & E × 250

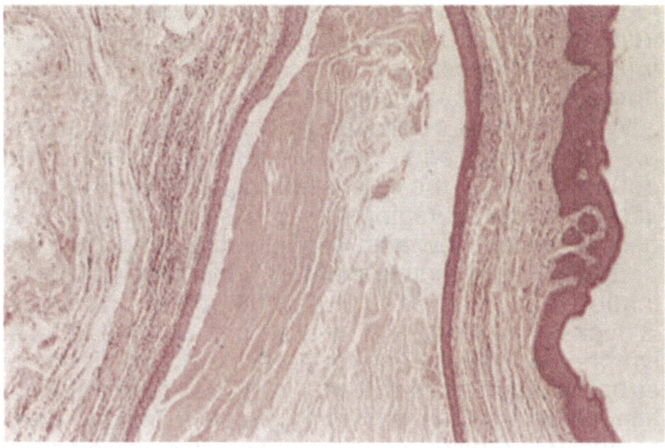

Figure 5.4 Vagina: epidermoid cyst. This cyst was removed from the lower, postero–lateral vaginal wall. It is lined by stratified squamous epithelium and contains laminated keratin. There is a mild chronic inflammatory cell infiltrate in the surrounding stroma. It occurred at the site of an episiotomy. H & E × 40

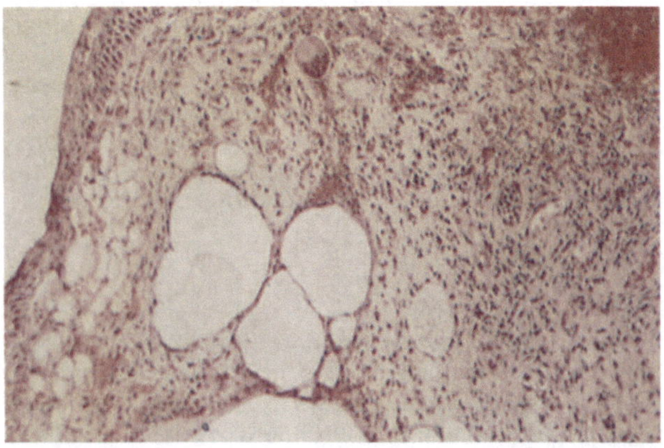

Figure 5.5 Vagina: emphysema. In the stroma beneath the vaginal epithelium there are several unlined cysts. The surrounding tissues are infiltrated by lymphocytes and occasional macrophages. A conspicuous macrophage giant cell is present centrally and above. H & E × 100

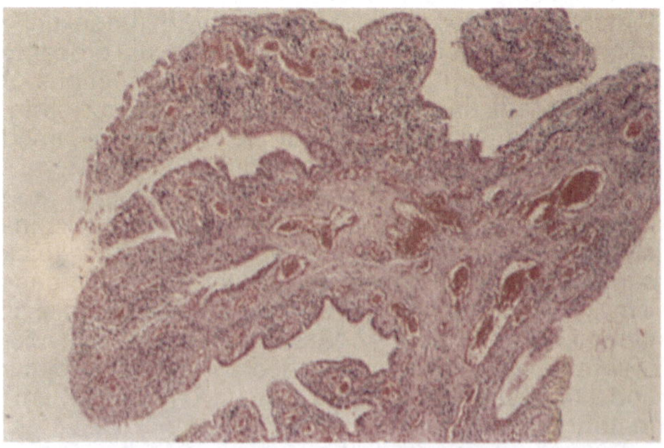

Figure 5.6 Vagina: prolapsed Fallopian tube. The tubal fimbria are congested and chronically inflamed. The covering epithelium shows non-specific reactive changes. H & E × 40

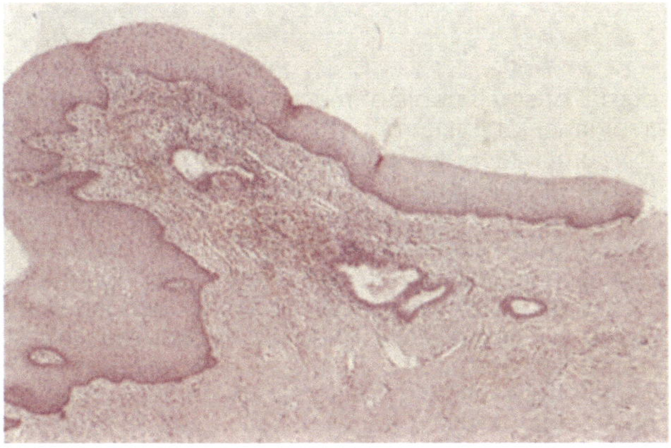

Figure 5.7 Vagina: adenosis. The vagina is lined by mature, metaplastic stratified squamous epithelium. In the stroma there are glands lined by mucus-secreting columnar epithelium. There is mild, non-specific, active chronic inflammation and hence mucus secretion is somewhat diminished. H & E x 40

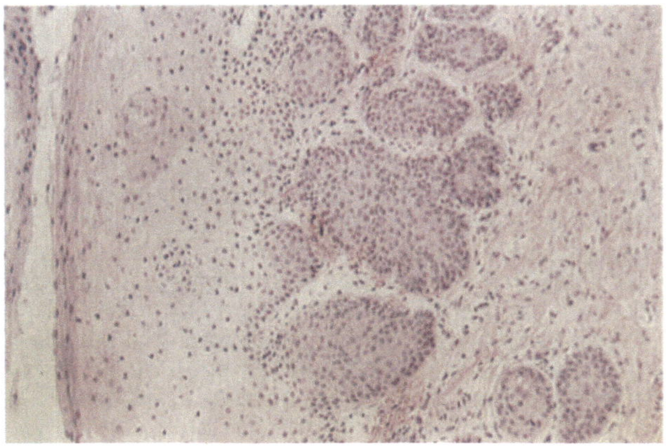

Figure 5.8 Vagina: squamous metaplasia in vaginal adenosis. Metaplasia has occurred in the surface epithelium (to the left) and in the glands. As a consequence nests of squamous epithelium, some showing keratinization lie within the vaginal stroma. There is a superficial resemblance to invasive squamous carcinoma but the deeply sited squamous epithelium shows no cytological atypia or abnormal mitotic activity. H & E x 100

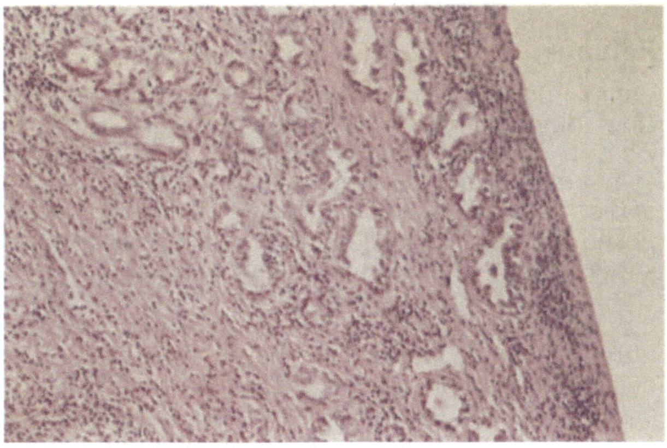

Figure 5.9 Vagina: adenosis with atypical features. The glandular acini in the vaginal wall are lined by cuboidal cells with large, rather pleomorphic, hyperchromatic nuclei. There are no atypical mitoses, and in this example the epithelium is not multilayered. The stroma is infiltrated by lymphocytes but there is no evidence of invasive neoplasia. H & E x 100

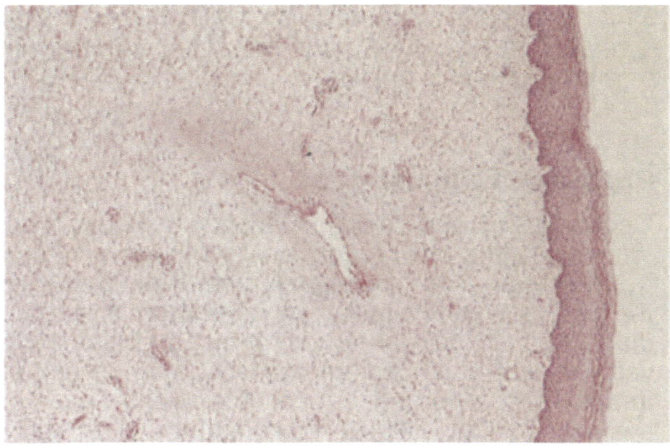

Figure 5.10 Vagina: fibroepithelial polyp. The stroma is composed of rather oedematous fibrous tissue in which there are many small, and occasional large, blood vessels. The covering epithelium is normal and in this example there is little or no inflammation. In other cases there may be a scattering, or aggregates, of lymphocytes. H & E x 40

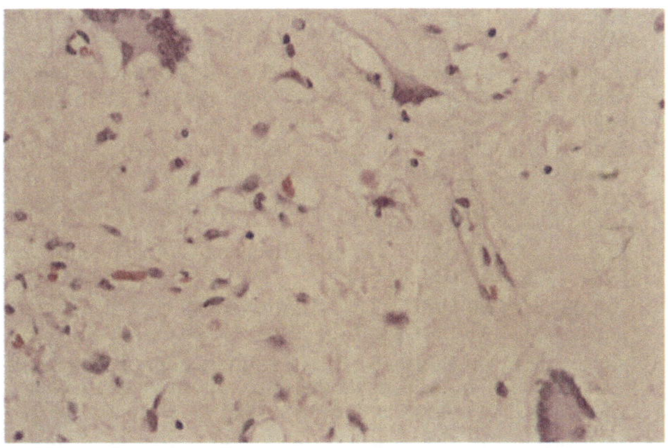

Figure 5.11 Vagina: fibroepithelial polyp. The stromal cells in this polyp show multinucleation and have abundant eosinophilic cytoplasm. The nuclei are pleomorphic and some are hyperchromatic but there are no mitoses. The polyp was removed from a woman of 54 years at the time of vaginal hysterectomy. She remains well 7 years later. H & E x 250

Cysts lined by endocervical, tubal or endometrial type epithelium can occur in the vagina[5] and it is possible that these paramesonephric (or Müllerian) cysts are derived from Müllerian remnants persisting after replacement of Müllerian epithelium by urogenital sinus squamous epithelium during vaginal development. Those lined by endometrial-type epithelium can be differentiated from endometriosis by the absence of any associated endometrial stroma.

Epidermoid cysts (Figure 5.4), lined by squamous epithelium and containing keratinous material, are most commonly found on the posterior vaginal wall and probably result from sequestration following obstetric trauma.

Emphysematous cysts of the vagina are distinctly uncommon: they occur as gas-filled blebs which elevate the overlying mucosa and, whilst often asymptomatic, may cause a vaginal discharge: occasionally, the cysts rupture and the patient complains of a popping noise emitting from the vagina. Microscopic examination (Figure 5.5) shows cystic spaces deep to the epithelium which are devoid of a lining and are surrounded by lymphocytes, histiocytes and foreign body giant cells. The pathogenesis of this condition is unknown.

Prolapsed Fallopian Tube

Occasionally a portion of the Fallopian tube prolapses into the vagina. This event usually follows a vaginal hysterectomy and presumably the tube prolapses through a small fistula. The condition is usually diagnosed clinically as florid granulation tissue in the vaginal vault, and histological examination reveals an initially disconcerting appearance which may be mistaken for metastatic tumour (Figure 5.6): this error is avoided if the absence of any cytological features of malignancy is appreciated and if this rare condition is borne in mind.

Adenosis

Vaginal adenosis, usually asymptomatic but occasionally associated with a mucoid discharge, appears to the naked eye as a reddish roughening of the vaginal mucosa, most commonly on the anterior wall of the upper vagina. Histologically, adenosis is characterized by the presence of glandular structures in the lamina propria of the vagina (Figure 5.7): these glands are lined, in most cases, by a mucinous epithelium of endocervical type but a minority of the glands may be lined by tubal or endometrial type epithelium. The glands can sometimes be seen opening into the vagina and their epithelial lining may extend onto the surface. The epithelium, both in the glands and on the surface, has a marked tendency to undergo squamous metaplasia (Figure 5.8) and the resultant multiple foci of squamous epithelium lying deep to the surface may give rise to a false suspicion of a squamous cell carcinoma: the lack of cytological and nuclear atypia and the presence, even in cases of apparently complete squamous metaplasia, of small pools of mucus in the foci help in the avoidance of this error.

Vaginal adenosis is thought to be due to a partial failure of the normally orderly process of Müllerian regression during the formation of the definitive vagina from the urogenital sinus, and is particularly common in individuals who have been prenatally exposed to diethylstilboestrol (DES), adenosis being found in about 70% of females exposed to this oestrogen before the 8th week of gestation. It is widely believed that clear cell adenocarcinomata of the vagina (see Chapter 6) usually develop from, and in, a preceding adenosis and atypical changes (Figure 5.9) in the glandular tissues, such as epithelial stratification, nuclear pleomorphism, hyperchromasia and an increased nucleo–cytoplasmic ratio, are thought to represent a transitional stage between benign adenosis and a frank adenocarcinoma[6]. It should perhaps be stressed, however, that a progression from histologically proven atypical adenosis to a clear cell adenocarcinoma has not yet been documented.

Polypi

Vaginal polypi are uncommon, can occur at any age (including infancy) and usually measure less than 2 cm in diameter. They are rubbery in consistency, sometimes pedunculated, greyish-white in colour and covered by vaginal mucosa. Their stroma is composed of loose, vascular connective tissue which may show varying degrees of oedema or myxoid change (Figure 5.10) and in which there is often a mild or moderate non-specific chronic inflammatory cell infiltrate. Scattered cells with abundant eosinophilic cytoplasm and pleomorphic, hyperchromatic nuclei are scattered throughout the stroma (Figure 5.11). Mitotic figures are very rare and a cambium layer is not seen, these features helping to differentiate the lesion from a sarcoma botyroides. It is not known whether these polypi are neoplastic in nature or not but they appear always to behave in a fully benign fashion[7].

References

1. Fleury, F. J. (1981). Adult vaginitis. *Clin. Obstet. Gynecol.*, **24**, 407–438
2. Vontver, L. A. and Eschenbach, D. A. (1981). The role of Gardnerella vaginalis in non-specific vaginitis. *Clin. Obstet. Gynecol.*, **24**, 439–460
3. Brown, W. J. (1978). Microbiol flora in infections of the vagina. In Hafez, E. S. E. and Evans, T. N. (eds.). *The Human Vagina*, pp. 423–434. (Amsterdam, New York and Oxford: North Holland Publ. Co.)
4. Friedrich, E. C. (1981). Tampon effects on vaginal health. *Clin. Obstet. Gynecol.*, **24**, 395–406
5. Deppisch, L. M. (1975). Cysts of the vagina: classification and clinical correlations. *Obstet. Gynecol.*, **45**, 632–637
6. Antonioli, D. A., Rosen, S., Burke, L. and Donahue, V. (1979). Glandular hyperplasia in diethylstilbestrol-associated vaginal adenosis: a case report and review of the literature. *Am. J. Clin. Pathol.*, **71**, 715–721
7. Chirayil, S. J. and Tobon, H. (1981). Polyps of the vagina: a clinico-pathologic study of 18 cases. *Cancer*, **47**, 2904–2907

Vagina: Neoplasms

6

Benign Neoplasms

Condyloma Acuminatum

This is the only common benign tumour of the vagina: it is often multiple and invariably associated with vulval and cervical lesions of similar type. The condylomata are usually small but occasionally attain a size sufficient to obstruct the vagina. Vaginal condylomata are histologically identical to those occurring in the vulva (see Chapter 4). Flat condylomata also occur in the vagina (Figure 6.1).

Rhabdomyoma

This rare tumour presents as a well defined nodule: histologically this is covered by squamous epithelium and is formed of large round, oval or elongated striated muscle cells set in a connective tissue stroma[1]: there is no pleomorphism or mitotic activity (Figure 6.2). These neoplasms can occur at any age and this benign neoplasm with its bland appearance must be differentiated from a rhabdomyosarcoma.

Mixed Tumour

These neoplasms are very rare but appear to be benign[2]. They present as well circumscribed, but not encapsulated, masses which histologically consist of islands of well glycogenated squamous epithelium set in a bland fibrous stroma (Figure 6.3).

Intraepithelial Neoplasia

Vaginal intraepithelial neoplasia (VAIN) is histologically identical to cervical intraepithelial neoplasia (see Chapter 8) and is similarly graded into VAIN I, VAIN II and VAIN III, the criteria for such grading being the same as those used for the cervical lesions (Figures 6.4 and 6.5). VAIN is frequently associated, either synchronously or asynchronously, with cervical or vulval intraepithelial neoplasia, the neoplasia may be invisible to the naked eye or can appear either as a sharply defined area of increased vascularity or as a whitish patch. VAIN requires to be differentiated from epithelial atrophy, from a flat condyloma and from reactive changes to inflammation.

The natural history of VAIN has not yet been defined, and although it is widely thought that VAIN can progress to an invasive carcinoma[3] the incidence of such a progression in untreated cases has not yet been established.

Malignant Neoplasms

Squamous Cell Carcinoma

This tumour accounts for between 1 and 2% of female genital tract cancer. However, the true incidence is difficult to determine for there is often some clinical doubt as to whether a neoplasm is truly arising in the vagina; it being a rule of thumb that a vaginal tumour extending to the external cervical os should be considered as a cervical carcinoma, and that one involving the vulva should be classified as a vulval carcinoma. The position is further complicated by the fact that a proportion of women who appear to have been successfully treated for cervical carcinoma later develop an apparently independent vaginal squamous carcinoma: in such instances it can be virtually impossible to distinguish between a recurrence of the cervical carcinoma and the development of a second primary tumour.

Vaginal squamous cell carcinomata occur most commonly between the ages of 55 and 70, develop particularly in the upper third of the vagina and arise predominantly on the anterior or posterior walls. Macroscopically they may assume an exophytic nodulo–papillary form or appear as an ulcerated endophytic lesion. Histologically, the neoplasm is a typical squamous cell carcinoma (Figure 6.6), most being rather poorly differentiated but a minority being well differentiated and forming squamous pearls.

The neoplasm tends to infiltrate locally, directly invading the paravaginal and parametrial tissues, the rectovaginal septum and either the bladder or rectum. Lymphatic spread from tumours in the upper third of the vagina is to the pelvic nodes whilst neoplasms in the middle and lower thirds also metastasize to the inguinal nodes. Blood borne spread, principally to bones and lungs, occurs late.

The overall 5 year survival rate for patients with a vaginal squamous cell carcinoma is 50%, the prognosis being almost entirely dependent upon the extent of spread at the time of initial diagnosis.

Adenocarcinoma

Vaginal adenocarcinoma was, until a decade ago, one of the rarest tumours of the female genital tract and, indeed, still is in Great Britain. Some years ago, however, it became apparent that there was, in certain parts of the United States, a significant increase in the incidence of clear cell adenocarcinomata of the vagina, this increase being entirely in young girls who had been exposed prenatally to diethylstilboestrol (DES). This association has now been fully confirmed and, currently, over 400 cases have accumulated[4],

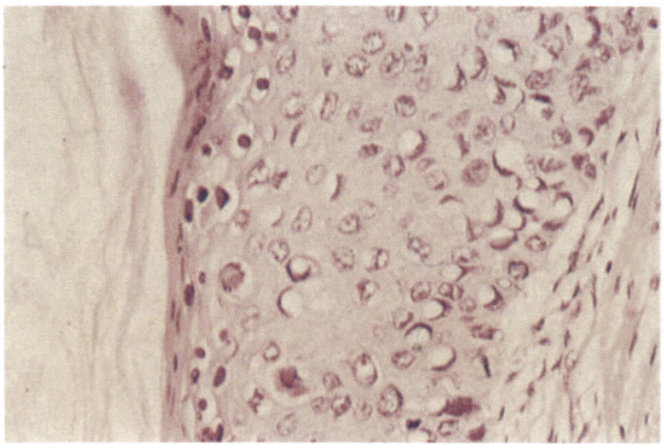

Figure 6.1 Vagina: flat condyloma. This vaginal biopsy came from a patient who had already had intraepithelial neoplasia of the cervix and vulva. It shows a flat condyloma acuminatum; the epithelial cells are enlarged and their nuclei moderately pleomorphic. The superficial cells, to the left, have perinuclear haloes, koilocytosis. H & E × 250

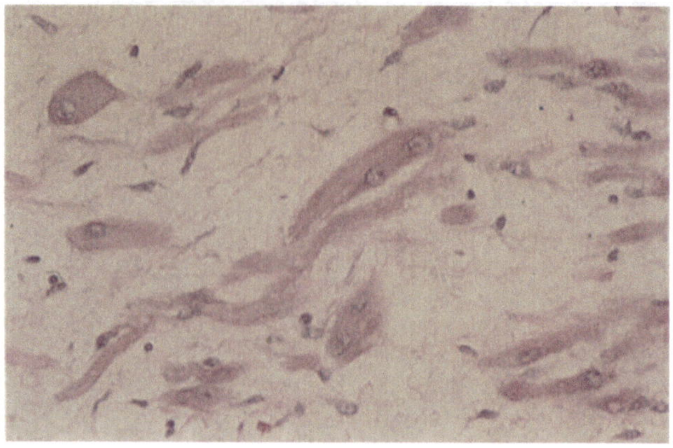

Figure 6.2 Vagina: rhabdomyoma. The nodule has a fine connective tissue stroma in which there are elongated and short oval or plump round striated muscle cells. The nuclei are round and their chromatin evenly dispersed; mitoses are absent. H & E × 250

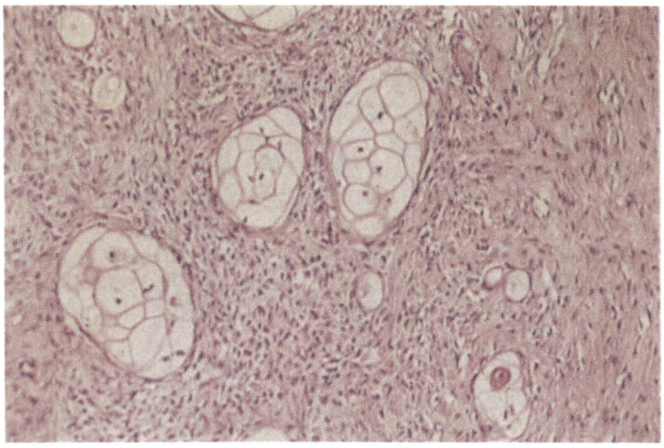

Figure 6.3 Vagina: mixed tumour. Well glycogenated islands of mature squamous epithelium with vacuolated cytoplasm lie in a cellular fibrous stroma. Centrally the stromal cells have little cytoplasm and round or oval nuclei; there is scanty collagen. To the right of the field, the stromal cells have more copious cytoplasm, smaller nuclei, reduced nucleo–cytoplasmic ratios and are arranged in interlacing bundles. H & E × 100

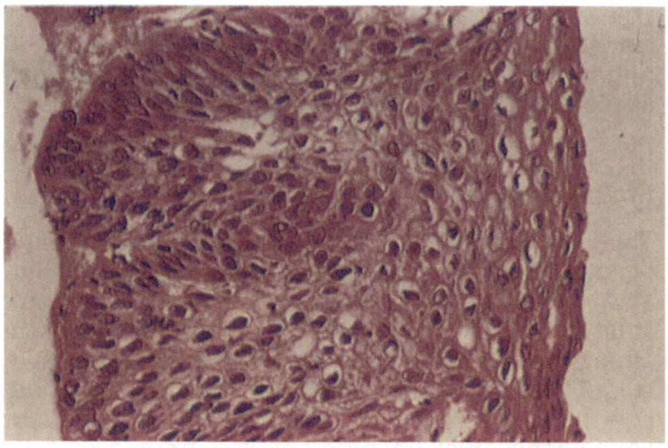

Figure 6.4 Vagina: squamous intraepithelial neoplasia grades I and II (VAIN I and II). This colposcopic biopsy (basal layer to the left) shows undifferentiated basaloid cells occupying between one third and half the depth of the epithelium. The presence of perinuclear haloes (koilocytosis) suggests that the lesion has a viral aetiology. H & E × 250

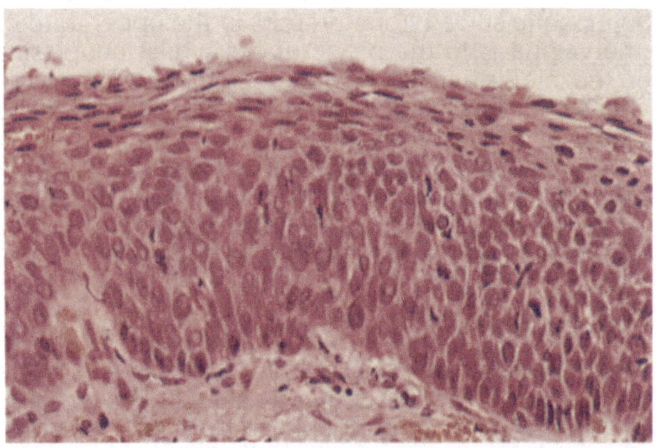

Figure 6.5 Vagina: squamous intraepithelial neoplasia grade III (VAIN III). In this colposcopic biopsy rather more than the lower two thirds of the depth of the epithelium are occupied by basaloid cells with high nucleo–cytoplasmic ratios and frequent mitoses. There is an absence of normal stratification and maturation. H & E × 250

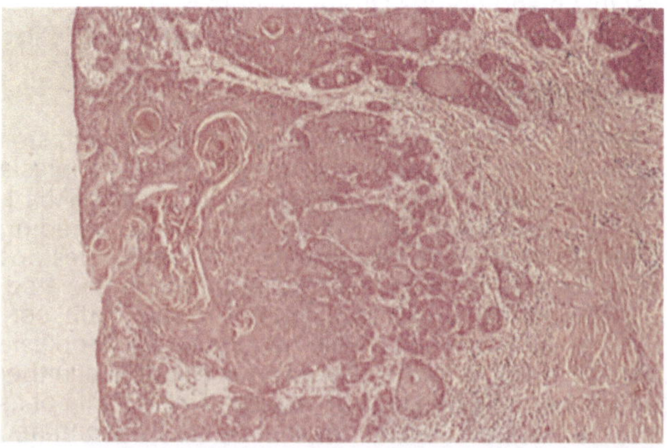

Figure 6.6 Vagina: squamous carcinoma. A well-differentiated squamous carcinoma is arising from the vaginal epithelium and penetrating the adjacent stroma in infiltrating islands. A high power view of a similar tumour is seen in Figure 4.3. H & E × 40

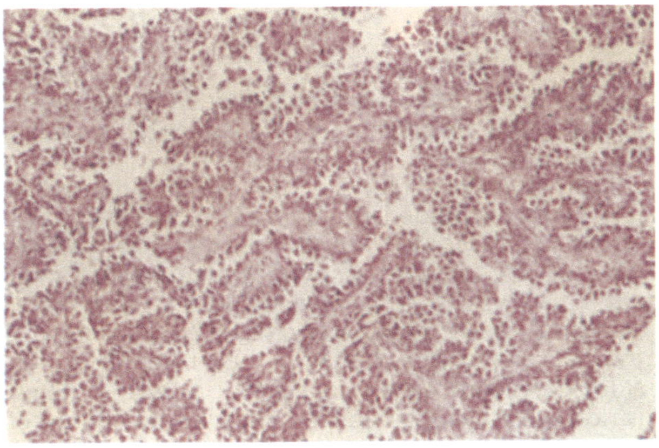

Figure 6.7 Vagina: clear cell carcinoma. A papillary area of tumour showing fine fibro-vascular connective tissue cores covered by large, pleomorphic cells which bud from the surface of the papillae. H & E × 100

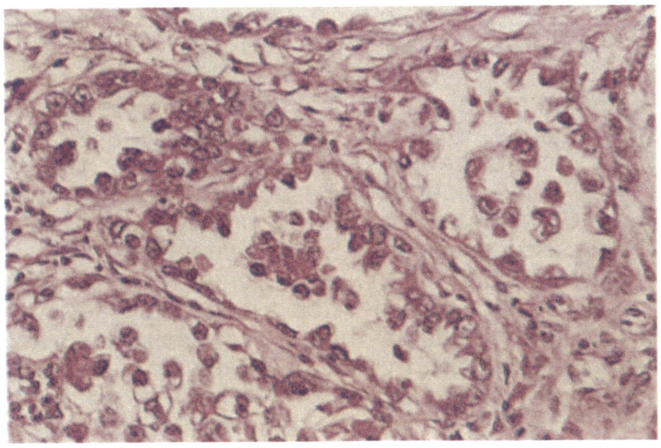

Figure 6.8 Vagina: clear cell carcinoma. These are acini or tubules of clear cell carcinoma lined by cells with large, prominent pleomorphic nuclei and pale eosinophilic cytoplasm, 'hobnail cells'. Note that although the tumour is termed 'clear cell carcinoma', the cytoplasm of the constituent cells is often granular or eosinophilic and not always clear. H & E × 250

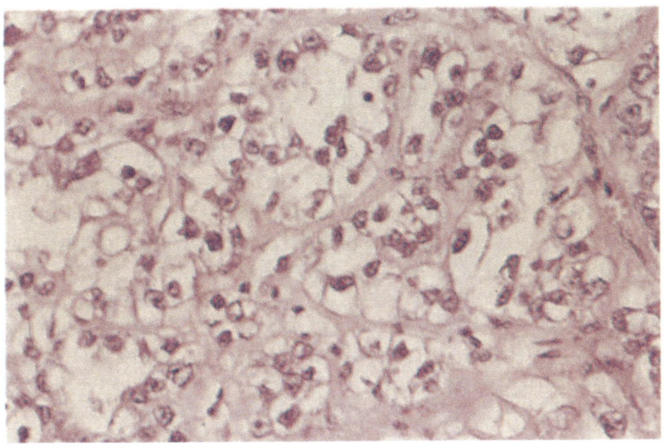

Figure 6.9 Vagina: clear cell carcinoma. Sheets of large cells with clear cytoplasm, well-defined cell boundaries and prominent pleomorphic nuclei are forming poorly defined acini. H & E × 250

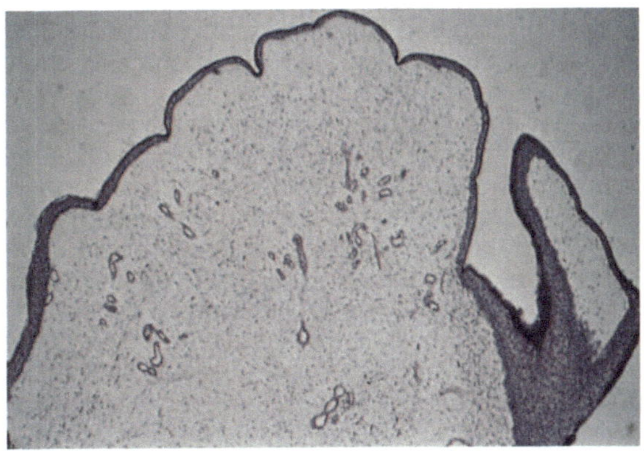

Figure 6.10 Vagina: sarcoma botyroides. The tumour is composed of a loose myxoid stroma in which there are small thin-walled blood vessels. The covering epithelium is squamous. There is very little condensation of the stromal cells beneath the surface epithelium except to the right where a hint of cambium layer can be seen. PTAH × 40

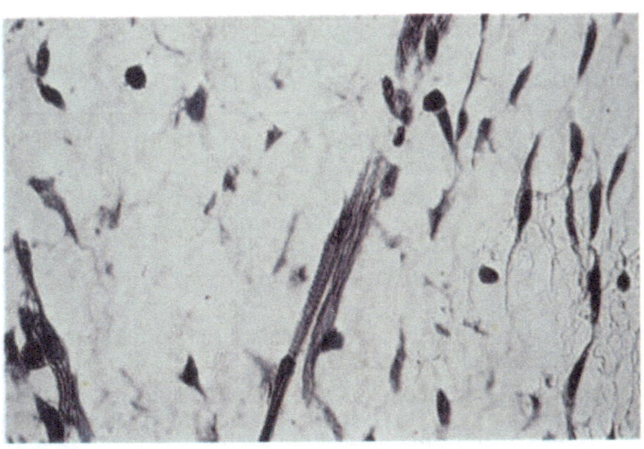

Figure 6.11 Vagina: sarcoma botyroides. Well-differentiated striated muscle fibres such as this or rhabdomyoblasts are frequently found in the stroma. PTAH × 250

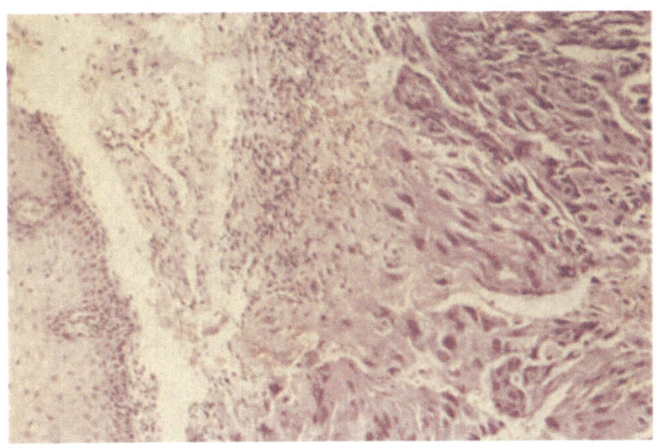

Figure 6.12 Vagina: metastatic choriocarcinoma. Beneath the vaginal squamous epithelium (to the left) there is an infiltrating mass of trophoblastic tissue. The absence of villi distinguishes the lesion from invasive hydatidiform mole. H & E × 100

common to most of which was the administration to the patient's mother of a synthetic oestrogen, usually DES, before the 18th week of pregnancy. Only 4 cases of this neoplasm have, however, been reported from Great Britain[5] and this is probably a reflection of the lesser usage of DES in this country.

Approximately 1 in 2000 women exposed prenatally to DES will develop a clear cell adenocarcinoma of the vagina, the tumour usually becoming apparent between the age of 14 and 23 years, most commonly in girls aged 17–19 years. The neoplasm almost certainly develops from pre-existing vaginal adenosis and is of Müllerian origin. It has, of course, to be borne in mind that very occasional instances of vaginal clear cell carcinoma occurred before the introduction of DES and that some examples will still present in non-exposed women, such cases usually, however, developing at a later age.

A clear cell adenocarcinoma usually develops in the upper third of the vagina, most commonly on the anterior wall: however, by the time of diagnosis it may form a bulky mass which fills the entire length of the vagina. Earlier cases may present as a polypoid, nodular or papillary mass though occasionally the neoplasm is flat or ulcerated. Histologically, there is a complex mixture of solid, papillary, tubular and cystic patterns (Figures 6.7, 6.8 and 6.9), the solid areas being formed of sheets of cells with clear cytoplasm and the tubules often being lined by 'hob-nail' cells which are characterized by their scanty cytoplasm and large, apparently naked, nuclei which protrude into the lumen. The cystic spaces tend to be lined by rather nondescript flattened cells.

The tumour spreads by local extension, by the lymphatics and by the blood stream and there is a surprisingly high incidence of spread to the supraclavicular nodes. The overall 5 year survival rate is approximately 80%, but a large tumour and deep invasion of the vaginal wall are both associated with a relatively poor prognosis.

Malignant Melanoma

The vagina is a rare site for this tumour: those that do occur are identical to their vulval counterparts (see Chapter 4), arise from the scattered melanoblasts normally present in the vagina and form pigmented nodules.

Leiomyosarcoma

This neoplasm, though extremely rare in the vagina, is nevertheless the commonest sarcoma to occur in the vagina of adult women[6]. It forms a bulky tumour which probably originates in the rectovaginal septum and ulcerates into the vagina. The histological appearances are similar to those of leiomyosarcomata in other sites and, typically, there are more than 10 mitotic figures per 10 high power fields. The prognosis is poor.

Sarcoma Botyroides

This is an uncommon vaginal neoplasm which usually arises during the first 5 years of life, principally during the first 2 years. The tumour is usually bulky at the time of presentation and forms a lobulated, soft, friable, polypoid mass of greyish-red somewhat gelatinous tissue which fills, and may protrude from, the vagina. Study of early cases has indicated that the tumour arises, often multifocally, deep to the vaginal epithelium, most commonly on the anterior wall of the upper vagina.

Histologically (Figures 6.10 and 6.11), the tumour is covered by thinned, often focally ulcerated, vaginal epithelium that dips down into the clefts between the lobules. The tumour has a very oedematous, myxoid stroma in which cells may be sparse and widely scattered or abundant and closely packed: most of the cells are spindle shaped or round and show considerable pleomorphism and mitotic activity, but there is nearly always a proportion of cells showing differentiation into either rhabdomyoblasts or striated muscle fibres. The neoplastic cells tend to be condensed below the covering epithelium to form a 'cambium' layer. The tumour tends to invade locally but lymphatic and blood borne spread occurs late and death, which is currently the rule, is due principally to the effects of pelvic infiltration.

The sarcoma botyroides is thought to be an embryonal rhabdomyosarcoma which originates from undifferentiated embryonic mesenchyme in the subepithelial vaginal sheath[7].

Endodermal Sinus Tumour

This extremely rare neoplasm of the vagina[8] occurs in young children and tends to resemble a sarcoma botyroides in its gross appearance. Histologically, the appearances are identical to those of the endodermal sinus tumour (yolk sac tumour) of the ovary (see Chapter 28), and it is assumed that these neoplasms arise from germ cells which have gone astray during their early embryonic transit from the foregut to the developing gonad.

Metastatic Tumours

A tumour in the vagina is more likely to be due to infiltration from a neoplasm in a neighbouring organ or to a metastasis than to a primary lesion. Spread to the vagina is principally from the cervix, endometrium, bladder, rectum, ovary and kidney whilst the vagina is a particularly common site of metastasis for choriocarcinoma (Figure 6.12).

References

1. Chabrel, C. M. and Beilby, J. O. W. (1980). Vaginal rhabdomyoma. *Histopathology*, **4**, 645–652
2. Sirota, R. L., Dickersin, G. R. and Scully, R. E. (1981). Mixed tumors of the vagina: a clinicopathological analysis of eight cases. *Am. J. Surg. Pathol.* **5**, 413–422
3. Woodruff, J. D. (1981). Carcinoma *in situ* of the vagina. *Clin. Obstet. Gynecol.*, **24**, 485–501
4. Herbst, A. L. (1981). Diethylstilboestrol and other sex hormones during pregnancy. *Obstet. Gynecol.*, **58**, 395–405
5. Buckley, C. H., Butler, E. B., Donnai, P., Fouracres, M., Fox, H. and Stanbridge, C. M. (1982). A fatal case of DES-associated clear cell adenocarcinoma of the vagina. *J. Obstet. Gynaecol.*, **3**, 126–127
6. Tavassoli, F. A. and Norris, H. J. (1979). Smooth muscle tumors of the vagina. *Obstet. Gynecol.*, **53**, 689–693
7. Huffman, J. W., Dewhurst, C. J. and Capraro, V. J. (1981). *The Gynecology of Childhood and Adolescence*. 2nd edn. (Philadelphia, London, Toronto: W. B. Saunders)
8. Rezaizadeh, M. M. and Woodruff, J. D. (1978). Endodermal sinus tumor of the vagina. *Gynecol. Oncol.*, **6**, 459–463

Cervix: Inflammatory Disease and Miscellaneous Non-Neoplastic Conditions

7

Non-specific Inflammation

Normally the cervical stroma contains a population of plasma cells, lymphocytes, eosinophils and histiocytes which is concentrated immediately beneath the surface epithelium: a failure to recognize this as a normal phenomenon frequently leads to an unwarranted diagnosis of cervical inflammation.

True inflammation of the cervix may accompany prolapse, ectopy or cervical polyps, is sometimes seen in women using an IUCD or can follow cervical surgery or irradiation: relatively rarely, cervical inflammation is due to infection.

The acutely inflamed cervix is swollen and congested: histologically, the stroma is oedematous and infiltrated by neutrophil polymorphs which often also accumulate within the cervical crypts. The squamous epithelium is poorly glycogenated and there is nuclear enlargement of uniform chromatin dispersal: characteristically, there is a paucity of mucin within endocervical cells and some degree of nucleomegaly may also be seen in the epithelial cells. Severe inflammation can result in granulation tissue formation within the stroma, and the adjacent epithelium may show squamous metaplasia. If the inflammatory process evolves into a chronic phase there may be stromal fibrosis with an accompanying stromal infiltrate of plasma cells, lymphocytes and histiocytes: neutrophil polymorphs sometimes persist in the crypts and in an immediately subepithelial position. In a proportion of cases there are clearly defined lymphoid follicles with typical germinal centres: this condition, known as 'follicular cervicitis' (Figure 7.1) is thought to be due to *Chlamydial* infection[1], and this diagnosis is strengthened if intracytoplasmic inclusions with clear halos are seen in cervical epithelial cells.

Specific Inflammation

Herpes Virus Infection

Herpetic infection of the cervix is usually associated with vulval and vaginal infection, the severity of which may mask the cervical lesions.

In the early stages the cervix is congested and inflamed[2], but within 24–48 hours vesiculation appears which is rapidly followed by superficial ulceration: rarely, a fungating necrotic mass may develop[3]. Histologically, the nuclei of the squamous epithelium become enlarged in the initial stages of infection and acquire a 'ground glass' appearance due to the presence of intranuclear virus particles[4]: multinucleate cells form in both the squamous and endocervical columnar epithelium (Figure 7.2). Spongiosis in the ectocervical epithelium is followed by intraepithelial vesiculation. Neutrophil polymorphs migrate through the epithelium and accumulate, together with degenerate epithelial cells, in the vesicle: sloughing of the superficial epithelial cells leads to ulceration but healing usually occurs without scarring.

Trichomonas Infection

Infection of the cervix with *Trichomonas vaginalis* is invariably associated with vaginal infection. The cervix is oedematous and, in severe cases, is covered by red spots which correspond to dilated capillaries in the stromal papillae. Histologically, the surface layers of the ectocervical squamous epithelium show degeneration and neutrophil polymorph infiltration (Figure 7.3) whilst in the deeper layers of the epithelium there is intracellular oedema and basal cell hyperplasia. The stroma may show an active, non-specific, chronic inflammatory cell infiltration but it is not uncommon for there to be a marked contrast between the intense epithelial inflammation and the paucity of the stromal cell infiltrate.

Cervical Ectopy and Squamous Metaplasia

A hormonally-induced increase in the bulk of the cervix occurs at puberty, during pregnancy and in women using oral steroid contraceptives: this results in an unfolding of the cervix and an eversion of the distal endocervical epithelium out on to what is anatomically the ectocervix. This condition of cervical ectopy is seen macroscopically as a red velvety area around the external os, the rubicund appearance reflecting the relative transparency of the thin endocervical epithelium which permits the subepithelial vasculature to be apparent. The exposure of the delicate endocervical epithelium to the acidity of the vagina results in its replacement by more robust metaplastic squamous epithelium, a process which commences peripherally and gradually results in an entire replacement of the columnar epithelium of the ectopy by squamous epithelium: an ectopy undergoing squamous metaplasia is often referred to as a 'transformation zone'.

Histologically, the surface of an ectopy has a characteristic villous-like pattern of columnar epithelium (Figure 7.4), small capillaries entering each of the villi: the stroma frequently shows a mild non-specific chronic inflammatory cell infiltration. As squamous metaplasia begins the villi become tightly packed and fuse, the metaplastic process being first apparent at the villous tips and in the adjacent crypts

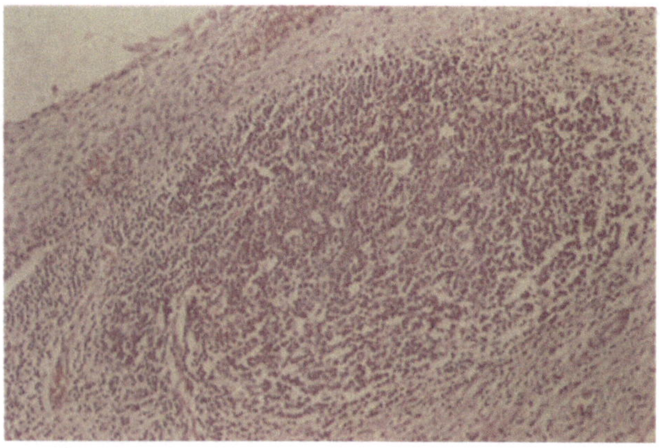

Figure 7.1 Cervix: follicular cervicitis. The squamous epithelium of the portio vaginalis lies to the upper left and in the stroma immediately beneath it there is a well formed lymphoid follicle with a germinal centre. Should the epithelium over such a follicle become ulcerated, or traumatized, lymphoid cells may be found in a cervical smear and must be differentiated from a neoplastic condition. H & E × 100

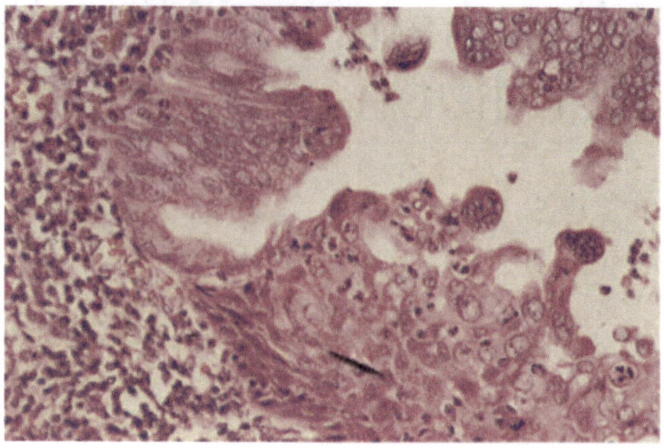

Figure 7.2 Cervix: herpes virus infection. A cervical crypt lined above and to the left by columnar epithelium showing reserve cell hyperplasia and below by rather immature squamous epithelium. Multinucleated cells are seen in the columnar and squamous cells and there is early intraepithelial vesiculation in the squamous epithelim where clusters of polymorphonuclear leukocytes have accumulated. H & E × 250

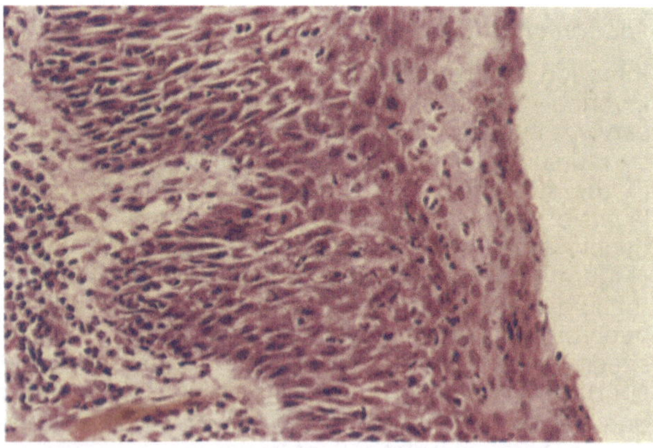

Figure 7.3 Cervix: *Trichomonas* infection. The superficial layers of the squamous epithelium of the ectocervix show degeneration and polymorphonuclear leukocyte infiltration. The deeper layers are minimally inflamed but frequent mitoses are present and the underlying stroma contains an infiltrate of lymphocytes and plasma cells. H & E × 250

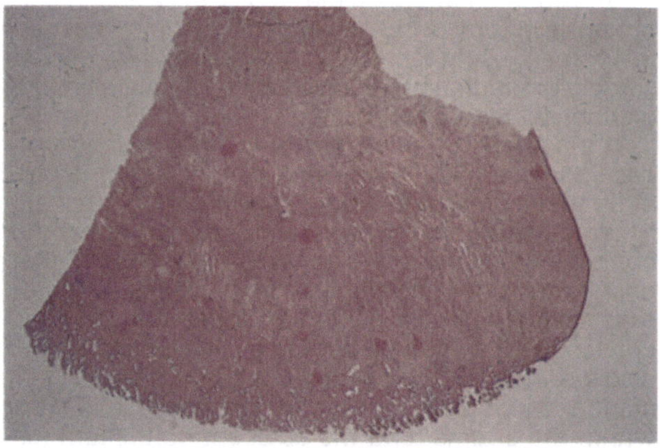

Figure 7.4 Cervix: ectopy. The squamous epithelium of the portio vaginalis is seen to the right and the surface of the endocervical canal below. In the area of the external os to the lower right there is an ectopy. Its surface has a villous configuration and the 'villi' are intensely congested and inflamed, appearing darkly stained in the section. H & E × 2.4

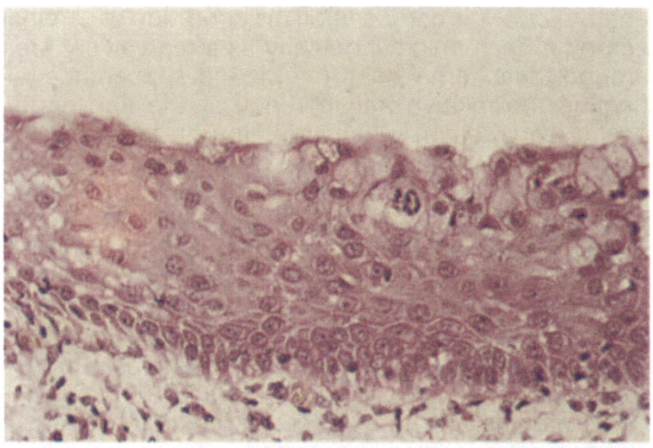

Figure 7.5 Cervix: reserve cell hyperplasia. The cervical stroma is covered by a stratified epithelium. The surface is formed by mucus-secreting columnar cells with copious, pale, faintly granular cytoplasm and the cells of the deeper layers are rounded, have distinct cell margins and large central nuclei. Already a differentiated layer of basal cells is apparent. H & E × 250

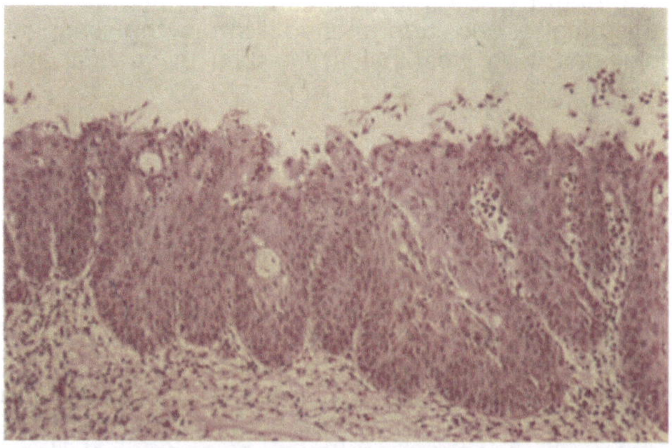

Figure 7.6 Cervix: immature squamous metaplasia. The process of metaplasia is more advanced than in Figure 7.5 but the 'villous' configuration of the endocervical crypt pattern is still apparent. The surface is covered by squamous epithelium showing stratification but incomplete maturation. This is distinguished from intraepithelial neoplasia by the absence of epithelial pleomorphism, nuclear chromatin abnormality, high nucleo-cytoplasmic ratios and abnormal mitoses. H & E × 10

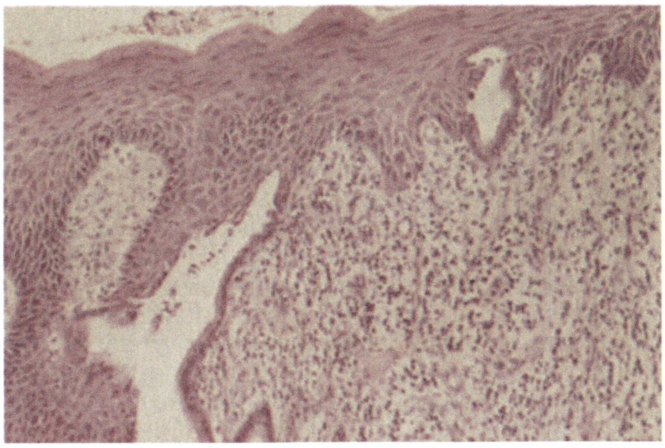

Figure 7.7 Cervix: prolapse. This patient has had an ectopy, the surface of which has undergone a process of squamous metaplasia. This is seen as a layer of slightly hyperkeratotic, mature squamous epithelium covering glandular cervical tissue. Residual cervical 'crypts are seen below the squamous epithelium. The stroma is chronically inflamed and young granulation tissue with thin-walled capillaries is seen. There is no ulceration in this example. H & E × 100

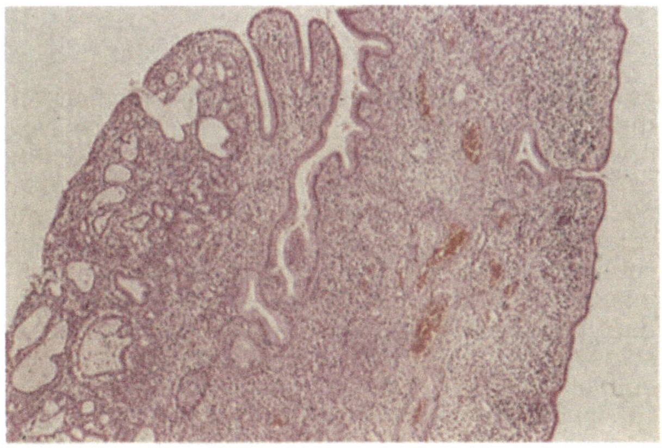

Figure 7.8 Cervix: simple polyp. This polyp is composed of endocervical tissue. The stroma is chronically inflamed and contains congested thick-walled, muscular arteries. The covering epithelium is tall and mucus-secreting in the crypt to the left but flattened; non-secretory and cubo–columnar to the right. On the left margin of the polyp there is focal microglandular hyperplasia (see Figure 7.10), a not uncommon finding. H & E × 40

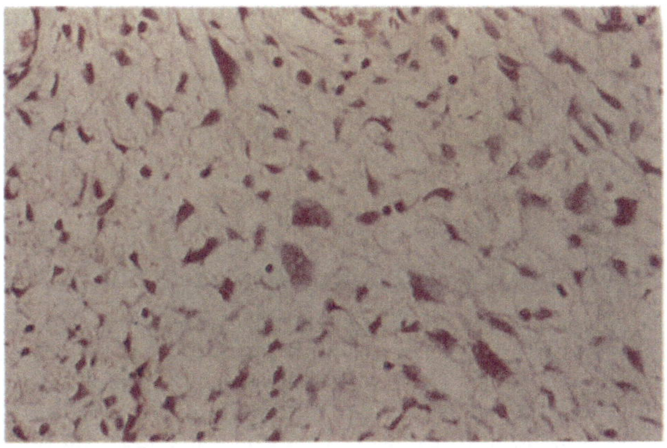

Figure 7.9 Cervix: simple polyp. The cells in the stroma of this cervical polyp are enlarged and pleomorphic and their nuclei are bizarre and angular. There are however no mitoses and the nuclear chromatin is finely distributed. H & E × 250

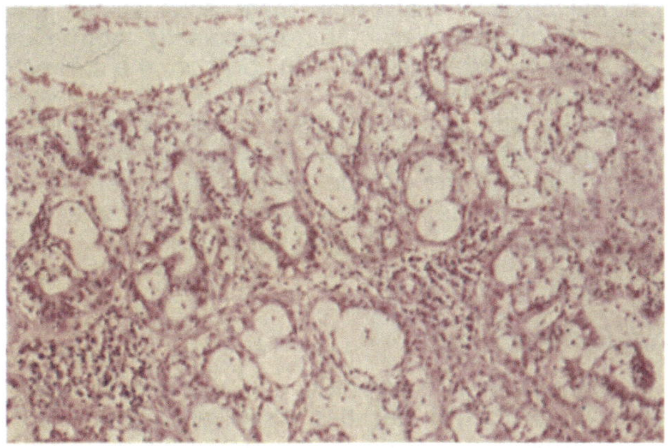

Figure 7.10 Cervix: microglandular hyperplasia. This lesion on a cervical ectopy is composed of closely packed glandular acini lined by flattened and cuboidal epithelium. Many of the acini contain polymorphonuclear leukocytes and there are dense clusters of lymphocytes in the underlying stroma. There is a little reserve cell hyperplasia to the right. Note the total absence of cytological atypia. H & E × 100

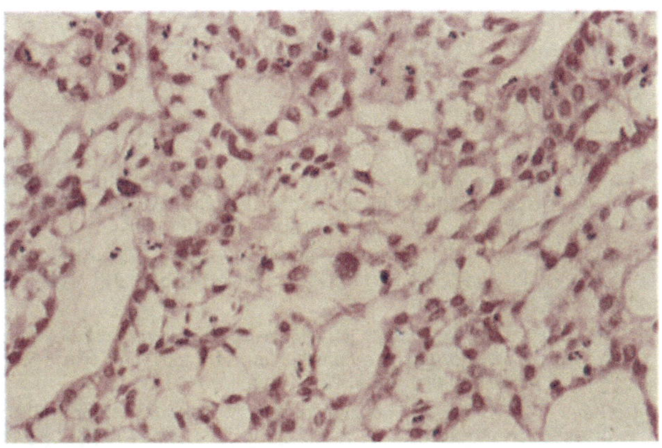

Figure 7.11 Cervix: microglandular hyperplasia. This florid, atypical focus of microglandular hyperplasia has a solid and reticular pattern with only minimal, abortive acinar formation. There is also cellular pleomorphism and nuclear hyperchromatism. There are, however, no abnormalities of nuclear chromatin dispersion and mitoses are infrequent. H & E × 250

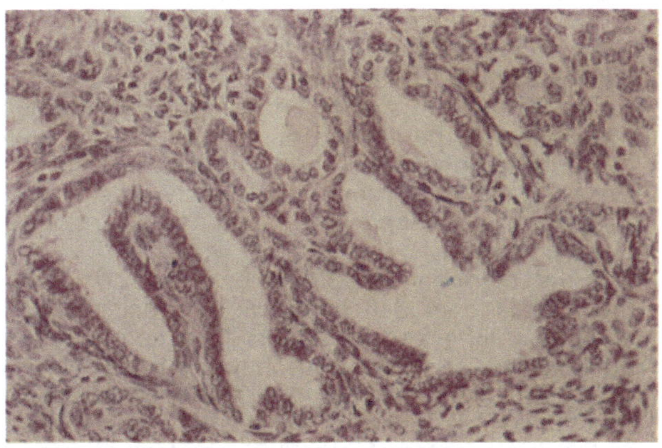

Figure 7.12 Cervix: Gartner's duct hyperplasia. It is not at all uncommon when examining the stroma of the lateral parts of the cervix to encounter ducts, isolated acini or branched ducts, lying directly in the fibro–muscular stroma. This example is typical of such ducts, the lining epithelium is flattened and cuboidal and scanty secretions may be seen within the lumena. H & E × 250

as a layer of cuboidal reserve cells which lie beneath the columnar epithelium (Figure 7.5). These cells gradually increase in number to produce the picture of 'reserve cell hyperplasia': their nuclei at first retain the characteristics of those of columnar cells, but the cytoplasm shows an increasing differentiation along squamous lines. The cytoplasm becomes more copious, stains eosinophilically and intercellular bridges become apparent: columnar cells may be retained for some time on the surface of the immature squamous epithelium. The morphology of the metaplastic squamous epithelium is distinctive as it retains the vascular pattern of the columnar endocervical epithelium until it reaches full maturity and even then the irregularity of the basal lamina may still indicate its metaplastic origin (Figure 7.6).

Uterine Prolapse

If the uterus prolapses the cervix descends and becomes elongated, there being a progressive eversion of the endocervical canal: there is usually striking squamous metaplasia, the metaplastic epithelium often being hyperkeratotic. In addition, the stroma is often congested, contains thick-walled blood vessels and often shows a non-specific chronic inflammatory cell infiltrate (Figure 7.7). Granulation tissue may form beneath the surface epithelium and there can be focal ulceration of the ectocervix, particularly if the cervix protrudes through the introitus.

Cervical Polyps

Cervical polyps are common, particularly between the fourth and sixth decades; they may cause intermenstrual or postcoital bleeding, but are quite commonly asymptomatic. They usually originate in the endocervix where an intercrypt fold gradually elongates and becomes polypoidal, usually reaching a length of between 0.5 and 2 cm: however, on rare occasions such polyps may assume enormous proportions and can measure 6–10 cm in diameter. Histologically, a fibrovascular stroma is covered by tall mucus-secreting epithelium of endocervical type: endocervical clefts are often included and these may develop a complex gland-like pattern or become cystic. The covering epithelium frequently shows reserve cell hyperplasia and squamous metaplasia whilst the stroma is often congested and inflamed, particularly at the leading tip of the polyp (Figure 7.8). Some polyps arise from the isthmic area and these contain intrastromal glands of endometrial type pattern whilst having a covering epithelium of endocervical type.

During pregnancy the stroma of a polyp sometimes shows focal decidual change, and on occasion this is sufficiently extensive to produce complete decidualization: an Arias–Stella change may occur in the crypt epithelium of the polyp. On other occasions the stromal fibroblasts may be enlarged, of bizarre shape and multinucleated (Figure 7.9): the lack of nuclear chromatin abnormalities and of mitotic figures distinguishes these cells from those seen in a sarcoma botyroides.

Microglandular Hyperplasia

This is a non-neoplastic lesion which develops in women using steroid contraceptives and during pregnancy. Clinically, it may be sufficiently extensive to form a polypoidal mass and cause postcoital bleeding, thus mimicking a neoplasm. Histologically, it may be focal, multifocal or extensive and polypoidal: it consists of closely packed glandular acini lined by a cuboidal or flattened epithelium which is poor in mucin: these foci may form along the endocervical canal, at the external os or adjacent to endocervical clefts. Foci of reserve cell hyperplasia and squamous metaplasia are common, and there is frequently an inflammatory cell infiltrate throughout the lesion (Figure 7.10). Usually the cells lining the acini are regular, whilst their nuclear chromatin is pale and uniformly dispersed: sometimes, however, the lesion is particularly florid and the glandular component arranged in a reticulated or solid pattern[5] (Figure 7.11). Under these circumstances the cells may have pleomorphic, hyperchromatic nuclei and the solid areas appear vacuolated due to cystic dilatation of the intercellular spaces: there can, therefore, be a resemblance to a clear cell adenocarcinoma from which, however, the lesion is distinguished by the absence of stromal invasion, irregular nuclear chromatin and mitotic activity.

Hyperplasia and Cysts of Gartner's Duct

Gartner's ducts (Wolffian or mesonephric ducts) are paired structures from which minor lateral branches emerge: they lie deep in the stroma of the lateral part of the cervix, are usually narrow and are lined by a low cuboidal epithelium. In some instances the duct becomes distended or cystic and the lining cells then tend to resemble those of the Fallopian tube. The associated acinar-like branches may also become more complex to form a gland-like structure deep in the lateral wall of the cervix (Figure 7.12): this can be distinguished from an invasive adenocarcinoma by the absence of cellular atypia and mitotic figures, and from endometriosis by the lack of stroma around the gland-like structures.

References

1. Hare, M. J., Toone, E., Taylor-Robinson, D., Evans, R. T., Furr, P. M., Cooper, P., and Oates, J. K. (1981). Follicular cervicitis – colposcopic appearances and association with *Chlamydia trachomatis*. *Br. J. Obstet. Gynaecol.*, **88**, 174–180
2. Skinner, G. (1976). Virus infections. In Jordan, J. A. and Singer, A. (eds.). *The Cervix*. (London, Philadelphia and Toronto: W. B. Saunders)
3. Ferenczy, A., (1982). Benign lesions of the cervix. In Blaustein, A. (ed.). *Pathology of the Female Genital Tract*. 2nd edn. (New York, Heidelberg and Berlin: Springer-Verlag)
4. Slavin, G. (1976). The pathology of cervical inflammatory disease. In Jordan, J. A. and Singer, A. (eds.). *The Cervix*. (London, Philadelphia and Toronto: W. B. Saunders)
5. Taylor, H. B., Irey, N. S. and Norris, H. J. (1967). Atypical endocervical hyperplasia in women taking oral contraceptives. *J. Am. Med. Assoc.*, **202**, 637–639

Cervix: Epithelial Abnormalities **8**

Cervical Intraepithelial Neoplasia (CIN)

This term is now used to encompass all cervical epithelial abnormalities previously classed either as 'dysplasia' or as 'carcinoma *in situ*'. The reasons for this change of terminology have been extensively discussed[1–3]: and need not be elaborated on here, it sufficing to say that CIN forms a single, continuous, neoplastic spectrum.

It is of value for descriptive and epidemiological purposes to subdivide CIN into various grades, but it is recognized not only that such grading is both arbitrary and subjective but is also devoid of long term prognostic value: it is true that, collectively, cases of CIN III are more likely to evolve into an invasive carcinoma than are cases of CIN I or II but on an individual basis a woman with CIN II may have as great a chance of eventually developing an invasive squamous cell carcinoma as does an individual patient with CIN III. One important correlate of grading is, however, that the probable time interval of progression varies, it generally taking much longer for cases of CIN I or II to evolve into an invasive tumour than will cases of CIN III. With modern therapeutic approaches to CIN, however, it is probably not so much the severity but the extent of the intraepithelial abnormality which poses the greatest threat to a woman, for a small sharply localized focus of CIN III is more easily treated than is an extensive area of CIN I or II[4].

CIN I

The essential feature of CIN I (Figure 8.1) is that whilst the cells throughout the full thickness of the epithelium show nuclear abnormalities those in the upper and middle thirds of the epithelium undergo cytoplasmic differentiation. At all levels of the epithelium the nuclei tend to have prominent nucleoli and to be moderately pleomorphic, enlarged and hyperchromatic. The cells in the lower third, or less, of the epithelium show no evidence of cytoplasmic differentiation or of orderly stratification, lack clearly defined boundaries and have a high nucleo–cytoplasmic ratio with nuclear crowding whilst those in the middle and upper thirds of the epithelium show evidence of stratification and cytoplasmic differentiation with a decreasing nucleo–cytoplasmic ratio. Mitotic figures are uncommon, are confined to the lower third of the epithelium and are usually of normal form.

CIN II

The histological features of CIN II (Figure 8.2) are similar to those of CIN I but undifferentiated, non-stratified cells with pleomorphic nuclei and a high nucleo–cytoplasmic ratio extend beyond the lower third of the epithelium but not into the upper third. The cells in the upper third of the epithelium show stratification and cytoplasmic differentiation. Mitotic figures are confined to the lower two thirds of the epithelium and are usually of normal form.

CIN III

In this condition (Figure 8.3) undifferentiated, non-stratified, basaloid cells showing nuclear crowding, indistinct cell boundaries and a high nucleo–cytoplasmic ratio occupy more than two thirds, or the full thickness, of the epithelium. The degree of nuclear pleomorphism is often greater than that seen in CIN I or II. Mitotic figures are frequently seen, are commonly present in the upper third of the epithelium and are often of abnormal form. CIN III of this pattern is often described as being of the 'small cell undifferentiated type' but it is recognized that other forms of CIN III also exist in which cells which are not totally undifferentiated, but are of similar appearance throughout, occupy most or all of the epithelial thickness: it is in these that a reliance on the proportion of the epithelial thickness occupied by undifferentiated cells breaks down, greater emphasis having to be placed on such features as lack of stratification, the site within the epithelium of mitotic figures and the normality or otherwise of the mitotic figures. Thus one variant of CIN III (Figure 8.4) is characterized by the presence of cells which although having nuclei of neoplastic type, showing no evidence of stratification and lacking clearly defined boundaries, are larger than undifferentiated basaloid cells and have a lower nucleo–cytoplasmic ratio: mitotic figures are usually abundant, are found at all levels within the epithelium and are frequently abnormal. The cells in this form of CIN III are thought to be of parabasaloid type. In a third variant of CIN III (Figure 8.5) the cells have a relatively low nucleo–cytoplasmic ratio and well defined cell boundaries: there is, however, a complete disorganization of growth pattern with lack of polarity and stratification. The nuclei are of neoplastic type whilst mitotic figures, commonly of abnormal form, are found with some frequency in all levels of the epithelium. This type of CIN III is known as the 'large cell keratinizing' variety.

Differential Diagnosis of CIN

Epithelial Atrophy

After the menopause the cervical squamous epithelium becomes thinned and atrophic (Figure 8.6): maturation is arrested in the middle zone of the epi-

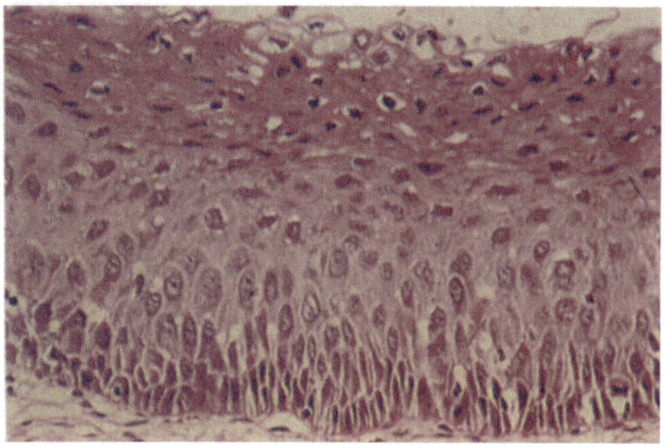

Figure 8.1 Cervix: cervical intraepithelial neoplasia Grade I (CIN I). A colposcopic cervical biopsy. The basal one third of the epithelium is occupied by cells with a high nucleo–cytoplasmic ratio. Nuclear abnormalities, pleomorphism, prominent nucleoli and irregularly dispersed chromatin occur at all levels of the epithelium, whilst cytoplasmic differentiation commences in the middle third, and the upper two thirds of the epithelium shows stratification and progressive cytoplasmic maturation. H & E × 250

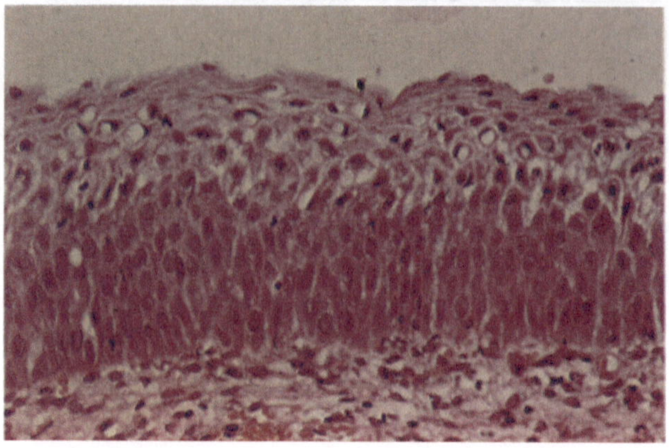

Figure 8.2 Cervix: cervical intraepithelial neoplasia grade II. In this example of CIN II, the cells in the lower half of the epithelium show a lack of stratification, are closely packed, have a high nucleo–cytoplasmic ratio and have irregularly dispersed chromatin. Stratification and cytoplasmic maturation commences in the upper half of the epithelium. H & E × 250

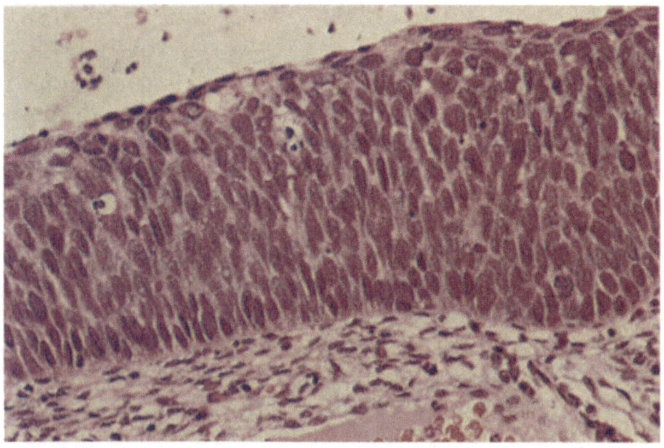

Figure 8.3 Cervix: cervical intraepithelial neoplasia grade III (CIN III). Virtually the full thickness of the epithelium is composed of undifferentiated, non-stratified basaloid cells. The cells are closely packed, have a high nucleo–cytoplasmic ratio and mitoses, which may or may not be normal, occur at all levels of the epithelium. The surface cells are flattened but show no evidence of stratification or cytoplasmic maturation. H & E × 250

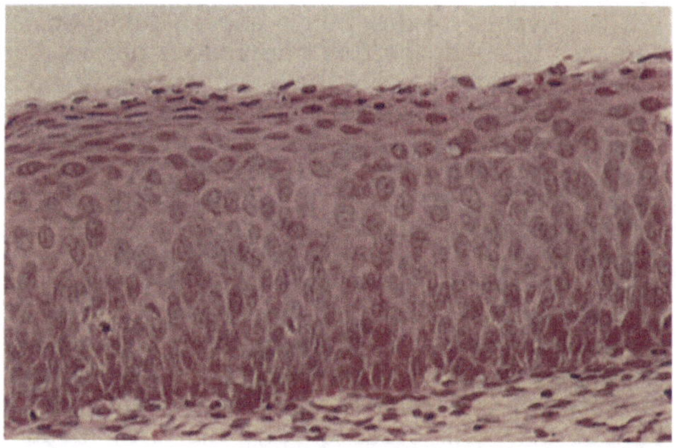

Figure 8.4 Cervix: intraepithelial neoplasia grade III (CIN III). Cells of parabasal type occupy just more than the basal two thirds of the epithelium. The cells are larger than those shown in Figure 8.3, and their nucleo–cytoplasmic ratio somewhat lower. Mitoses are seen in the midzone. Superficial cytoplasmic maturation is evident. H & E × 250

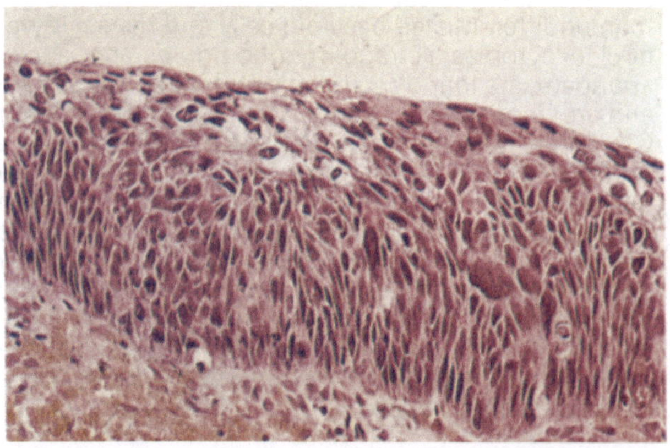

Figure 8.5 Cervix: intraepithelial neoplasia grade III (large cell, keratinizing). The epithelium is completely occupied by non-stratified, disordered cells with keratinized cytoplasm and large pleomorphic nuclei. H & E × 250

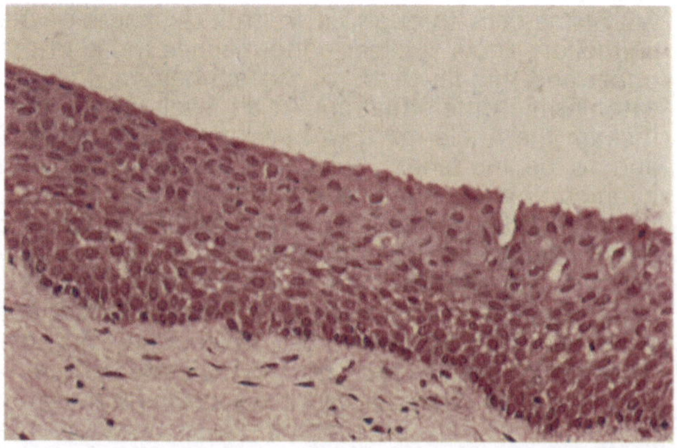

Figure 8.6 Cervix: atrophy. The epithelium is shallow, has a distinct basal layer and several parabasaloid layers. Maturation, whilst showing normal stratification, is arrested. The absence of nuclear atypia, mitoses and pleomorphism distinguishes the appearance from intra-epithelial neoplasia. H & E × 250

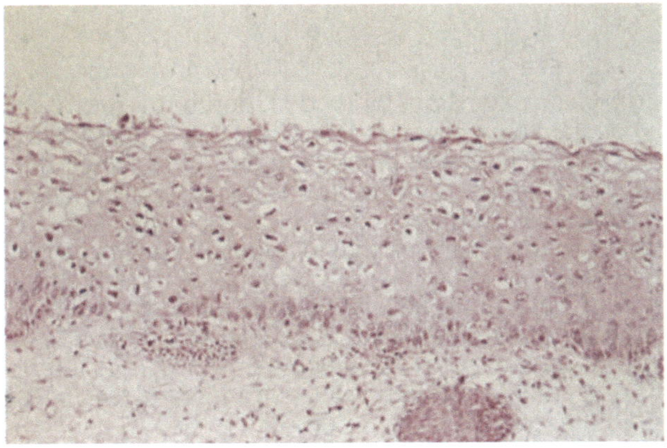

Figure 8.7 Cervix: flat condyloma acuminatum. The epithelium is of normal thickness. At all levels above the basal layer there is a mild disturbance of normal stratification. The cells are a little pleomorphic and there are clear perinuclear vacuoles (koilocytosis). H & E × 100

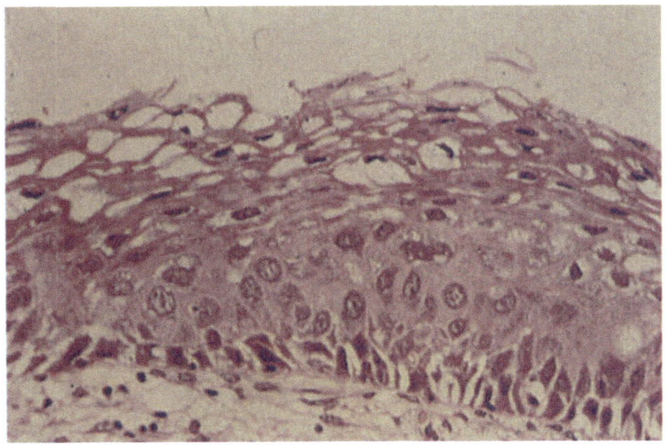

Figure 8.8 Cervix: flat condyloma acuminatum with intraepithelial neoplasia. In the upper layers of the epithelium there is nuclear pleomorphism and koilocytosis is seen. In the lower third of the epithelium, there are abnormalities of nuclear chromatin dispersion and whilst there is cytoplasmic maturation in the upper epithelium, the nuclear atypia persists. H & E × 250

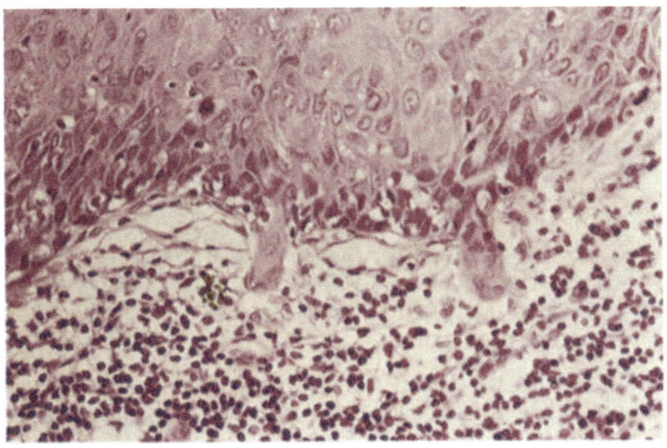

Figure 8.9 Cervix: microinvasive squamous carcinoma – early stromal invasion. Two tongues of atypical squamous cells showing marked cytoplasmic maturation have breached the basal layer of the squamous epithelium and penetrated the stroma. The overlying squamous epithelium shows a large cell keratinizing CIN. Note the intense stromal lymphocytic infiltrate in the area of invasion. H & E × 250

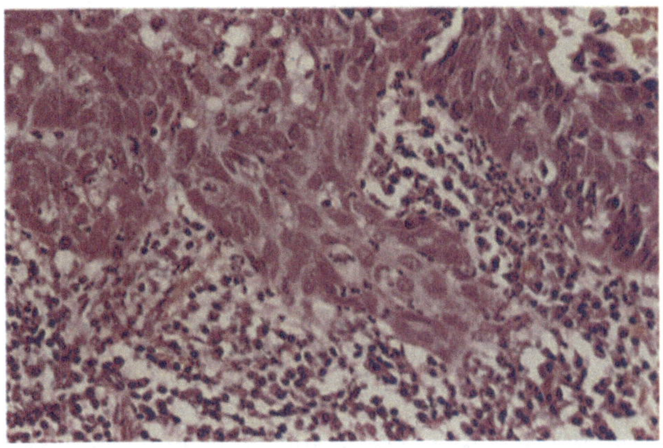

Figure 8.10 Cervix: microinvasive squamous carcinoma. A larger focus of microinvasive carcinoma than that seen in Figure 8.9. The epithelium from which the tumour arises shows CIN III and lies to the upper right. The infiltrating tongues show greater cytoplasmic maturation than the epithelium from which they arise and are infiltrated by polymorphonuclear leukocytes: the stroma contains polymorphonuclear leukoyctes, plasma cells and lymphocytes. H & E × 250

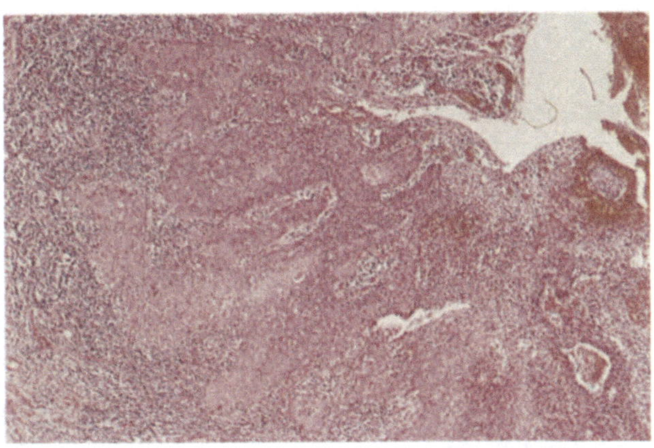

Figure 8.11 Cervix: microcarcinoma (occult invasive squamous carcinoma). A small, confluent, focally keratinizing squamous carcinoma arises from an epithelium showing intraepithelial neoplasia. Tumour penetrates to the left and there is an intense, peripheral lymphocytic infiltrate. The tumour measures 0.5 × 0.5 × 0.3 cm. H & E × 40

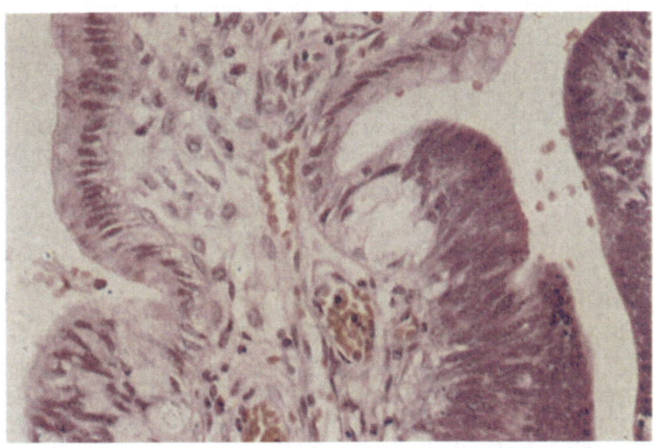

Figure 8.12 Cervix: adenocarcinoma *in situ*. The cervical crypt to the left is lined by tall, mucus-secreting columnar cells whilst in that to the right the epithelium is multilayered, shows a lack of cytoplasmic mucus, has a high nucleo-cytoplasmic ratio and hyperchromatic nuclei. These latter features are those of adenocarcinoma *in situ*. The unusual degree of cytoplasmic vacuolation in the normal epithelium to the lower left is due to the fact that the patient was pregnant. H & E × 250

thelium which consists, therefore, of only three or four layers of basaloid or parabasaloid cells which have scanty cytoplasm and large dense, often somewhat irregular, nuclei. This picture may be mistaken for CIN but the thinness of the epithelium, the presence of mitotic figures only in the basal layer and the absence of neoplastic nuclear abnormalities are all of help in achieving the correct diagnosis.

Immature Squamous Metaplasia

Squamous metaplasia has been discussed in Chapter 7: during the immature phase of such metaplasia there may be little or no differentiation of the squamous cells, but the condition can be distinguished from CIN by the lack of nuclear pleomorphism, the low nucleo-cytoplasmic ratio, the absence of abnormal mitotic figures and, often, the presence of columnar mucus-secreting cells on the surface. However CIN can develop in immature metaplastic squamous epithelium and the two diagnoses are not mutually exclusive. The development of CIN in such cases is revealed most clearly by the presence of nuclear atypia.

Flat Condyloma

It is now recognized that many condylomatous lesions of the cervix are of the flat variety and do not form the typical polypoid wart-like lesions of a condyloma acuminatum[5]. These flat lesions are not visible to the naked eye and cannot be distinguished colposcopically from a focus of CIN. The squamous epithelium at the site of a flat condyloma (Figure 8.7) may be of normal thickness, thinned or of increased thickness. The characteristic feature of a flat condyloma is the presence of koilocytic cells: these are found in the upper part of the epithelium and have a large, clear perinuclear halo with irregular but sharp boundaries. The nuclei often show degenerative changes such as break up or margination of chromatin or pyknosis. Other typical features include elongation and widening of the dermal papillae with accentuation of the rete ridges, individual cell keratinization and multinucleation: there is often a minor degree of nuclear atypia and there may be some superficial hyperkeratosis. An 'atypical' flat condyloma has been described[6] in which there is a combination of condylomatous features and both nuclear and cytological atypia (Figure 8.8): it would probably be more correct to regard such a lesion as a condyloma in which CIN is developing. If CIN supervenes in a flat condyloma the typical condylomatous features tend to be progressively lost.

Microinvasive Carcinoma

There have been great difficulties in arriving at an acceptable definition of a microinvasive carcinoma of the cervix, but that which has been most widely used in the last few years defines this lesion as 'one in which single or multiple, non-confluent tongues of neoplastic cells have breached the basement membrane of an epithelium showing CIN, and are extending into the stroma to a depth of not more than 3 mm from the base of the epithelium, whether this be on the surface or within a crypt: there should be no invasion of vascular-like spaces'. It will be recognized that this definition implies that confluence of invading tongues, extension beyond a depth of 3 mm and vascular space involvement all negate a diagnosis of microinvasive carcinoma, the tumour in such circumstances being referred to as an 'occult invasive carcinoma'. In recent years it has, however, been increasingly recognized that included under the general heading of 'microinvasive carcinoma' are two different entities, one being that in which tongues of squamous carcinoma are just beginning to invade the stroma and the other in which a small invasive tumour is present. Microinvasive lesions are therefore divided into two groups[7]:

(1) *Early stromal invasion*. In this condition invasive buds of neoplastic squamous cells are present which are either in continuity with an epithelium showing CIN or may be apparently separated from the epithelium (Figure 8.9): the invading cells do not extend beyond a depth of more than 1 mm from the nearest surface or crypt membrane. Aids in recognizing this very early invasive lesion include the better differentiation in the invading tissue than in the epithelium from which it has arisen, and well marked stromal lymphocytic infiltration and oedema at the site of invasion (Figure 8.10).

(2) *Microcarcinoma*. This is a measurable small carcinoma and should be measured in two dimensions (Figure 8.11). The depth should be measured from the base of the epithelium from which the tumour develops and should not exceed 5 mm and the largest diameter should not exceed 10 mm in the section which shows the greatest extent.

It should be noted that in both these categories it should be stated whether vascular-like spaces are involved or not.

Adenocarcinoma *in situ*

This is characterized by varying degrees of cellular atypia within the endocervical cells (Figure 8.12) and, although its natural history has not yet been fully elucidated, it must be assumed that in a proportion of cases an adenocarcinoma *in situ* is a precursor of an invasive adenocarcinoma.

References

1. Richart, R. M. (1973). Cervical intraepithelial neoplasia: a review. *Pathol. Ann.*, **8**, 301–328
2. Koss, L. G. (1978). Dysplasia: a real concept or a misnomer? *Obstet. Gynecol.*, **51**, 374–379
3. Buckley, C. H., Butler, E. B. and Fox, H. (1982). Cervical intraepithelial neoplasia. *J. Clin. Pathol.*, **35**, 1–13
4. Richart, R. M. (1980). The patient with an abnormal PAP smear – screening techniques and management. *N. Engl. J. Med.*, **302**, 312–314
5. Meisels, A., Morin, C. and Casas-Cordero, M. (1982). Human papillomavirus infection of the uterine cervix. *Int. J. Gynecol. Pathol.*, **1**, 75–94
6. Meisels, A., Roy, M., Fortier, M., Morin, C., Casas-Cordero, M., Shah, K. V. and Turgeon, H. (1981). Human papillomavirus infection of the cervix: the atypical condyloma. *Acta Cytol.*, **25**, 7–16
7. Burghardt, E. (1982). Microinvasive and occult invasive carcinoma: pathology. In Jordan, J. A., Sharp, F. and Singer, A. (eds.). *Pre-clinical Neoplasia of the Cervix*. pp. 239–254. (London: Royal College of Obstetricians and Gynaecologists)

Cervix: Neoplasms

9

Squamous Cell Carcinoma

Between 80 and 85% of malignant cervical neoplasms are of this type. An early squamous cell carcinoma may appear as an area of roughening, as a focal induration or as a shallow ulcer, whilst the more advanced lesions may grow in either an endophytic or an exophytic manner: the endophytic tumours form either hard nodular masses or excavating ulcers with raised, indurated, margins, whilst the exophytic form presents as a bulky, friable, polypoid or papillary mass which protrudes into the vagina.

Histologically, squamous cell carcinomata infiltrate the cervical stroma as a network of anastomosing bands which appear on transection as irregular islands with spiky or angular edges. About 20% are of the well differentiated (or 'large cell keratinizing') type (Figure 9.1): intercellular bridges are readily apparent and there is a conspicuous formation of keratin pearls. The moderately differentiated (or 'large cell non-keratinizing') tumours account for about 60% of squamous cell carcinomata and are formed of cells which, though recognizably of squamous type, have larger and more irregular nuclei than in the well differentiated form (Figure 9.2). The remaining 20% of cervical squamous cell carcinomata are poorly differentiated ('small cell non-keratinizing type') (Figure 9.3): foci of abortive squamous differentiation are occasionally apparent.

Uncommon histological variants of cervical squamous cell carcinoma are a spindle cell form which mimics a sarcoma, and a glycogen rich, clear celled type of well differentiated tumour (Figure 9.4). The poorly differentiated small cell carcinomata may bear a close resemblance to the malignant carcinoid tumour of the cervix, and all such neoplasms should be subjected to a silver stain.

Verrucous Carcinoma

Tumours of this type occasionally occur in the cervix, they are identical to those which develop in the vulva (see Chapter 4).

Basaloid Carcinoma

This is a rare neoplasm which tends to occur in elderly women as an ulcerated infiltrating mass[1]. Histologically, small cells with scanty cytoplasm and regular hyperchromatic nulclei form nests or cords; prominent palisading is seen at the periphery of the tumour nests (Figure 9.5). No squamous differentiation is seen and, as the tumours are usually in close apposition to the cervical squamous epithelium, it is possible that these neoplasms should be regarded as basal cell carcinomata.

Adenocarcinoma

Approximately 10% of cervical carcinomata are of this type. These neoplasms may adopt an exophytic, nodular, polypoid or ulceroinfiltrative form but in some cases of deep-seated intracryptal adenocarcinoma the cervix may appear normal to the naked eye.

Histologically, there are a number of differing types of adenocarcinoma and these are classified by cell type[2]:

(1) *Endocervical type.* This is the commonest form, accounting for about 75% of cases. Adenocarcinomata of this type almost certainly arise from endocervical reserve cells and are formed of columnar cells which, although showing atypia and mitotic activity, retain a resemblance to normal endocervical epithelium (Figure 9.6): Mucus secretion is a constant feature and is sometimes excessive, pools of mucus being formed which disrupt the acini and spill over into the stroma to produce a 'colloid' or 'mucoid' carcinoma: squamous metaplasia is sometimes seen and is of no significance.

Endocervical-type adenocarcinomata are frequently well differentiated and are at times confused with a microglandular hyperplasia: the presence of large, hyperchromatic nuclei, abnormal mitotic figures, marked cellular atypia and stromal infiltration aid in distinguishing between these two conditions. A small proportion of these neoplasms are, however, exceptionally well differentiated and closely resemble normal endocervical epithelium (Figure 9.7), these being known as 'adenoma malignum' or 'minimal deviation adenocarcinomata'[3]. Features indicative of the true nature of such a lesion include bizarre angulated outpouchings from the apparent crypts, the presence of mitotic figures and the deep penetration into the cervical stroma. The prognosis of these uncommon tumours does not appear to differ substantially from that of a more conventional endocervical adenocarcinoma.

(2) *Endometrioid type.* These are histologically identical to an endometrial adenocarcinoma (Figure 9.8) with well formed glandular acini lined by cuboidal endometrial type cells, little or no mucus production and, quite commonly, foci of squamous metaplasia. A minority of such tumours may arise from foci of cervical endometriosis but most are probably derived from endocervical reserve cells which have a potentiality for differentiating along a variety of Müllerian pathways.

(3) *Serous adenocarcinoma.* Any cervical adenocarcinoma may grow in a papillary fashion, but

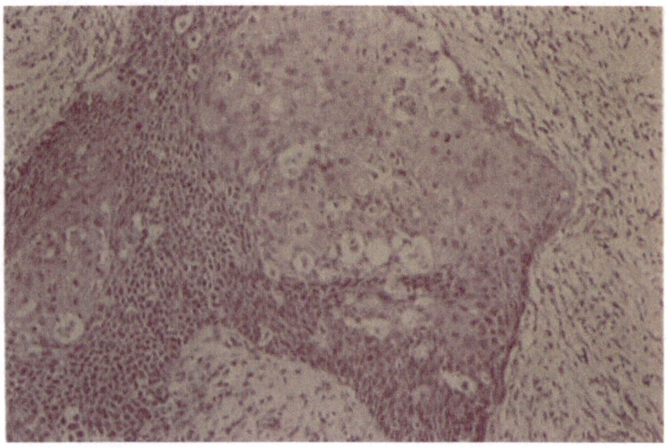

Figure 9.1 Cervix: squamous cell carcinoma. This irregular island of well-differentiated infiltrating tumour shows tightly packed cells with extensive cytoplasmic maturation (keratinization) nuclear hyperchromatism and little nuclear pleomorphism. The larger keratinized cells contrast with the smaller, non-keratinized basal cells below and to the left. H & E × 100

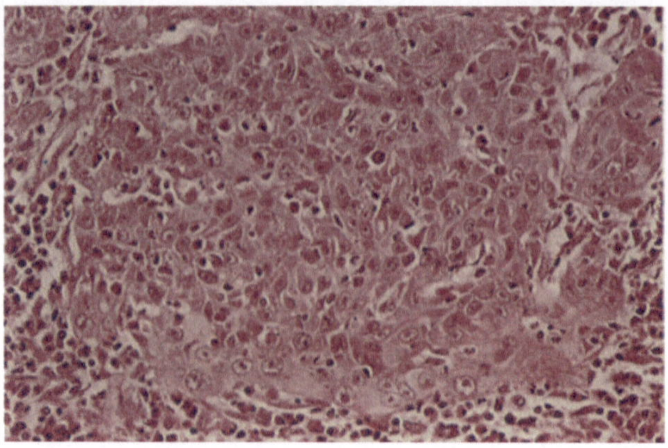

Figure 9.2 Cervix: moderately differentiated (large cell non-keratinizing) squamous cell carcinoma. The tumour cells are large, have plentiful eosinophilic cytoplasm and rather pleomorphic nuclei. Intercellular bridges are rarely seen and keratin pearls are absent. H & E × 250

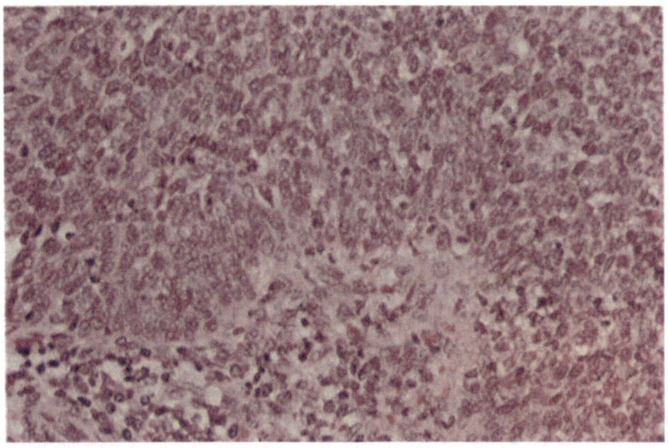

Figure 9.3 Cervix: squamous cell carcinoma. A poorly differentiated, small cell, non-keratinizing tumour which is composed of sheets of pleomorphic cells with high nucleo–cytoplasmic ratios, and markedly hyperchromatic nuclei in which there are numerous mitoses. An inflammatory infiltrate is seen below at the advancing margin of the tumour. H & E × 250

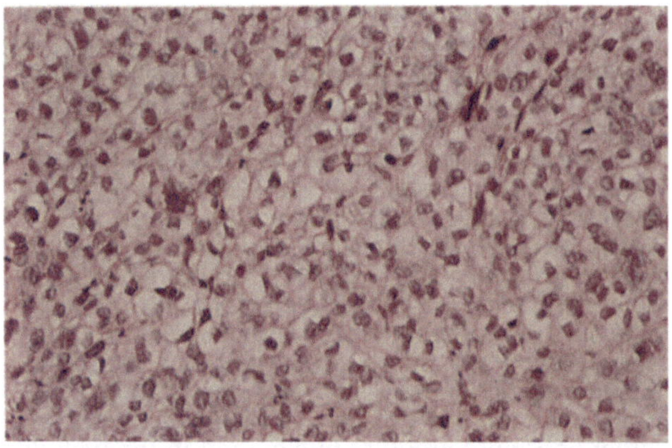

Figure 9.4 Cervix: clear-celled squamous cell carcinoma. The cytoplasm appears clear in these tumour cells due to an accumulation of glycogen. The nuclei are large, rather irregular in outline, moderately pleomorphic and hyperchromatic. Cell boundaries are well-defined. H & E × 250

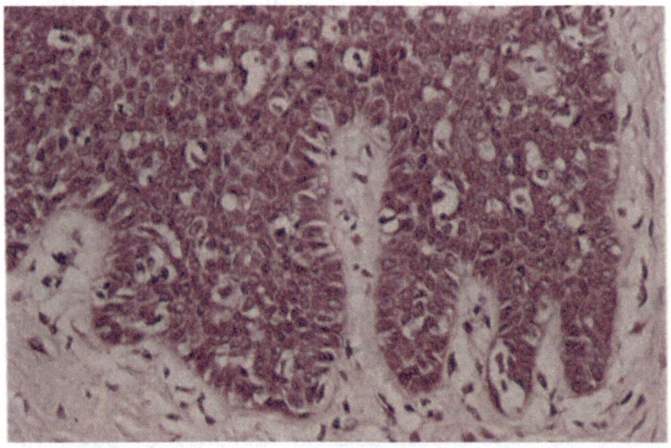

Figure 9.5 Cervix: basaloid carcinoma. The tumour is composed of regular and irregular nests of small, darkly staining basaloid cells with hyperchromatic nuclei and very high nucleo–cytoplasmic ratios. Note the palisading of the peripheral cells. H & E × 250

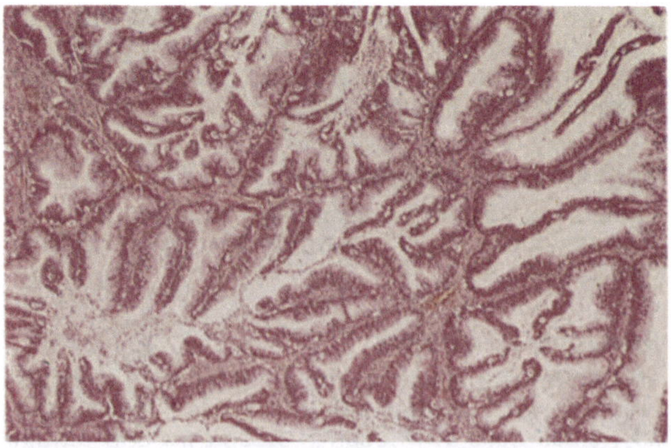

Figure 9.6 Cervix: adenocarcinoma of endocervical type. The well formed glandular acini have a very characteristic branching or arborescent pattern. The glands are lined by tall, mucus-secreting epithelium of endocervical type. H & E × 40

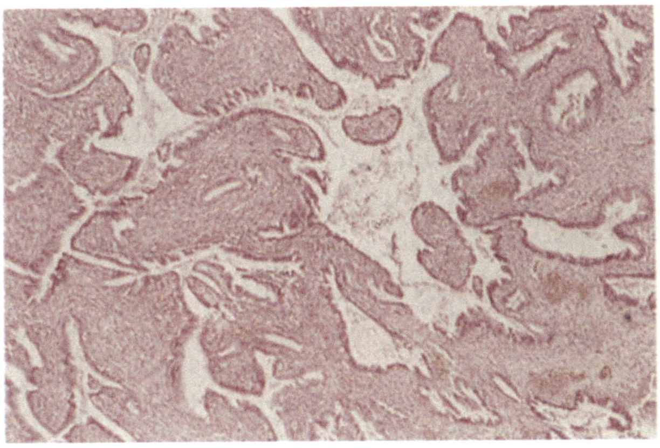

Figure 9.7 Cervix: adenoma malignum,'a very well differentiated adenocarcinoma of endocervical type. The irregular branching crypts are lined by tall mucus-secreting epithelium of endocervical type, the arborization of the crypts exceeding that seen in the normal cervix. Although mitoses are present there is little cytological atypia. H & E × 40

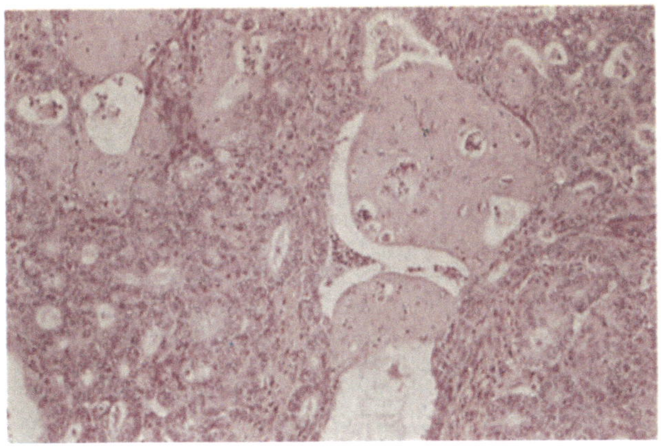

Figure 9.8 Cervix: endometrioid adenocarcinoma. This well differentiated tumour is composed of small round glandular acini lined by cuboidal cells showing fairly extensive squamous metaplasia. The foci of metaplastic epithelium have small, regular nuclei and eosinophilic cytoplasm; they form nodules which protrude into individual tumour acini. H & E × 100

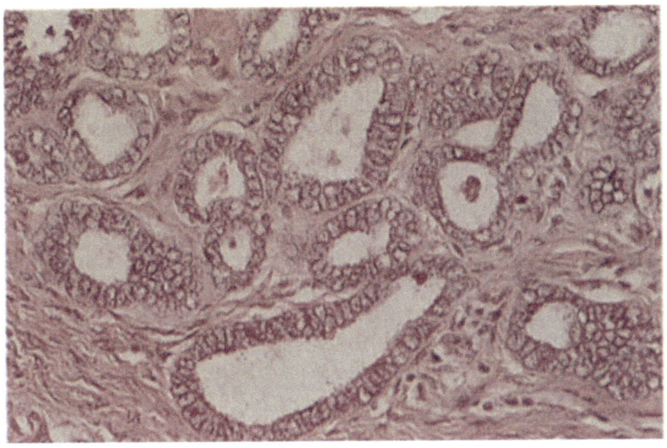

Figure 9.9 Cervix: mesonephric adenocarcinoma. The cervical stroma is infiltrated by small glands, tubules and acini lined by remarkably uniform cuboidal cells showing only minimal multilayering. In some areas the tubules may be scanty or focally clustered and in a small biopsy difficult to distinguish from a focus of hyperplastic Gartner's duct (Figure 7.12). H & E × 250

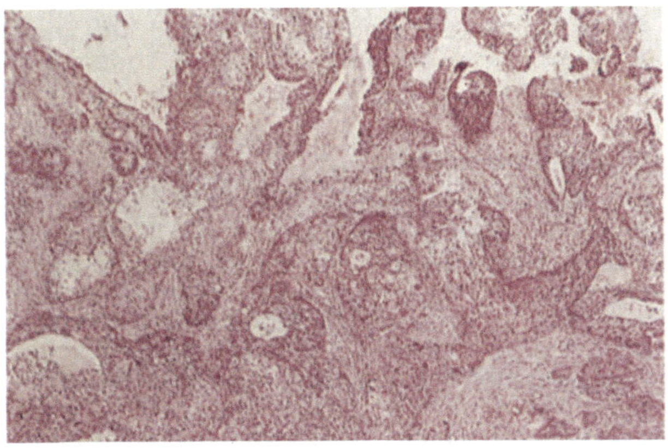

Figure 9.10 Cervix: mucoepidermoid carcinoma. The tumour comprises infiltrating sheets of poorly differentiated, non-keratinizing squamous epithelium. The centres of many of the cellular islands show degeneration cellular vacuolation and mucus accumulation. H & E × 40

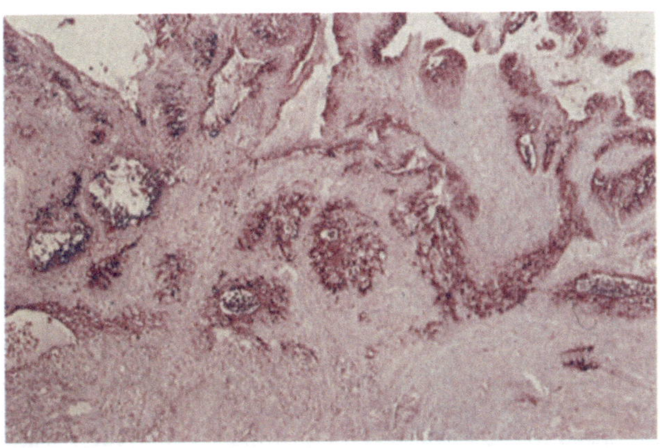

Figure 9.11 Cervix: mucoepidermoid carcinoma. A sequential section of the tumour shown in Figure 9.10 stained with PAS (after diastase digestion) and Alcian blue. It shows that the vacuolated cells contain mucus and confirms the presence of mucus pools in the centres of the tumour lobules. PASD and Alcian blue × 40

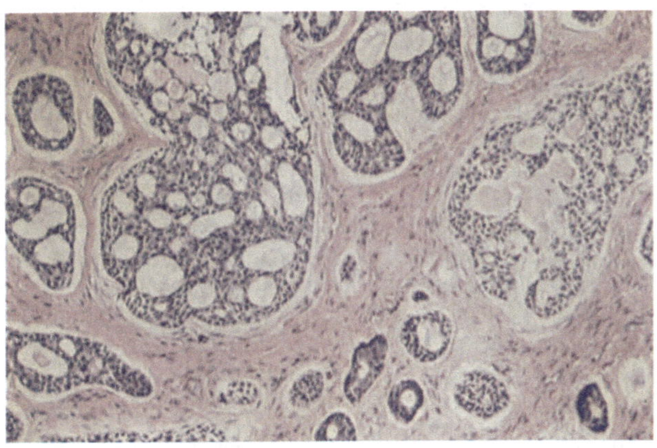

Figure 9.12 Cervix: adenoid cystic carcinoma. Nests of darkly staining basaloid cells lie in a fibrous stroma. Within the nests there are cylindrical hyaline bodies, which appear round on cross-section, and small acini creating a sieve-like appearance. H & E × 100

occasionally a papillary cervical adenocarcinoma histologically mimics an ovarian serous or a tubal adenocarcinoma. Such neoplasms indicate yet again the competence of the endocervical reserve cells to pursue differing Müllerian pathways of differentiation.

(4) *Clear cell adenocarcinoma.* These tumours are of Müllerian origin, are identical to the clear cell adenocarcinoma of the vagina (see Chapter 6) and, as is the case with their vaginal counterparts, usually, though not invariably, arise in girls who have been exposed prenatally to DES.

(5) *Intestinal type.* Very rarely a cervical adenocarcinoma is histologically similar to an intestinal adenocarcinoma and contains goblet, Paneth and argyrophil cells, such neoplasms probably arising from a focus of intestinal metaplasia.

(6) *Mesonephric* (*Wolffian type*). These very uncommon neoplasms are formed of tubular glands which are arranged in an irregular fashion and are lined by cubo–columnar cells[4]: the glands bear a distinct resemblance to the remnants of Gartner's duct (Figure 9.9) and, like these, occur deep compared to normal endocervical epithelium.

Mixed Carcinomata

A number of neoplasms are included within this category[5]: all are probably derived from pluripotential reserve cells, and it is by no means certain that each represents a distinct entity rather than a variation on a common theme which is due to differences in growth rate and degree of differentiation. All tend to behave in a rather aggressive fashion and have a poor prognosis.

(1) *Adenosquamous carcinoma.* These tumours contain an admixture of adenocarcinoma and squamous cell carcinoma, and are distinguished from a collision tumour by the intimate intermingling and blending of the two components, and from an endocervical adenocarcinoma with squamous metaplasia by the clearly malignant nature of the squamous tissue.

(2) *Muco-epidermoid carcinoma.* For the most part these neoplasms resemble a squamous cell carcinoma from which they differ, however, by the presence of mucus both intracellularly and, as small pools, in extracellular sites (Figures 9.10 and 9.11). Glandular acini are absent though the cells immediately surrounding a mucus pool may adopt a cuboidal or columnar shape.

(3) *Glassy cell carcinoma.* This uncommon neoplasm is formed of uniform, large, polygonal cells with abundant granular or 'ground glass' cytoplasm, centrally placed round vesicular nuclei with large nucleoli and distinct cell boundaries. The cells are arranged in nests or sheets but abortive squamous pearls or inadequately formed glandular acini are sometimes seen, and these neoplasms are regarded as poorly differentiated adenosquamous carcinomata[6].

(4) *Adenoid cystic carcinoma.* These rare tumours tend to develop at a relatively late age and are formed of uniform, small, basaloid cells with scanty cytoplasm and densely staining nuclei[7]: the cells are arranged in sheets, masses or anastomosing cords and the solid masses have a cribriform appearance which is produced by the presence of rounded spaces containing hyaline material (Figure 9.12). In at least 75% of cases an adenoid cystic carcinoma is either admix with a squamous cell carcinoma or an adenocarcinoma or is associated with CIN: this finding can be interpreted either as indicating that the adenoid cystic pattern is a non-specific one which may be adopted by squamous or glandular carcinomata, or that the tumour is one of pluripotential cells which can partially differentiate into either squamous or adenocarcinoma, or both.

Carcinoid Tumours

Carcinoid tumours (also known as 'apudomata' or 'argyrophil tumours') of the cervix are rare, and have a wide histological spectrum which ranges from a well differentiated neoplasm which closely resembles a gastrointestinal carcinoid tumour, to an anaplastic form which is very similar to a bronchial oat cell carcinoma[8]. The well differentiated tumours may show an insular, trabecular, ribbon or festooned pattern and, occasionally, amyloid is present in the stroma. A Grimelius stain will reveal a variably sized population of argyrophil cells and neurosecretory granules are seen on electron microscopy. The well differentiated tumours are of relatively low grade malignancy but the anaplastic form is a highly aggressive neoplasm.

Malignant Melanoma

This is an extremely rare tumour in the cervix and may arise either from the very sparse stromal melanocytes or in a focus of epidermal metaplasia.

Sarcoma

Cervical sarcomata are notably rare but leiomyosarcomata or cervical stromal sarcomata are occasionally encountered. The various forms of mixed Müllerian tumours (see Chapter 16) can all occur in the cervix as can the embryonal rhabdomyosarcoma of childhood.

References

1. Daroca, P. J. and Dhurandhar, H. N. (1980). Basaloid carcinoma of uterine cervix. *Am. J. Surg. Pathol.*, **4**, 235–239

2. Langley, F. A. and Fox, H. (1981). Pathology of clinical invasive carcinoma of cervix. In Coppleson, M. (ed.). *Gynecologic Oncology* pp. 465–474. (Edinburgh, London, Melbourne and New York: Churchill-Livingstone)

3. Silverberg, S. G. and Hurt, W. G. (1975). Minimal deviation adenocarcinoma ('adenoma malignum') of the cervix: a reappraisal. *Am. J. Obstet. Gynecol.*, **121**, 971–975

4. Buntine, D. W. (1979). Adenocarcinoma of the uterine cervix of probable Wolffian origin. *Histopathology*, **11**, 713–718

5. Abell, M. R. (1973). Invasive carcinomas of the uterine cervix. In Norris, H. J., Hertig, A. T. and Abell, M. R. (eds.). *The Uterus, International Academy of Pathology Monographs in Pathology.* pp. 413–456. (Baltimore: Williams and Wilkins)

6. Zaino, R. J., Nahhas, W. A. and Morter, R. (1982). Glassy cell carcinoma of the uterine cervix: an ultra-structural study and a review. *Arch. Pathol. Lab. Med.*, **106**, 250–254

7. Hoskins, W. J., Averette, H. E., Ng, A. B. P. and Yon, J. L. (1979). Adenoid cystic carcinoma of the cervix uteri: report of six cases and review of the literature. *Gynecol. Oncol.*, **7**, 371–384

8. Albores-Saavedra, J., Rodriguez-Martinez, H. A. and Larraza-Hernandez, O. (1979). Carcinoid tumors of the cervix. *Pathol. Ann.*, **14**, 273–291

Endometrium: Normal Cyclical Changes

10

The endometrium consists of simple tubular glands set in a vascular, cellular stroma. Lymphocytes and lymphoid aggregates are present throughout the cycle and neutrophil polymorphs are present in the stroma immediately before, and during, menstruation. Only the functional superficial compact and spongy layers of the corpus reflect the cyclical changes of ovarian function, the basal (Figure 10.1) and isthmic endometrium (Figure 10.2) remaining hormonally unresponsive in the normal cycle. The demarcation between functionalis and basalis is abrupt, although somewhat irregular, whilst that between the basalis and myometrium is rather ill-defined.

The menstrual cycle is the recurrent priming of the endometrium in preparation for the implantation of a fertilized ovum, and menstruation follows the abrupt fall in progesterone levels which occurs, in the absence of pregnancy, at the end of the cycle. Bleeding does not occur at this stage of the cycle in other primates in which luteal decay is less abrupt[1].

The menstrual cycle varies in length from 22 to 34 days and it is customary in Britain to date the cycle from the first day of menstruation, though in many countries, particularly in North America, the date of ovulation is taken as day 1 of the cycle. This latter form is sometimes preferred because variations in the length of the normal cycle are usually due to changes in the length of the pre-ovulatory phase, the time from ovulation to menstruation being remarkably constant.

Recognition of the individual components of the endometrial changes are a prerequisite to the understanding and assessment of the adequacy and quality of the cyclical response. In the proliferative phase the somewhat limited range of histological features permits recognition only of the early, mid and late proliferative phase, whilst the changes following ovulation are so specific in the normal cycle that it is possible to recognize the interval since ovulation with an accuracy of 24–48 hours. It goes without saying that such judgement can be made only on a sample of functionalis[2,3].

Proliferative (Follicular or Pre-ovulatory) Phase (days 5–14)

The increasing levels of oestrogen in the follicular phase of the cycle cause an increase in the height of the functional endometrium, due to the co-ordinated growth of the glands and stroma, and also induce the development of progesterone receptors. Thus, as oestrogen levels rise, progesterone receptors increase, to a peak in the pre-ovulatory phase, and the adequacy of oestrogen stimulation in the follicular phase controls the potential of the endometrium to respond to progesterone released from the corpus luteum after ovulation.

Regeneration of the endometrium commences from the basal layers, and surface epithelial regrowth may be complete, before the cessation of menstruation.

(1) *Early proliferative phase* (*days 5–7*). The glands are small, straight, tubular and round in cross-section; their epithelium is cubo–columnar and moderately basophilic, occasional mitotic figures are present. The stromal cells are elongated and compact whilst their cytoplasm is indistinct and remains so until the mid-secretory phase; stromal mitoses are frequent.

(2) *Mid-proliferative phase* (*days 8–10*). As oestrogen levels rise, the glands multiply and increase in length; their epithelium becomes taller and pseudo-stratified, whilst mitotic figures are more frequent in both glands and stroma. A minor degree of transient stromal oedema is common and capillaries are numerous although arterioles and arteries remain inconspicuous (Figure 10.3).

(3) *Late proliferative phase* (*days 11–14*). Glandular growth now outstrips that of the stroma, and as a result the glands become twisted and slightly tortuous. Glandular epithelial stratification persists but mitoses diminish in both glands and stroma. Endometrial growth has now reached its maximum and the endometrium is about 7 mm deep.

Secretory (Post-ovulatory) Phase (days 15–28)

Following ovulation, maturation and secretory transformation of the endometrium occur, under the combined influence of oestrogen and progesterone, in preparation for the implantation of the fertilized ovum. Menstruation follows the abrupt fall in progesterone levels which commences on the 26th day of the cycle in the absence of pregnancy.

(1) *Interval phase* (*day 15*). Ovulation has occurred but hormonal changes are not usually reflected in the endometrium until 36 hours post-ovulation.

(2) *Transition from proliferative to secretory phase* (*day 16*). Between 36 and 48 hours after ovulation subnuclear glycogen vacuoles appear in the glandular epithelium, these reaching a peak between 17 and 18 days (Figure 10.4). Pseudo-stratification and mitoses diminish and the glands dilate a little. Individual epithelial cells are

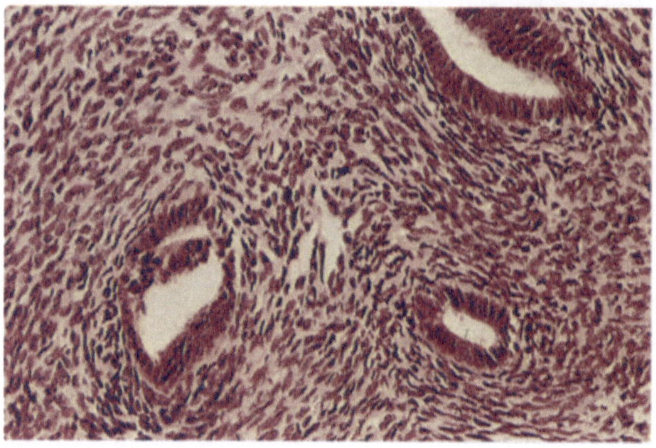

Figure 10.1 Endometrium: basal layer. The basal endometrium is hormonally unresponsive and the tissue remains similar in appearance to this throughout the cycle. The glands are lined by columnar cells with tall, thin, closely packed nuclei and scanty cytoplasm; they show neither secretory nor proliferative activity. The stroma is composed of closely packed cells with a relatively high nucleo–cytoplasmic ratio. H & E × 250

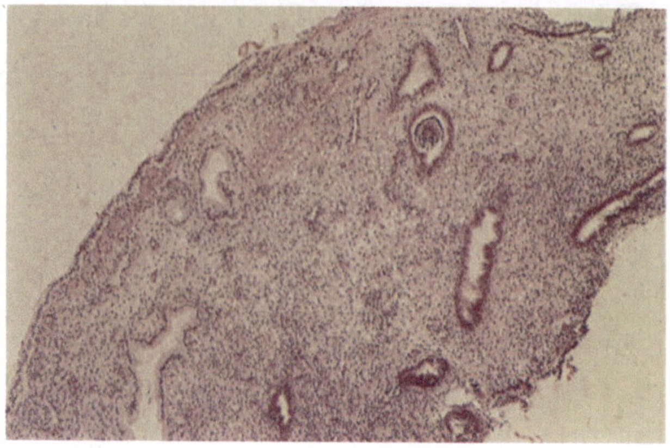

Figure 10.2 Endometrium: isthmus. This is a fairly typical example of isthmic tissue as it appears in endometrial curettings. The uterine surface lies to the upper left and is covered by tall mucus-secreting cells of endocervical type; the immediately adjacent crypts are lined by similar cells. The more deeply placed glands to the right are lined by epithelium of endometrial type and resemble those seen in the basal endometrium (see Figure 10.1). The transition from cervical to endometrial epithelium at the isthmus is gradual, endometrial epithelium first appearing in the deeply sited glands, next the superficial glands and finally the surface epithelium. H & E × 40

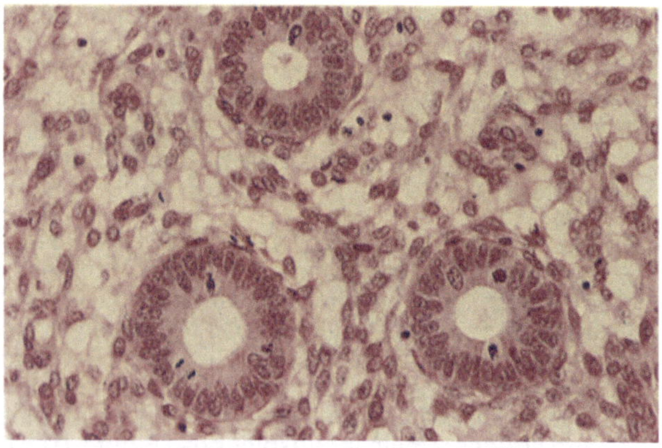

Figure 10.3 Endometrium: mid proliferative phase. The glands are straight, tubular and round on transverse section. Their epithelium is multi-layered, cubo–columnar and contains numerous mitoses. The stroma is cellular, and mitoses are present. The stromal cells have ovoid or elongated nuclei, their cytoplasm is scanty and eosinophilic whilst cell boundaries are indistinct. H & E × 250

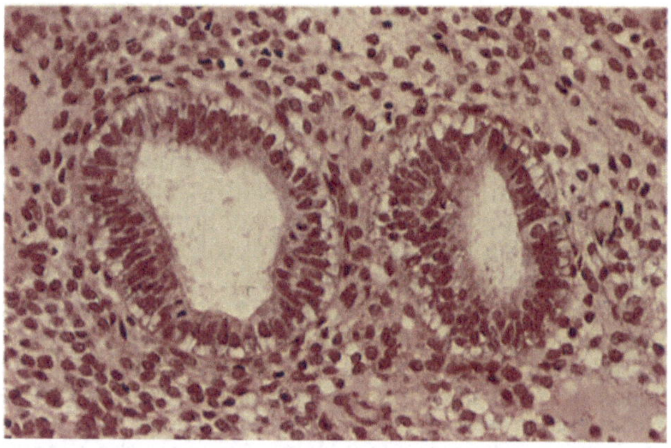

Figure 10.4 Endometrium: transition from proliferative to secretory phase. (16th day of cycle, second post-ovulatory day.) The glandular epithelium remains multilayered but subnuclear vacuoles are present in their cytoplasm. The stromal cells are similar to those seen in the follicular phase but there is a little stromal oedema. H & E × 250

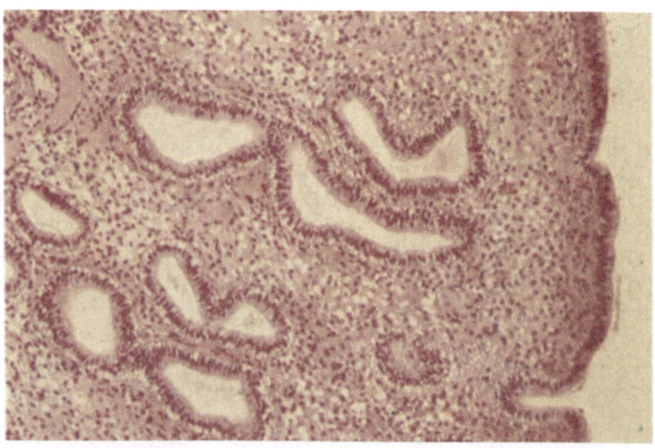

Figure 10.5 Endometrium: early secretory phase (17th–18th day of cycle, 3rd and 4th post-ovulatory days). The glands are mildly tortuous, there is uniform subnuclear vacuolation in the glandular epithelium and the stroma is mildly oedematous. Such an appearance is presumptive evidence that ovulation has occurred. H & E × 100

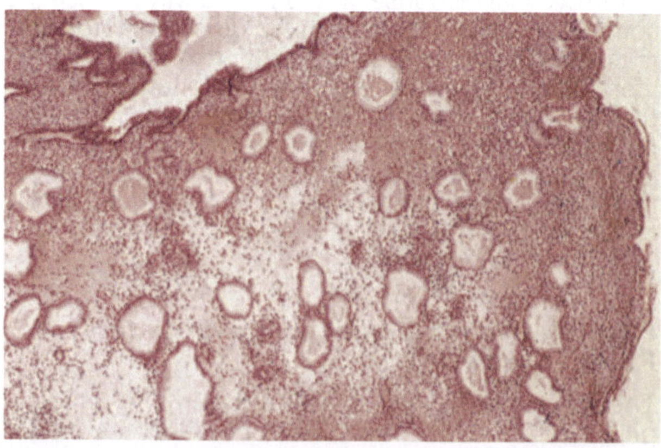

Figure 10.6 Endometrium: mid secretory phase (20th day of cycle, 6th post-ovulatory day). The glands appear somewhat angular on section and their lumena are distended by pink staining secretion; the epithelium is mono-layered and pale staining. The stroma is congested and oedematous. Spiral arteries are conspicuous and their walls are muscularized. Note that these changes are occurring in a uniform manner throughout the tissue. H & E × 40

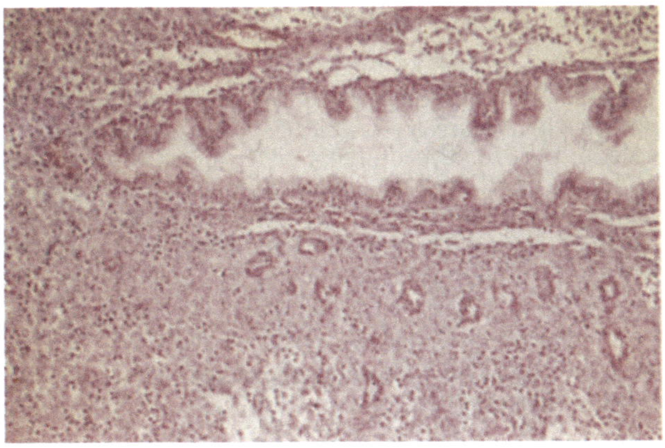

Figure 10.7 Endometrium: late secretory phase (27th day of cycle, 13th post-ovulatory day). The gland in the upper half of the field is lined by a single layer of folded epithelium formed by pale-staining cubo–columnar cells with basal nuclei. A trace of secretion remains within the gland lumen but secretory activity is exhausted. The spiral artery, in the lower half of the field, is well muscularized and surrounded by a mantle of stromal cells which have undergone a pre-decidual change, i.e. their cytoplasm has become more copious and more densely eosinophilic and their cell boundaries more distinct. There is a stromal infiltrate of macrophages or K-cells which have darkly-staining irregular nuclei which are somewhat pyknotic in appearance. H & E × 100

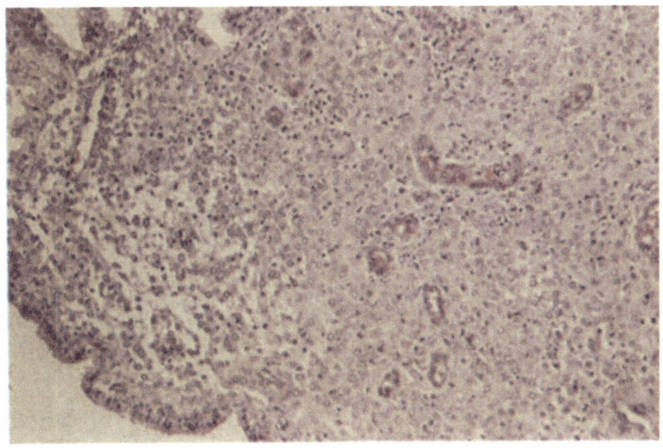

Figure 10.8 Endometrium: late secretory phase (27th day of cycle, 13th post-ovulatory day). This field, which is taken from the compact, superficial layer of the endometrium, shows pre-decidual change (Figure 10.7) beneath the surface epithelium and around spiral arteries; K-cell infiltration is marked. H & E × 100

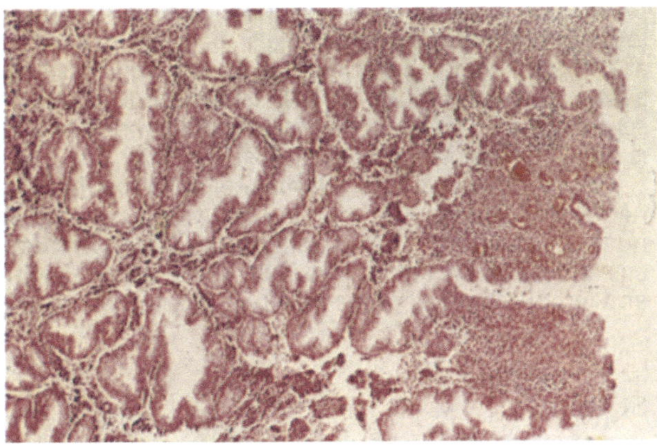

Figure 10.9 Endometrium: menstrual phase (1st day of cycle). The field, from a hysterectomy specimen, shows the fully developed compact superficial layer to the right and the underlying spongy layer to the left. The pre-decidualized compact layer contains small congested blood vessels, immediately deep to which there is crumbling stromal breakdown and haemorrhage indicative of the onset of menstruation. The exhausted secretory glands are serrated and collapsed. H & E × 40

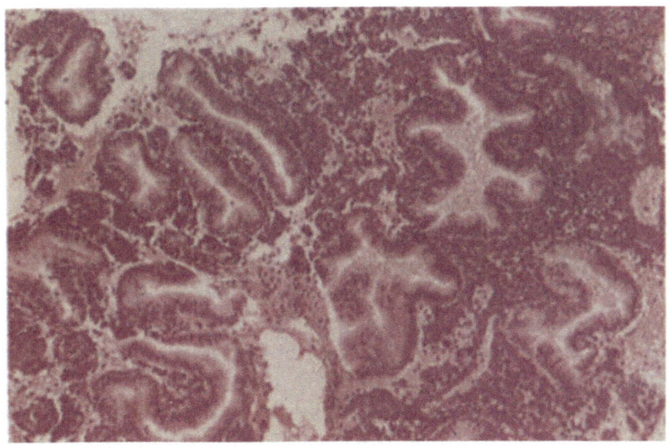

Figure 10.10 Endometrium: menstrual phase. This is menstrual endometrium as seen in curettings. It consists of fragments of closely compacted stromal cells, blood and serrated collapsed glands. The condensation of the tissue may lead to a spurious back-to-back appearance of the glands and there may be confusion with a neoplasm. H & E × 100

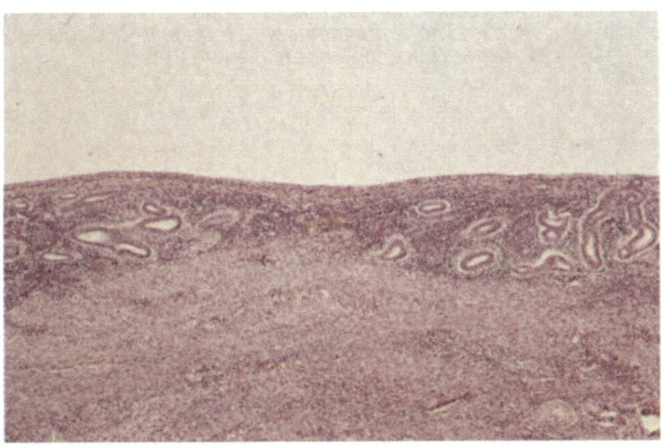

Figure 10.11 Endometrium: post-menopause. The endometrium in this post-menopausal hysterectomy specimen is shallow; the stroma is compact and densely cellular whilst the glands which are lined by cubo–columnar cells, are small and tubular. There is neither secretory nor proliferative activity and there is a resemblance to normal basal endometrium (Figure 10.1). H & E × 40

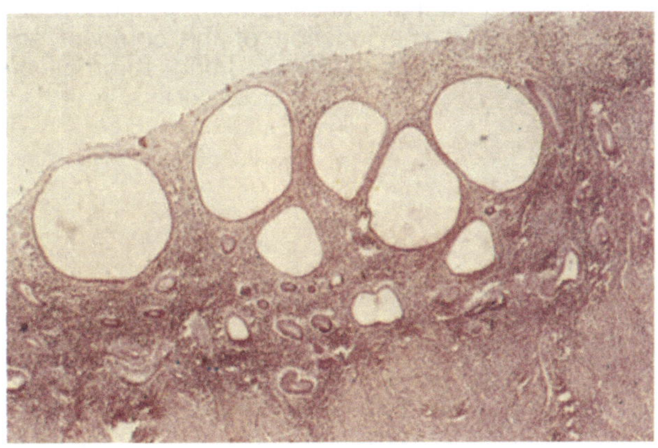

Figure 10.12 Endometrium: senile cystic atrophy. The endometrium from this post-menopausal hysterectomy specimen contains large, cystically dilated glands lined by a single layer of flattened epithelium which shows neither secretory nor proliferative activity. The remaining small, non-cystic glands are similar to those seen in Figure 10.11 and the stroma is compact. H & E × 40

domed on their lumenal surface. These changes when seen uniformly in more than 50% of glands indicate that progesterone levels are rising and are presumptive evidence of ovulation. Scanty, ill-formed subnuclear vacuoles may be seen in the presence only of oestrogen secretion.

(3) *Early secretory phase* (*days 17–18*). Glandular subnuclear vacuoles reach a peak, mitoses cease and the stroma is mildly oedematous (Figure 10.5).

(4) *Mid-secretory phase* (*days 19–23*). The nuclei of the glandular epithelium return to a basal position on days 19–20 as glycogen is secreted into the gland lumena, thus distending them, and the cell surface becomes ragged. Intraglandular secretion reaches a peak on day 21. Stromal oedema progressively increases, reaching a peak on days 22–23, and spiral artery development occurs under the influence of progesterone (Figure 10.6). The vessels proliferate, pericytes widen, myofibrils differentiate and, at the same time, the perivascular stromal cells show increasing eosinophilia and density; these are predecidual cells. The vessels are sensitive even to low levels of progesterone and hence only low, even otherwise inadequate, levels will cause vascular transformation[4].

(5) *Late secretory phase* (*days 24–28*). Glandular secretion diminishes, lumena narrow and the epithelium, which becomes more shallow, folds in a saw-toothed like manner into the glandular lumen. The spiral arteries become larger and thicker and their mantle of predecidual cells increases (Figure 10.7); at the same time a predecidual change is seen in the most superficial stroma, forming the compact layer (Figure 10.8). K-cells (stromal macrophages or granulocytes) increase in number and neutrophil polymorphs can be seen in the compact and spongy stroma by day 27. Stromal mitoses recommence.

Menstruation (days 1–5)

The onset of menstruation is signalled by glandular collapse and stromal condensation, crumbling and haemorrhage at the junction of the compact and spongy layers (Figure 10.9); fibrin thrombi are present. Between days 2–4 most of the compact and spongy layers are shed (Figure 10.10), but it is not uncommon for the deepest part of the functionalis to be retained and for these fragments of exhausted secretory glands to be incorporated into the regenerating endometrium. The postmenstrual endometrium is 1–2 mm thick.

Menopausal and Postmenopausal Endometrium

After the cessation of ovulation, which defines the menopause, oestrogen levels may decline rapidly producing an inactive endometrium with small glands lined by a single layer of cuboidal epithelium (Figure 10.11), or may fall more slowly, as indicated by slight multilayering of glandular epithelium in the absence of mitotic activity or by the presence of occasional glandular mitoses in the first two years after the menopause. The endometrium is shallow and usually the glands are straight and tubular. However, in a proportion of women the glands, lined by a single layer of flattened cuboidal cells, become distended and cystic, creating the picture recognized as senile cystic atrophy (Figure 10.12). This occurs as a consequence of blockage of the glandular orifices and is not due to regressed hyperplasia.

The cytoplasm of the stromal cells diminishes and hence the stroma appears unusually cellular due to nuclear crowding. The distinction between functionalis and basalis is lost. There is no spiral artery growth and lymphoid aggregates may be numerous.

References

1. Yen, S. S. C. and Jaffe, R. B. (eds.). (1978). *Reproductive Endocrinology*. (Philadelphia, London and Toronto: W. B. Saunders)
2. Noyes, R. W., Hertig, A. T., and Rock, J. (1950). Dating the endometrial biopsy. *Fertil. Steril.*, **1**, 3–25
3. Hendrickson, M. R. and Kempson, R. L. (1980). The normal endometrium. In *Surgical Pathology of the Uterine Corpus*. pp. 36–98. (Philadelphia, London, Toronto: W. B. Saunders)
4. de Brux, J. (1981). Evaluation of ovarian disturbances by endometrial biopsy. In de Brux, J., Mortel, R. and Gantray, J. P. (eds.). *The Endometrium: Hormonal Impacts*, pp. 107–121. (New York and London: Plenum Press)

Endometrium: Functional Disturbances

11

The endometrium is exquisitely sensitive to ovarian hormones, and disturbances of ovarian function are accurately reflected by changes in endometrial morphology. These latter changes often allow recognition of the nature of the endocrinological disorder providing that a full and accurate history, which includes details of the menstrual cycle, the date of the last menstrual period and information about administration of hormones or drugs, is made available to the pathologist. Some of the abnormalities discussed in this section occur in ovulatory cycles and others in anovulatory cycles but all, although often asymptomatic, can give rise to complaints of abnormal or irregular uterine bleeding or of infertility.

Functional Disorders Occurring in Ovulatory Cycles

Follicular Phase Abnormalities

There may be either an undue lengthening or an unusual shortening of the proliferative phase of the endometrial cycle to over 21 days or to less than 8 days. The endometrium is of normal morphology but appears unusually retarded or advanced in relationship to the last menstrual period, though normal in relation to the date of ovulation. Variations in the length of the follicular phase are not uncommon in the perimenarchal and perimenopausal years and, in the latter circumstances, a lengthening of the cycle may be an indication of impending ovarian failure.

Luteal Phase Abnormalities

Following ovulation, progesterone levels usually rise abruptly to a plateau which is sustained until about the 12th or 13th postovulatory day when, if pregnancy has not occurred, they fall abruptly and steeply. If any component of this normal pattern is faulty, e.g. if the initial rise in levels is too slow or occurs in a stepwise manner, the plateau levels too low or irregularly sustained or the final fall occurs too early, then a fully adequate secretory transformation of the endometrium will not be achieved. Causes of inadequate development, or poor maintenance, of the corpus luteum, include central defects in LH secretion, high prolactin levels or an impaired ability of the oocytes to organize follicular development. However, in some instances of apparent luteal phase defect the corpus luteum is functioning normally, but the endometrium will fail to respond fully to progesterone because of inadequate production of oestrogens during the follicular phase, with a resulting failure of induction of endometrial progesterone receptors.

Intermittent luteal phase deficiency is quite common and of no great significance but persistent luteal phase defect can lead to dysfunctional uterine bleeding, infertility or recurrent very early abortion. The endometrial abnormalities characteristic of this condition are detected most easily in samples obtained between the 8th and 10th postovulatory days when secretory activity is normally at its height.

The simplest histological appearance seen in luteal phase deficiency is one in which the glands and stroma mature synchronously, but the secretory changes in the endometrium are retarded relative to the date of ovulation (Figure 11.1), e.g. a biopsy taken on the 12th or 13th postovulatory day shows an appearance more typical of the 8th or 9th day after ovulation. This type of picture probably reflects an unusually slow rise in progesterone levels as the corpus luteum develops.

If the luteal phase deficiency is secondary to inadequate production of oestrogens during the follicular phase the secretory phase endometrium is usually thin with sparse, straight glands showing diminished glycogen secretion set in an immature stroma with poor or absent spiral artery development (Figure 11.2).

More commonly, luteal phase defects are found in women with a fully adequate follicular phase, and the resulting histological picture will be a variable one reflecting differing degrees of inadequate progesterone stimulation combined with oestrogen persistence or dominance during the secretory phase. The endometrium is, in such cases, usually thick: the stroma is dense and cellular and characteristically shows markedly diminished oedema in the mid mid-secretory phase, and poor or absent predecidual change in the late secretory phase (Figure 11.3). The glands often show a similarly generalized poor secretory transformation and remain few and narrow with little secretory activity. In addition, or alternatively, the glands may show widely differing degrees of maturation, with proliferative, mid-secretory and late secretory type glands co-existing in the same endometrium (Figure 11.4): this condition is termed 'irregular ripening' and, in an adequate sample, it may be possible to see that the glands showing the greatest maturity are those nearest to the spiral arteries, whilst those which are least mature are furthest away from these vessels[1]. In some cases the most striking feature is an asynchronous maturation of the glands and stroma, in which the glands, which may be generally inadequately transformed or may show irregular ripening, lag behind the stroma in their maturation. In all these variants of oestrogen persistence during the luteal phase it is usual to find spiral artery development appropriate to the stage of the

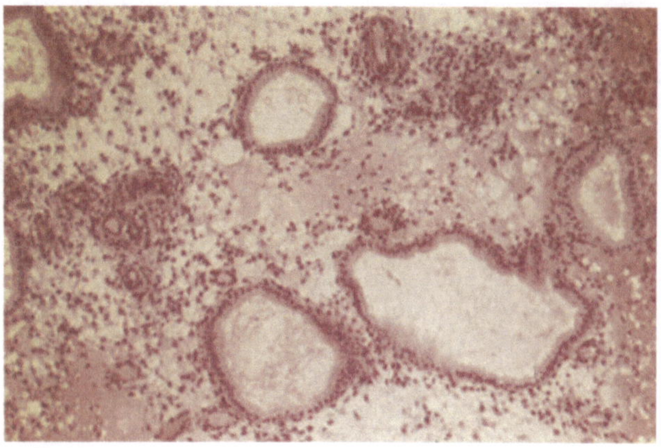

Figure 11.1 Endometrium: secretory retardation. The appearances of this endometrium are consistent with the 23rd day of a 28-day cycle (9th post-ovulatory day) and the glands and stroma are synchronously matured. Yet the biopsy was taken on the 27th day of the cycle in a woman who menstruated regularly every 28 days. H & E × 100

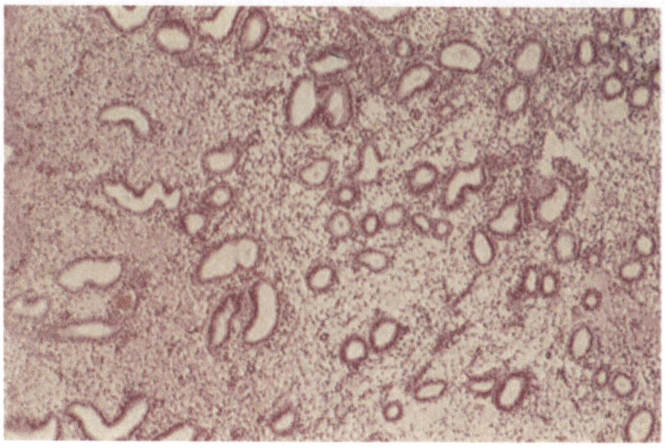

Figure 11.2 Endometrium: luteal phase insufficiency. This endometrium from the 23rd day of the cycle (9th post-ovulatory day) has small poorly developed glands showing rather irregular, inadequate early secretory activity. There is a little stromal oedema but no arterial growth. The appearances are those of luteal phase insufficiency secondary to an inadequate follicular phase. H & E × 40

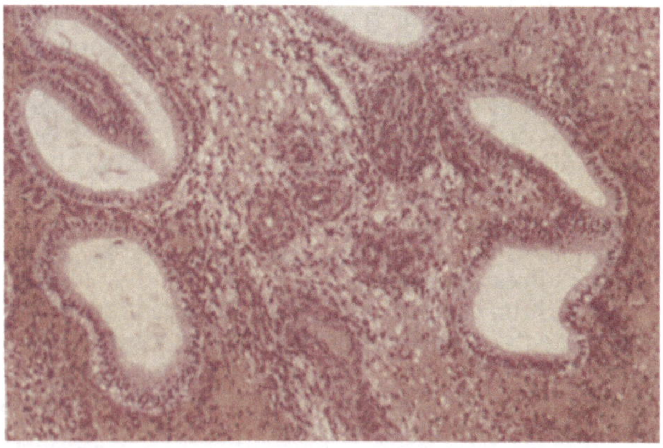

Figure 11.3 Endometrium: luteal phase insufficiency. Endometrium from the 22nd day of a cycle (8th post-ovulatory day). The glands which show very poor secretory transformation are only a little tortuous and the epithelium contains subnuclear vacuoles; there is virtually no intraglandular secretion. The stroma is cellular, and shows only a trace of oedema yet the spiral arteries are well developed and muscularized. The appearances are those of luteal phase insufficiency with oestrogen dominance. H & E × 100

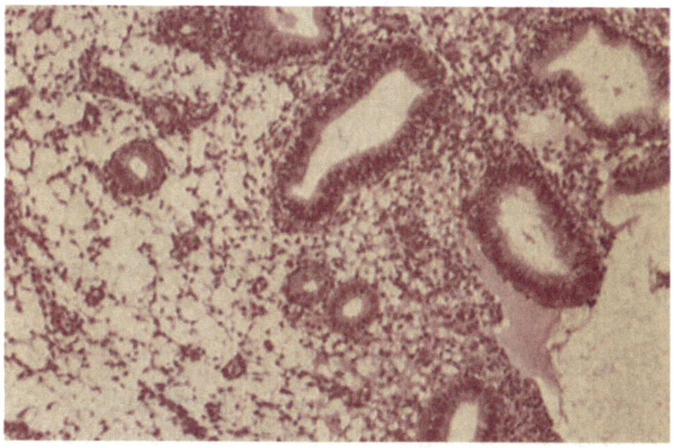

Figure 11.4 Endometrium: luteal phase insufficiency. The endometrium was taken on the 22nd day of the cycle (8th post-ovulatory day) from a patient with secondary infertility. The glands vary greatly in their size, maturation and secretory transformation. The one at the upper right corner shows established secretion whilst those at the lower left are tiny and of proliferative shape; the intermediate glands are in transition from proliferative to early secretory phase showing both mitoses and subnuclear vacuolation. The stroma is immature and spiral artery growth poor. The appearances are those of luteal phase insufficiency with irregular ripening. H & E × 100

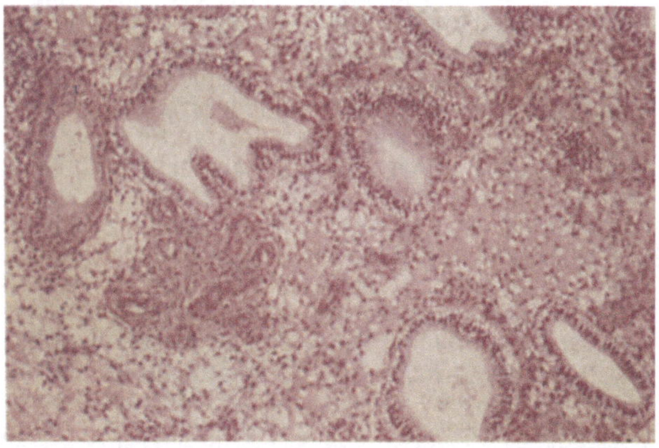

Figure 11.5 Endometrium: luteal phase insufficiency. This biopsy from an infertile patient was taken on the 23rd day of the cycle (9th post-ovulatory day). The stromal maturation is normal and adequate for the day of cycle, stromal oedema is copious and well-muscularized spiral arteries with very early perivascular decidual change are present. The glands, however, although of normal configuration and secretory transformation, are severely retarded in relation to stromal maturation, the discrepancy being about five days. H & E × 100

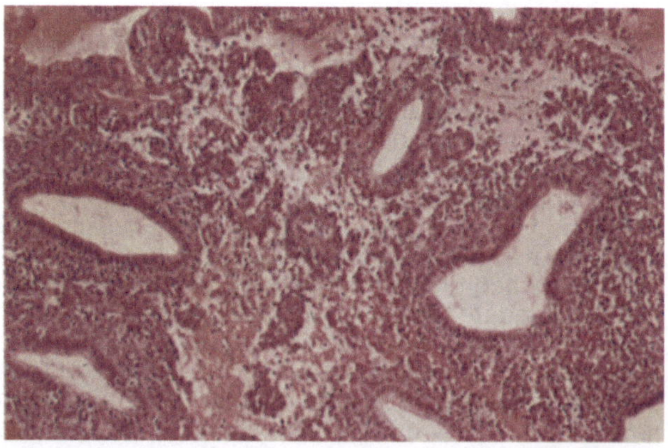

Figure 11.6 Endometrium: luteal phase insufficiency. Spontaneous stromal breakdown is seen in an endometrium showing poor secretory transformation. There is minimal stromal decidualization and the glands are straight, tubular and minimally secretory. The biopsy was obtained on the 24th day of the cycle (10th post-ovulatory day) and the glands are similar to those seen in Figure 11.3. H & E × 100

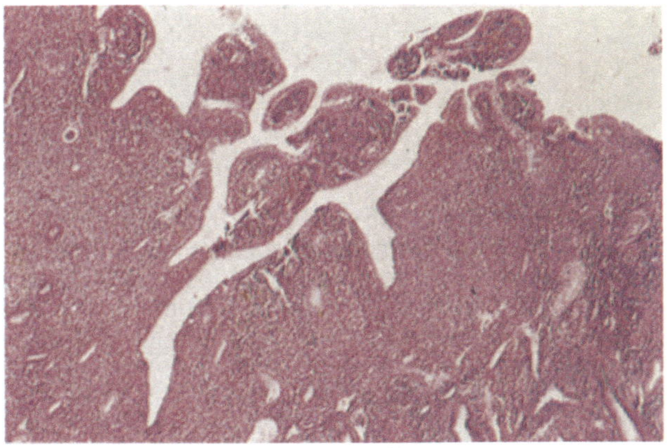

Figure 11.7 Endometrium: delayed (irregular) shedding. The varied endometrial pattern seen in this example explains the nature of the curettings obtained in patients with delayed shedding. To the lower left, there are small early proliferative glands and to the right, secretory glands. On the endometrial surface, condensed stromal fragments of menstrual type are covered by regenerating epithelium. The sample was obtained from a woman who had been bleeding for ten days. H & E × 40

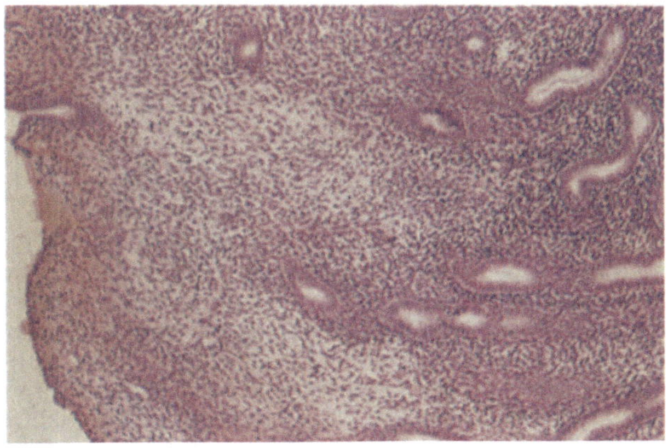

Figure 11.8 Endometrium: anovulatory cycle. The sample was obtained from a woman of 31 years who developed a premature menopause. The endometrium is shallow, the glands straight and tubular and the stroma rather compact. Only very occasional mitoses are present in the glandular epithelium. H & E × 100

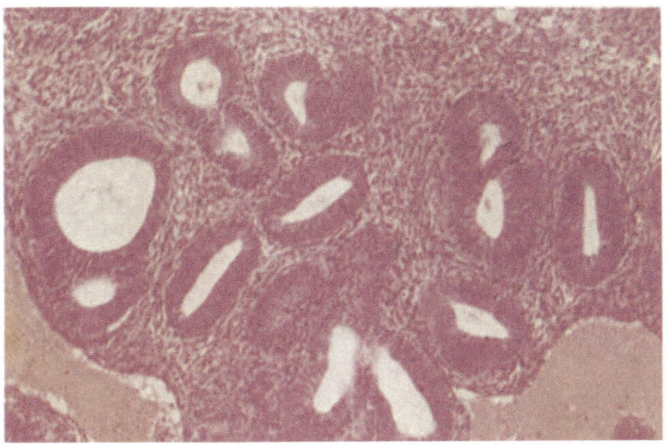

Figure 11.9 Endometrium: anovulatory cycle. An endometrial biopsy from a perimenopausal patient. The glands are lined by proliferative multilayered epithelium and are a little crowded; the stroma is cellular. There is no glandular dilatation or architectural atypia. This is the picture of irregular proliferation. H & E × 100

cycle[2] with thick walled vessels set in groups (Figure 11.5).

Premature involution of the corpus luteum, and hence an unusually short luteal phase, may occur in both adequate and inadequate corpora. In the former case breakdown occurs in a mid-secretory endometrium but in the latter, and much more common case premature breakdown occurs in an endometrium containing poorly matured secretory glands (Figure 11.6). Delayed endometrial shedding, with prolonged menstruation (i.e. longer than 5 days), may be preceded by a short luteal phase and prolongation of bleeding may simply be a reflection of the inability of a failing corpus luteum to maintain a secretory endometrium. More commonly, menstruation is prolonged because of an abnormally persistent corpus luteum[3]: persistence in such cases may, in some instances, be due to unrecognized pregnancy with very early abortion. In cases of delayed shedding a biopsy taken on the 6th or 7th day of menstruation will show a mixture of necrotic menstrual-type endometrium, endometrium containing collapsed, star-shaped secretory glands and normal proliferative endometrium (Figure 11.7).

Functional Disorders in Anovulatory Cycles

There are two forms of anovulation. The first is that in which there is an absence of developing follicles as in streak gonads or the formation of inadequate follicles, because of deficient FSH production. The resulting absent or low oestrogen levels result either in an atrophic or a weakly proliferative endometrium (Figure 11.8).

The second form of anovulation is that in which follicles develop normally but persist, such an event being possibly due to inadequate LH surges. Under these circumstances the endometrium in the late stage of the cycle tends to be unduly thick whilst the glands may show some degree of crowding, are convoluted and lined by an epithelium which shows a minor degree of multilayering: they are set in a moderately oedematous stroma (Figure 11.9). These appearances, sometimes referred to as 'irregular proliferation', will if there is a sequence of anovulatory cycles with persistent follicles, eventually evolve into a cystic glandular hyperplasia.

References

1. Dallenbach-Hellweg, G. (1981). *Histopathology of the Endometrium.* 3rd edn. (Berlin, Heidelberg and New York: Springer-Verlag)
2. de Brux, J. (1981). Evaluation of ovarian disturbances by endometrial biopsy. In de Brux J., Mortel R., and Gantray, J. P. (eds.). *The Endometrium: Hormonal Impacts.* pp. 107–121. (New York and London: Plenum Press)
3. Hendrickson, M. R. and Kempson, R. L. (1980). *Surgical Pathology of the Uterine Corpus.* (Philadelphia, London, Toronto: W. B. Saunders)

Endometrium: Inflammatory Disease 12

Inflammation can be difficult to recognize in the endometrium, a tissue with a normal complement of lymphocytes and which, during the luteal phase of the cycle, normally shows oedema, congestion, necrosis and, in the later stages, a neutrophil polymorphonuclear leukocyte infiltration. The presence, at any stage of the cycle, of plasma cells, or of neutrophil polymorphonuclear leukocytes at times other than the late secretory and premenstrual phase are, however, clear indications of an inflammatory process: tissue destruction, the formation of microabscesses and the presence of granulomata are equally definite hallmarks of true endometrial inflammation.

Non-infective Endometritis

Many examples of endometrial inflammation are non-infective in origin and represent a reaction to foreign bodies, e.g. an intrauterine contraceptive device, chemical substances injected to procure abortion, or to necrotic tissue such as retained products of conception, endometrial neoplasms, torted polypi or infarcted submucous leiomyomata. Some degree of non-infective endometritis is a normal feature of the pregnant uterus, is constantly present in the puerperium and regularly occurs after uterine irradiation.

In most cases of non-infective endometritis the histological features are quite non-specific, there usually being a plasma cell and/or polymorph infiltrate (Figure 12.1): postirradiation endometritis is however, characterized not only by a plasma cell infiltrate but also by stromal fibroblastic atypia, a vasculitis which progresses to vascular hyalinization and, rarely, stromal granulomata.

Histiocytic Endometritis

This is a particular variant of non-infective endometritis and appears to be usually the end result of a sterile pyometra or haematometra[1]. The endometrium is partially or completely replaced by sheets of mono- or multinucleated macrophages which are intermingled with plasma cells and lymphocytes (Figure 12.2): the macrophages have granular, PAS-positive cytoplasm which contains lipid and, if there has been a haematometra, haemosiderin. This condition closely resembles malakoplakia from which, however, it can be distinguished by the absence of Michaelis–Gutmann bodies.

Infective Endometritis

Infection of the endometrium is uncommon, a fact attributable to the combination of an effective cervical mucus barrier, the adequacy of natural uterine drainage and, during the reproductive years, the regular shedding of the endometrial tissue. Modification of any of these factors may result in infection: thus, inadequate production of cervical mucus because of overenthusiastic conization or cautery, cessation of regular endometrial loss and obstruction to natural drainage all predispose to infection[2]. In most cases the infection is an ascending one and polymicrobiol in type. Mild infections are characterized only by a scattering of plasma cells, neutrophil polymorphonuclear leukocytes and eosinophils, but in more severe infections there may be a marked periglandular aggregation of stromal plasma cells, an accumulation of acute inflammatory cells within glandular lumena (Figure 12.3), granulation tissue formation and fibrosis. In these severe inflammatory disorders hormone receptor development is inhibited with a resulting loss of the normal cyclical changes in the endometrium (Figure 12.4) whilst both the surface and glandular epithelium may show marked reactive changes with nuclear enlargement and pleomorphism without, however, any hyperchromatism or abnormal mitotic activity (Figure 12.5).

Granulomatous Endometritis

Tuberculosis

Tuberculous infection of the endometrium is now uncommon in Great Britain, although still an important disease in many less affluent parts of the world: it is nearly always secondary to tubal tuberculosis, about 50% of women with tubal tuberculosis having an accompanying endometrial infection. Tuberculosis often, but not invariably, either has no effect on the normal cyclical changes in this tissue or only limits their full expression: hence during the reproductive years, the histological recognition of endometrial tuberculosis may pose a diagnostic problem, for the regular shedding of the tissue prevents the full development of granulomata and their progression to caseation. In the typical case there may be, from about the 20th day of the cycle, collections of intraglandular neutrophil polymorphonuclear leukocytes without any stromal inflammation (Figure 12.6), an appearance which mimics, and may be confused with, that seen in some IUCD wearers. Subsequently, loose clusters of epithelioid macrophages accumulate in the stroma and are surrounded

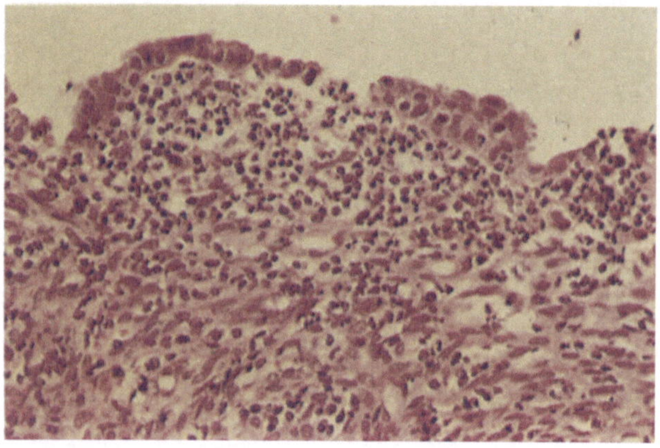

Figure 12.1 Endometrium: acute non-specific endometritis. In this biopsy the superficial part of the stroma is infiltrated by polymorphonuclear leukocytes and an occasional plasma cell. H & E × 250

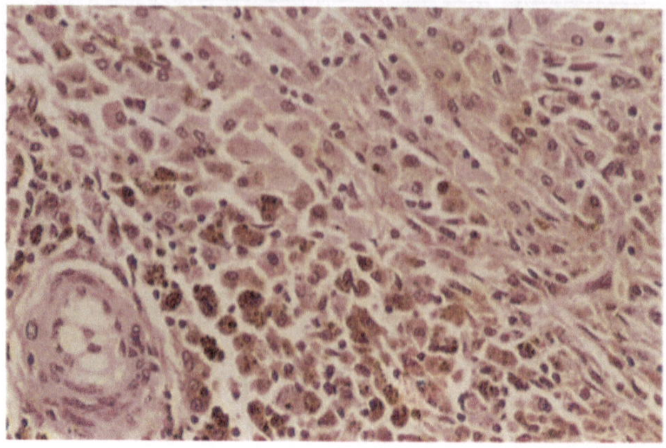

Figure 12.2 Endometrium: histiocytic endometritis. The entire endometrium is replaced by sheets of macrophages with copious, pale, granular cytoplasm interspersed with lymphocytes. To the lower left many of the macrophages contain typical golden brown haemosiderin. There are no Michaelis–Gutmann bodies. H & E × 250

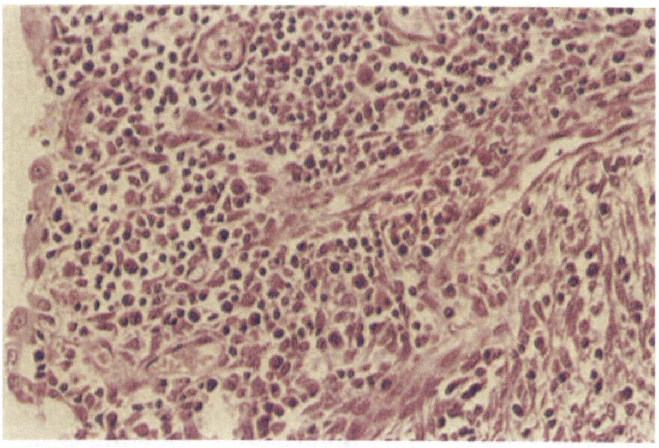

Figure 12.3 Endometrium: non-specific infective endometritis. The endometrial stroma is heavily infiltrated by plasma cells, histiocytes and lymphocytes and there is early granulation tissue formation with fibroblasts and thin-walled capillaries. The surface epithelial cells are pleomorphic and show nuclear enlargement, a non-specific reactive change (see also Figure 12.5). H & E × 250

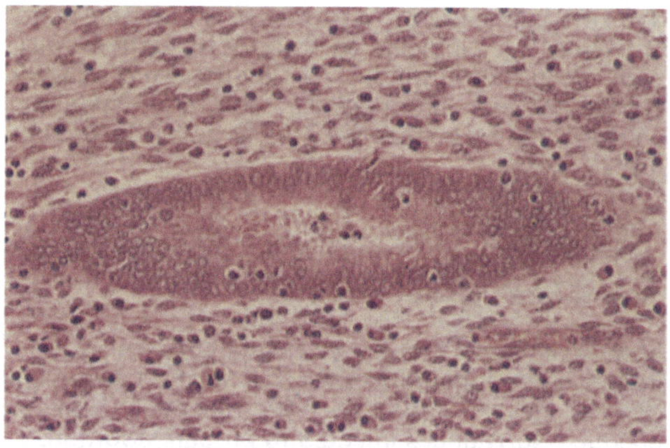

Figure 12.4 Endometrium: non-specific infective endometritis. The gland in the centre of the field is lined by epithelium with neither proliferative nor secretory activity, and therefore showing no evidence of normal cyclical changes. The stroma is inflamed and inflammatory cells lie within the glandular epithelium. The sample demonstrates the effect of impairment of hormone receptor site development in severe endometritis. H & E × 250

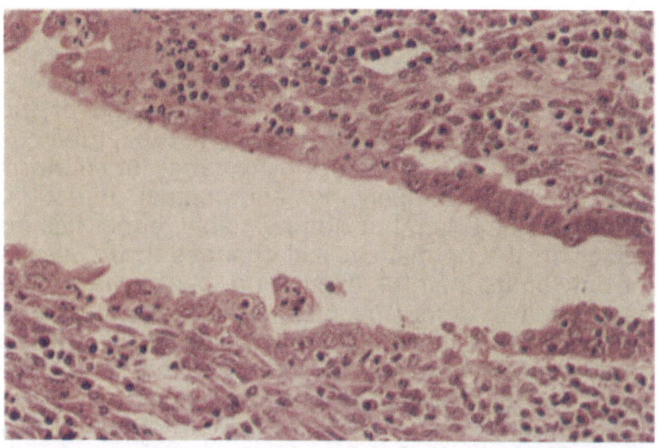

Figure 12.5 Endometrium: non-specific infective endometritis. The glandular epithelium in this case shows not only an absence of normal cyclical changes but also severe reactive atypia with cellular pleomorphism, nuclear enlargement and loss of nuclear polarity. H & E × 250

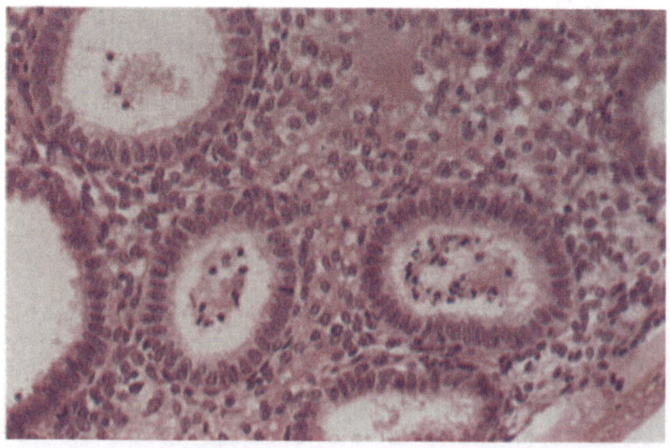

Figure 12.6 Endometrium: tuberculosis. In this biopsy there are many glands in which polymorphonuclear leukocytes and macrophages are seen; cultures were positive for *Mycobacterium* tuberculosis. Often an appearance such as this is combined with intrastromal granuloma formation but in this patient there was no other evidence of infection. H & E × 100

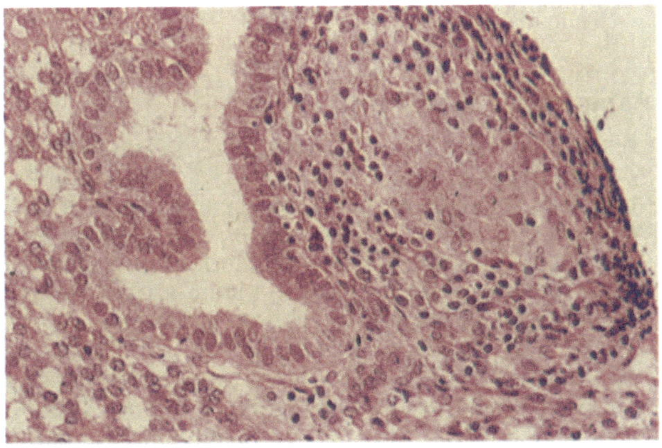

Figure 12.7 Endometrium: tuberculosis. An ill-formed granuloma composed of a cluster of epithelioid cells surrounded by lymphocytes lies to the right of a gland in the late secretory phase. There are no giant cells or caseation and this appearance is typical of that which is encountered in endometrial curettings in the reproductive years. H & E × 250

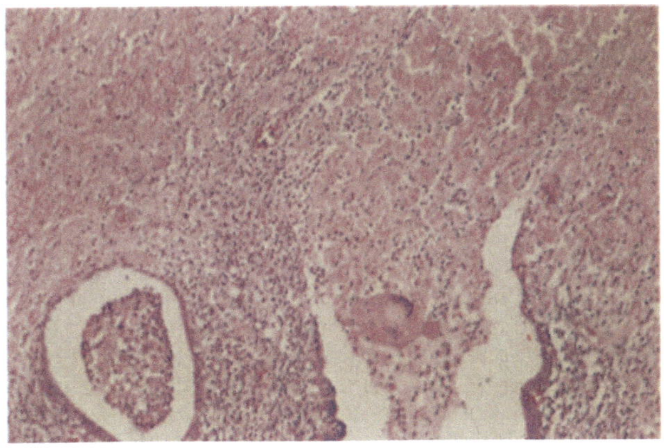

Figure 12.8 Endometrium: tuberculosis. In the postmenopausal patient, a more typical picture of caseating tuberculosis is seen. In the lower half of the field there are endometrial glands whilst the uterine cavity, above, contains caseous material; note the Langhans giant cell in the gland lumen. H & E × 100

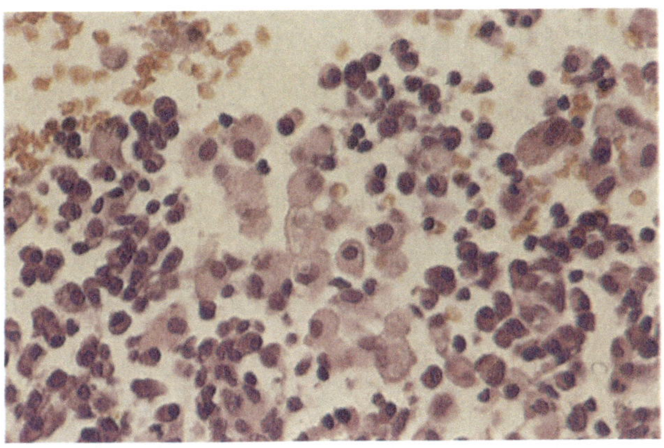

Figure 12.9 Endometrium: malakoplakia. The endometrium in this sample was largely replaced by sheets of macrophages and plasma cells. The macrophages in the centre of the field contain the 'target-like' Michaelis–Gutmann bodies. H & E × 400

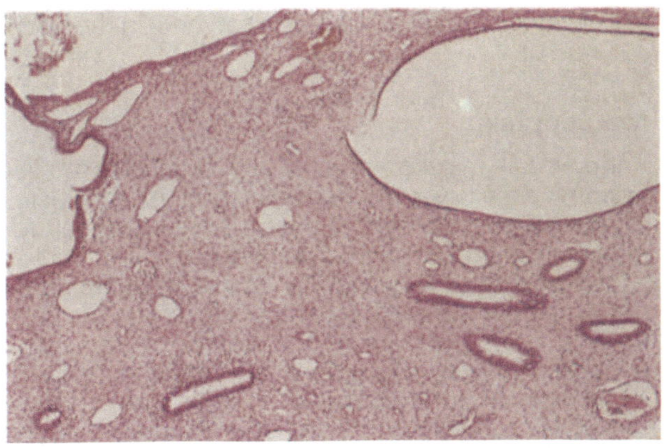

Figure 12.10 Endometrium: Asherman's syndrome. The atrophic endometrium, in the lower half of the field, contains scanty, poorly developed glands in a fibrous stroma. Synechiae lie in the upper half of the field and are composed of fibrous stroma covered by epithelium of endometrial type. Elsewhere in the corpus uteri there were foci of more normal proliferative endometrium. H & E × 40

by a cuff of lymphocytes: occasional Langhans' giant cells may be formed and recognizably tuberculous granulomata (Figure 12.7), usually few in number, may be found in the immediately premenstrual phase. Even when the histological picture strongly suggests tuberculosis it is distinctly unusual for a Ziehl–Neelsen stain to be positive and microbiological studies are essential in every suspected case.

After the menopause there is, of course, no bar to the development of typical tuberculous granulomata and, indeed, a fully developed fibro–caseous tuberculosis is often seen with, sometimes, the uterine cavity being lined by tuberculous granulation tissue and filled with caseous material (Figure 12.8).

Non-tuberculous Granulomatous Endometritis

Granulomata may be seen in the endometrium in response to foreign material and may be seen in fungal, mycoplasmal or bilharzial infections. Sarcoidosis can affect the endometrium[3] though this diagnosis should probably not be entertained unless there is clear evidence of the disease elsewhere in the body.

Malakoplakia

Endometrial malakoplakia is rare but can, on occasion, cause postmenopausal bleeding[4]. The histological picture is similar to that of a histiocytic endometritis, differing only by the presence of Michaelis–Gutmann bodies (Figure 12.9): these latter are small, round, laminated calcospherites which may be seen both in the cytoplasm of the macrophages and in extracellular sites. Malakoplakia is thought to be an expression of an abnormal immunological response to bacteria, usually *E. coli*: the organisms are retained within the phagolysosomes of the macrophages but are not digested.

Asherman's Syndrome

This condition is characterized by the formation of adhesions between the two surfaces of the endometrium: these may be single or multiple and can, in extreme cases, obliterate the cavity. Intrauterine adhesions usually occur as a complication of post-abortal or puerperal curettage though a small proportion of cases follow myomectomy. Whether trauma alone is responsible for the formation of the adhesions or whether there must always be a superadded infective endometritis[5] is debatable: certainly this syndrome, often in a severe form, can complicate endometrial tuberculosis[6]. The bands joining the two endometrial surfaces consist of a core of partially fibrotic or hyalinized endometrial stroma (Figure 12.10) covered by cells similar to those of the endometrial surface epithelium: occasionally the bands contain smooth muscle fibres or foci of calcification. The uninvolved endometrium may show normal cyclical changes, inadequate secretory change or be completely inactive and atrophic.

References

1. Buckley, C. H. and Fox, H. (1980). Histiocytic endometritis. *Histopathology*, **4**, 105–110
2. Rotterdam, H. (1978). Chronic endometritis: a clinicopathologic study. *Pathol. Ann.*, **13**, 209–231
3. Ho, K. H. (1979). Sarcoidosis of the uterus. *Hum. Pathol.*, **10**, 219–222
4. Thomas, W. Jr., Sadeghieh, B., Fresco, R., Rubenstone, A. I., Stepto, R. C. and Carasso, B. (1978). Malacoplakia of the endometrium, a probable cause of post-menopausal bleeding. *Am. J. Clin. Pathol.*, **69**, 637–641
5. Czernobilsky, B. (1979). Endometritis and infertility. In Wallach, E. E. and Kempera, R. D. (eds.). *Modern Trends in Infertility and Conception Control.* pp. 54–65 (Baltimore: Williams and Wilkins)
6. Schenker, J.G. and Margalioth, E.J. (1982). Intrauterine adhesions: an updated appraisal. *Fertil. Steril.*, **37**, 593–610

Endometrium: Metaplasia and Polypi 13

Metaplasia

Metaplasia, the process whereby one mature tissue is replaced by another foreign to the anatomical area, may occur in the normal, atrophic, hyperplastic or neoplastic endometrium[1, 2]. The endometrial epithelium is usually replaced by another epithelium of Müllerian type, this reflecting the latent capacity of indifferent endometrial cells to differentiate along a variety of alternative Müllerian pathways.

Squamous Metaplasia

The term 'squamous metaplasia' is used to encompass not only the replacement of endometrial epithelium by easily recognizable keratinizing squamous epithelium but also the development of intraglandular morules, these latter being sheets of cells which have vaguely squamoid features but which lack the defining light microscopic features of squamous tissue[3].

Typical keratinizing squamous metaplasia (Figures 13.1 and 13.2) is common and occurs in patients with endometritis, endometrial hyperplasia or endometrial neoplasia: it is also seen in women wearing an IUCD, in patients receiving postmenopausal oestrogen replacement therapy and has a particular tendency to complicate a chronic pyometra. It must be emphasized, however, that squamous metaplasia can also occur in normal endometria and, indeed, it has been maintained that diligent search will reveal occasional foci of such metaplasia in the endometria of the vast majority of healthy premenopausal women[4]. The process of squamous metaplasia in the endometrium closely mirrors that occurring in the cervix, and may similarly involve both the surface epithelium and that of the glands: the foci of intraglandular squamous metaplasia may merge imperceptibly with morules. Replacement of the entire endometrium by keratinizing squamous epithelium is known as ichthyosis uteri: this can complicate a chronic pyometra but sometimes occurs spontaneously in elderly women in whom it can, because of ulceration, cause postmenopausal bleeding.

Morules form nodular cell clusters which characteristically protrude into glandular lumena (Figure 13.3): they are seen most frequently in hyperplastic endometria. The morules may become aggregated to form sheets and necrosis is not uncommon in the centre of large morules. The cells forming the morules have regular, ovoid, vesicular nuclei with finely dispersed chromatin, a moderate amount of eosinophilic cytoplasm and indistinct cell boundaries: intercellular bridges, keratinization and nuclear pyknosis are not seen but, nevertheless, morules are best considered as foci of immature squamous metaplasia.

It is recognized that most instances of the very rare squamous cell carcinoma of the endometrium arise in an ichthyotic uterus but focal squamous metaplasia is, in itself, of no importance and its presence in nonmalignant endometria does not have any malign implications.

Ciliated Cell (Tubal) Metaplasia

Strictly, the term 'metaplasia' should not be used to describe the presence of ciliated cells in the endometrium for these are a normal constituent of this tissue. The term is, however, applied to the condition in which there is a predominance of pyramidal ciliated cells, with eosinophilic and often vacuolated cytoplasm, in the lining of a gland or group of glands. There is a tendency for these ciliated cells to become stratified and, in some instances, form intraglandular tufts or papillae: the bland nature of the nuclei and the lack of mitotic figures help in dispelling a false impression of neoplasia when encountering this pattern. Ciliated cell metaplasia is seen quite commonly both in normal proliferative and hyperplastic endometria.

Eosinophilic Metaplasia (Figure 13.4)

In this condition, cells resembling those seen in ciliated cell metaplasia, but lacking cilia and having more strikingly eosinophilic (and sometimes granular) cytoplasm, are seen lining a gland or group of glands. This form of metaplasia is often noted in hyperplastic endometria and in polypi.

Mucinous Metaplasia (Figure 13.5)

This occurs most commonly after the menopause, and in its most typical form glandular epithelium is replaced by endocervical-type columnar epithelium: this change is usually focal but rarely the whole endometrium undergoes mucinous metaplasia, a phenomenon that can result in a mucometra. When mucinous metaplasia occurs in a hyperplastic endometrium the overall appearances may bear a close resemblance to those seen in ovarian mucinous tumours of borderline malignancy.

Papillary Metaplasia

Occasionally, there may be branching and budding of the endometrial surface epithelium to form papillary aggregates of cells with indistinct margins and central nuclei (Figure 13.6): in some instances there is an apparent formation of a syncytium (Figure 13.7). This abnormality, which would be better termed papillary

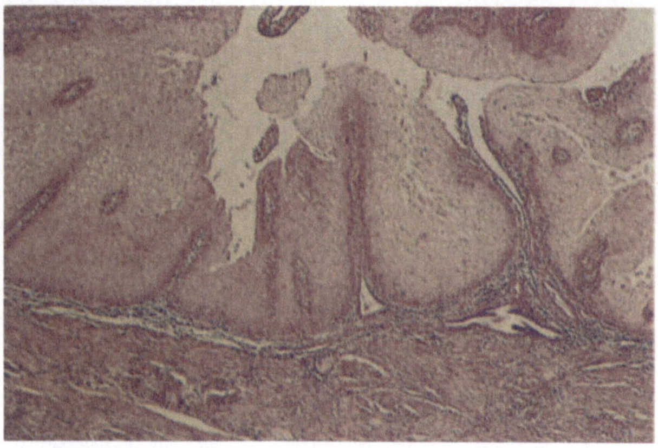

Figure 13.1 Endometrium: squamous metaplasia. This is an example of *ichthyosis uteri*; the endometrium is almost completely replaced by mature metaplastic squamous epithelium beneath which basal glands can still be distinguished. H & E × 40

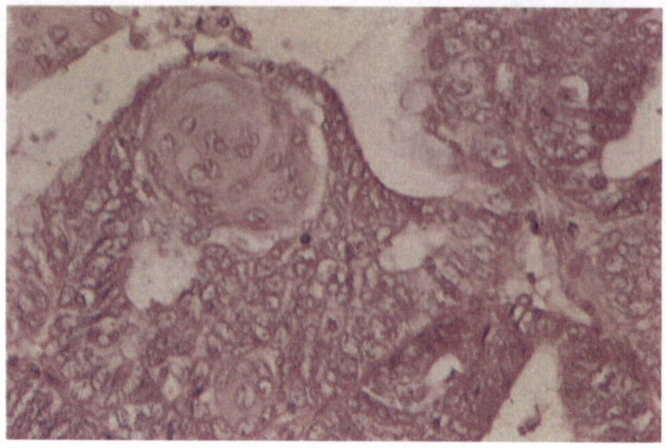

Figure 13.2 Endometrium: squamous metaplasia. A well formed squamous epithelial pearl (upper left) is seen in this endometrial adenocarcinoma. H & E × 250

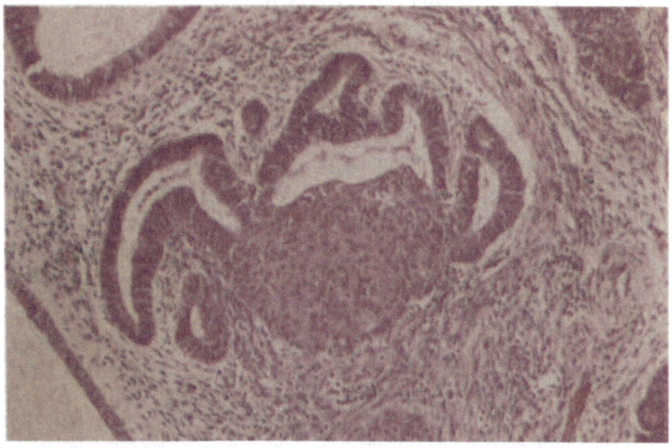

Figure 13.3 Endometrium: squamous metaplasia. A morule is formed by large, non-keratinizing squamoid cells with small regular ovoid nuclei and copious eosinophilic cytoplasm. It has formed deep to the columnar epithelium which lies attenuated over its surface as it protrudes into the lumen of a gland showing mild architectural atypia. H & E × 100

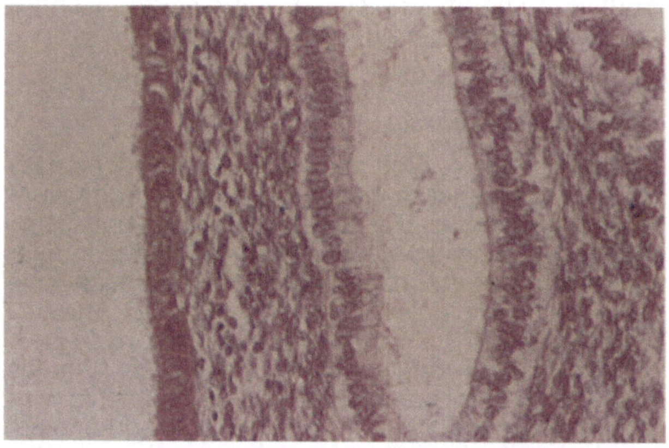

Figure 13.4 Endometrium: eosinophilic metaplasia. The glands to the right are of normal configuration and are lined by columnar cells in which there are subnuclear vacuoles. To the left, the gland is lined by a uniform population of short, columnar cells with round, rather pleomorphic nuclei and granular eosinophilic cytoplasm. H & E × 250

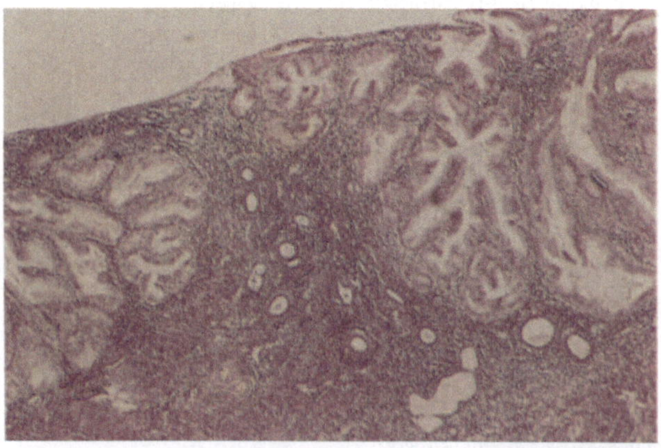

Figure 13.5 Endometrium: mucinous metaplasia. In the endometrium of this post-menopausal woman there were several areas similar to those shown here. Foci of hyperplastic glands are lined by tall mucus-secreting columnar cells with small regular nuclei. Between and below the hyperplastic foci there is atrophic endometrium. H & E × 40

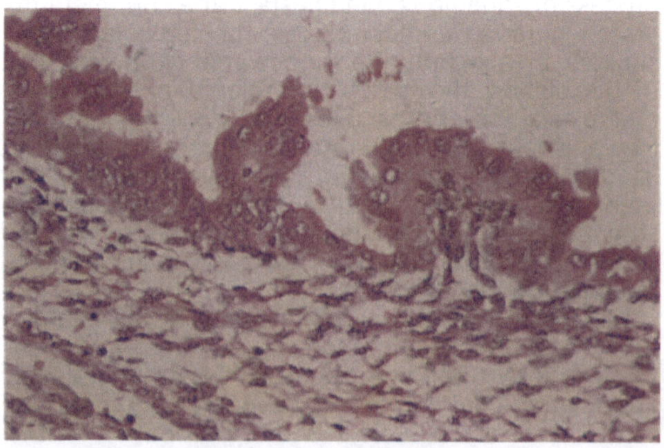

Figure 13.6 Endometrium: papillary metaplasia. The surface epithelium forms papillary projections and tufts. H & E × 250

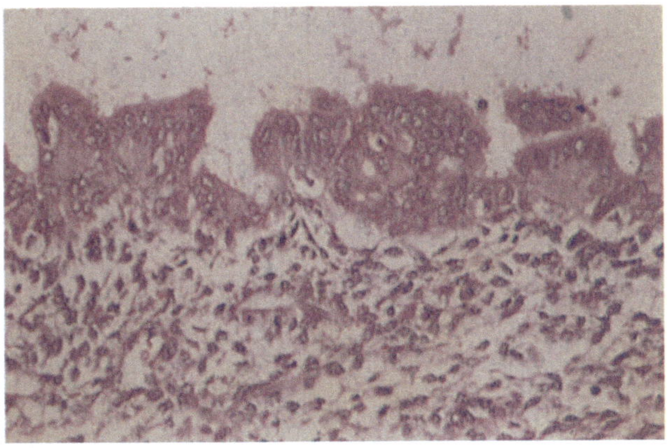

Figure 13.7 Endometrium: syncytial metaplasia. In this field, taken from the same sample as Figure 13.6, the papillary surface projections appear to be forming a syncytium. H & E × 250

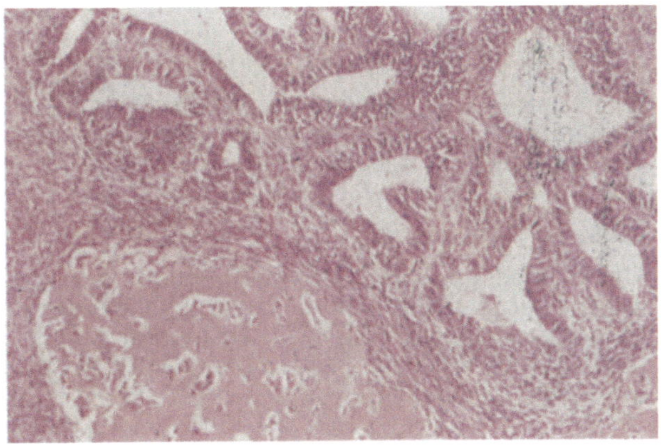

Figure 13.8 Endometrium: stromal metaplasia. The stroma in this hyperplastic endometrium shows osseous metaplasia. To the lower left, there is an irregular focus of pink-staining osteoid whilst to the right the glands are crowded and show mild architectural atypia. H & E × 100

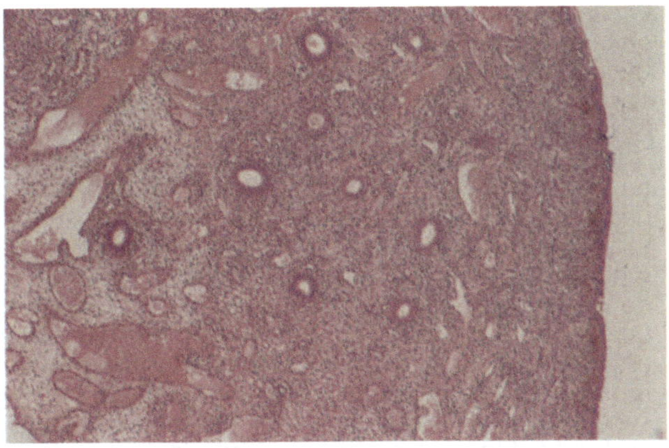

Figure 13.9 Endometrium: polyp. The polyp is composed of small tubular endometrial glands, showing neither secretory nor proliferative activity, in a rather fibrous stroma. The polyp is covered by a single layer of cubo–columnar epithelium (to the right) beneath which there is a focal haemorrhage. In other cases the tip of the polyp may show inflammation and ulceration. Note the large dilated stromal vessels. H & E × 40

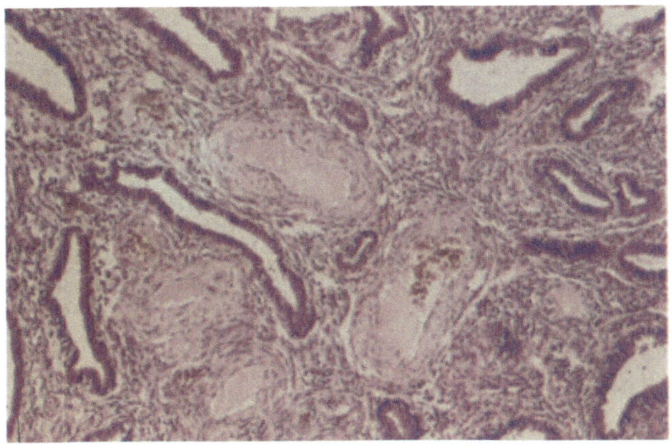

Figure 13.10 Endometrium: polyp. The thick-walled, muscular arteries amidst the basal glands are typical of those seen in the pedicle and core of a large proportion of endometrial polypi. H & E × 100

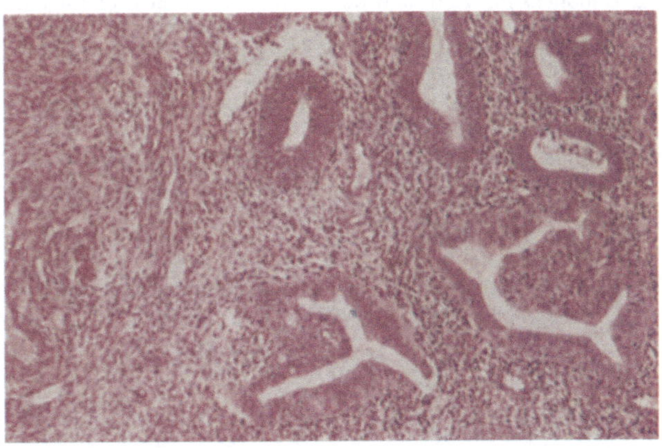

Figure 13.11 Endometrium: adenomyomatous polyp. The stroma is predominantly fibrous but to the left well formed bands of smooth muscle can be seen. The glands show a mild degree of architectural atypia. In the two at the bottom of the field there is epithelial cytological atypia characterized by loss of nuclear polarity, an increased nucleo–cytoplasmic ratio and nuclear pleomorphism. H & E × 100

change rather than papillary metaplasia, is particularly frequent in the endometria of postmenopausal women receiving oestrogens.

'Hob-nail' Metaplasia

This change, usually seen in conjunction with other metaplastic epithelia, is characterized by the presence of tear-drop shaped cells, with eosinophilic or clear cytoplasm, which have their apices directed towards the basement membrane.

Clear Cell Metaplasia

In some otherwise unremarkable postmenopausal endometria occasional glands are lined by cubo-columnar cells with clear cytoplasm which contains glycogen and a trace of mucin: these cells are reminiscent of those seen in an Arias-Stella reaction but lack the nuclear atypia which is a feature of that hypersecretory change.

Stromal Metaplasia

Although most metaplastic processes in the endometrium are confined to the epithelial component there may, rarely, be cartilaginous, osseous, fatty or smooth muscle metaplasia within the stroma (Figure 13.8). Stromal metaplasia of these various types can be distinguished from fetal remnants by the merging with normal stroma at their periphery and from malignant mixed Müllerian tumours by their bland histological appearances.

Polypi

The term 'polyp' is purely descriptive and does not, in itself, denote any specific pathological process: thus an endometrial neoplasm may well present as a uterine polyp. Conventionally, however, the term 'endometrial polyp' is generally taken as meaning a focal, circumscribed overgrowth of the mucosa, usually of the basal portion, which protrudes into the uterine cavity. Such polypi can occur at any age after puberty but are most common during the fifth and sixth decades: they arise most frequently in the fundus, may be pedunculated or sessile, usually measure 0.5–3 cm in their longest diameter and are pinkish, fleshy and smooth surfaced. Histologically, a typical polyp consists of endometrial glands and stroma covered by a single layer of cuboidal epithelium (Figure 13.9). Usually the glands do not share in the normal cyclical activity of the endometrium and are either atrophic or only weakly proliferative; architectural atypia is not uncommon whilst sometimes the glands in a polyp show either a cystic glandular hyperplasia or a hyperplasia with cellular atypia: in postmenopausal women the glands often show senile cystic change. In a few polypi secretory change may occur in the glands but this is usually patchy and irregular. The stroma of a polyp almost invariably contains some fibrous tissue and this, together with the presence of thick-walled vessels (Figure 13.10) both in the stalk and in the polyp, is of diagnostic help in recognizing a polyp in uterine curettings. It should be noted that reliance, for making this diagnosis, on the presence of surface epithelium on all sides of an endometrial fragment is unfounded, for a similar appearance can be seen in polypoidal fragments of normal endometrium[1].

In some polypi, classed as 'adenofibromatous polypi' the stroma consists largely of fibrous tissue whilst in others, known as 'adenomyomatous polypi', interlacing bands of smooth muscle fibres are present in the stroma: in some adenomyomatous polypi the glandular component shows a degree of cytological atypia[5] and such polypi (Figure 13.11) can be mistaken either for an adenocarcinoma which is infiltrating the myometrium or for a malignant mixed Müllerian tumour: the small size of the lesion, its occurrence in relatively young women and the presence of smooth muscle are all of aid in the recognition of this type of polyp. Sometimes an endometrial polyp consists solely of endometrial stroma, these 'stromatous' polypi being very uncommon.

Malignant change in a polyp is distinctly unusual, and most cases in which it has been thought that a benign polyp has undergone malignant transformation have, in fact, been polypoid adenocarcinomata which were malignant from the outset. This is not to deny that an adenocarcinoma may, on occasion, develop in a polyp for such a change has been well documented[6]: however, to establish this diagnosis it is necessary to show that the malignant tumour is separated from a normal endometrium by the base and stalk of the polyp, the latter showing no evidence of malignancy.

References

1. Hendrickson, M. R. and Kempson, R. L. (1980). *Surgical Pathology of the Uterine Corpus.* (Philadelphia, London, Toronto: W. B. Saunders)
2. Hendrickson, M. R. and Kempson, R. L. (1980). Endometrial epithelial metaplasias: proliferations frequently misdiagnosed as adenocarcinoma. Report of 89 cases and proposed classification. *Am. J. Surg. Pathol.*, **4**, 525–542
3. Dutra, F. (1959). Intraglandular morules of the endometrium. *Am. J. Clin. Pathol.*, **31**, 60–65
4. Baggish, M. S. and Woodruff, J. D. (1967). The occurrence of squamous epithelium in the endometrium. *Obstet. Gynecol. Surv.*, **22**, 69–115
5. Mazur, M. T. (1981). Atypical polypoid adenomyomas of the endometrium. *Am. J. Surg. Pathol.*, **5**, 473–482
6. Salm, R. (1972). The incidence and significance of early carcinomas in endometrial polyps. *J. Pathol.*, **108**, 47–54

Endometrium: Hyperplasia and Intraendometrial Neoplasia

14

Hyperplasia

Endometrial hyperplasia is not a single entity, and to use this term without any qualifying adjective not only denies the existence of a variety of hyperplastic conditions of the endometrium but also conceals their independent, and vastly different, relationships to the subsequent development of an endometrial adenocarcinoma.

A useful histological classification of endometrial hyperplasias, based largely on that of Welch and Scully[1], allows for the recognition of four forms:

(1) *Cystic glandular hyperplasia*. This involves the whole endometrium with the distinction between functional and basal zones being lost. The glands are markedly variable in size, some being unduly large, others of normal calibre and yet others unusually small (Figure 14.1). The glands are usually rounded but there may be some budding into the surrounding stroma: the glandular lining is formed of regular tall cuboidal, or columnar, cells with basophilic cytoplasm and round basal or central nuclei (Figure 14.2): multilayering is not uncommon. The ratio of glands to stroma is normal, for the stroma shares in the hyperplastic process and tends to be markedly hypercellular, often showing the 'naked nuclei' appearance characteristic of a proliferative phase endometrium. Mitotic figures may be common or sparse, are seen in both glands and stroma and are invariably of normal form.

(2) *Adenomatoid hyperplasia*. This is rare and invariably focal: this form of hyperplasia sometimes appears to be localized to a polyp, but this is possibly because this localized lesion tends to become polypoid. There is a simple excess of glands which, whilst of somewhat variable calibre, are usually of approximately normal size (Figure 14.3). The glands are round with a regular single-layered lining epithelium, and the condition differs from a normal proliferative endometrium only by the marked excess of glands and the reduction, though not the complete disappearance, of the intervening stroma.

(3) *Glandular hyperplasia with architectural atypia*. This form of hyperplasia is restricted to the glandular component of the endometrium, and is usually focal rather than diffuse. The glands, though variable in size, tend to be larger than normal and are more numerous, the stroma being reduced by the glandular crowding. There is an abnormal pattern of glandular growth with outpouchings, or budding, of the glandular epithelium into the stroma to produce the 'finger in glove' appearance (Figure 14.4). Papillary projections of epithelial cells, with connective tissue cores, into the glandular lumena are not uncommon and sometimes solid buds of cells project into the glands. The glandular epithelium is regular and formed of tall cuboidal cells with rounded or ovoid nuclei which are basally or centrally placed. Mitotic figures may be present in the glandular epithelium and are of normal form.

(4) *Glandular hyperplasia with cellular atypia*. This is always focal and the hyperplastic process is restricted to the glands. There is crowding of the glands with a reduction in the amount of interglandular stroma and, in severe cases, the stroma may be either reduced to a thin wisp between the glands, often only detectable with a reticulin stain, or completely obliterated with the glands assuming a 'back to back' pattern (Figure 14.5). The glands are usually markedly irregular in shape and the cells lining the glands show varying degrees of nuclear and cytoplasmic atypia (Figure 14.6). In the milder forms the nucleo–cytoplasmic ratio is either normal or only slightly increased, the nuclei are ovoid or sausage-shaped, nuclear polarity is retained, there is no significant enlargement of the nucleoli and the nuclear chromatin pattern is normal. In more severe cases the nucleo–cytoplasmic ratio is increased, the nuclei tend to be rounded, the nucleoli are enlarged, nuclear polarity is disturbed or lost and the nuclear chromatin may be either clumped or cleared. With progressively severe cellular atypia there is an increasing degree of multilayering of the glandular epithelium and of intraluminal budding and tufting (Figure 14.7): the intraluminal tufting can, in severe forms, be of a complex nature and the tufts may fuse to give a cribriform pattern within the gland though the apparent 'bridges' thus formed retain a stromal support, albeit one which may be revealed only with the help of a trichrome or reticulin stain. Mitotic figures are uncommon in cases of mild atypia but tend to be more numerous as the degree of atypia increases: they are usually, however, of normal form.

Intraendometrial Adenocarcinoma

The term 'adenocarcinoma *in situ* of the endometrium' has been used very loosely, and can be taken to indicate either a neoplasm which is not invading the

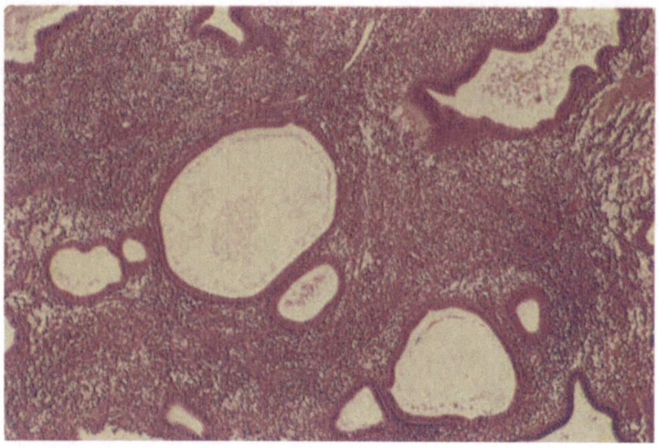

Figure 14.1 Endometrium: cystic glandular hyperplasia. The glands vary in size, some being almost normal whilst others are large and cystically dilated; there is no secretion. The stroma is intensely cellular. H & E × 40

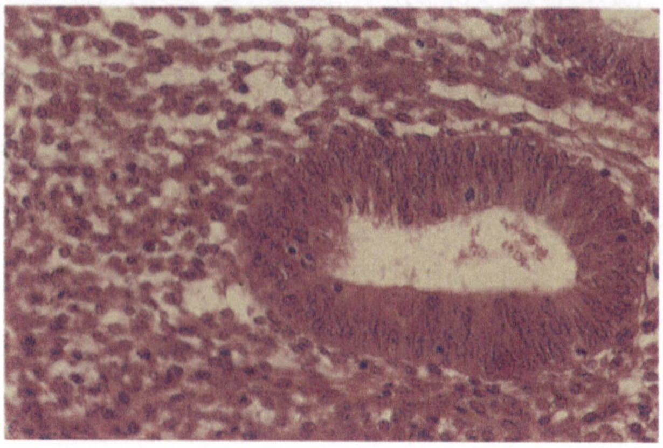

Figure 14.2 Endometrium: cystic glandular hyperplasia. The gland is lined by multilayered tall columnar cells in which occasional normal mitoses can be seen. The stroma, in which mitoses are also present, is cellular; the nuclei are round or ovoid and the cell boundaries ill-defined. H & E × 250

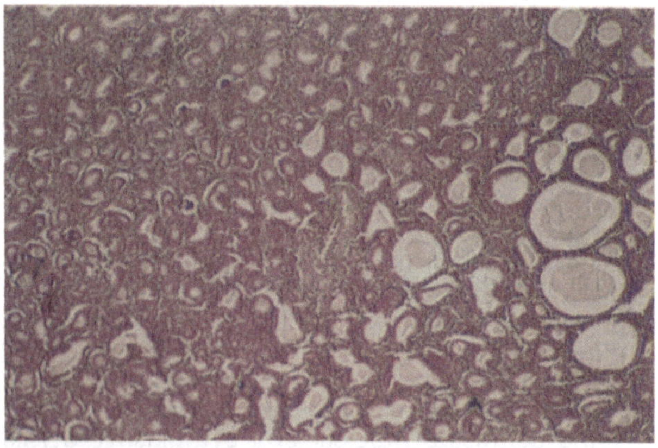

Figure 14.3 Endometrium: adenomatoid hyperplasia. The lesion, which was polypoidal, is composed of closely packed glands some of which are of normal calibre whilst others are cystically dilated. The glandular epithelium shows no multilayering or cytological atypia. H & E × 40

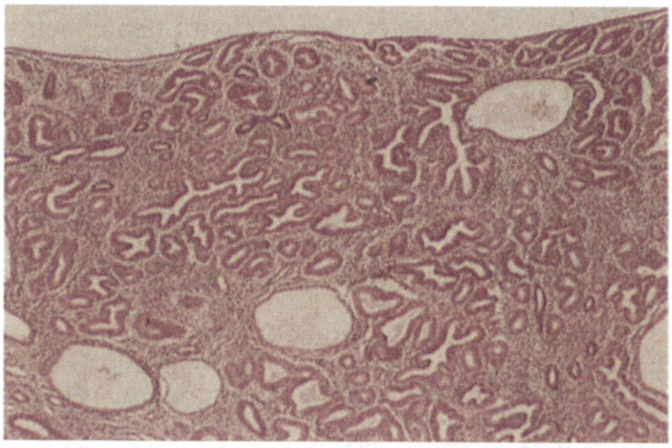

Figure 14.4 Endometrium: glandular hyperplasia with architectural atypia. The tissue was from a woman of 52 years who had a hysterectomy following the detection of atypical hyperplasia in curettings taken to investigate perimenopausal bleeding. The endometrium is deep, occasional glands are cystically dilated but the majority are rather closely packed with little intervening stroma and several are branched and show irregular infoldings of their epithelium. There is no secretion. The stroma is of proliferative type. This is a moderate degree of architectural atypia. H & E × 40

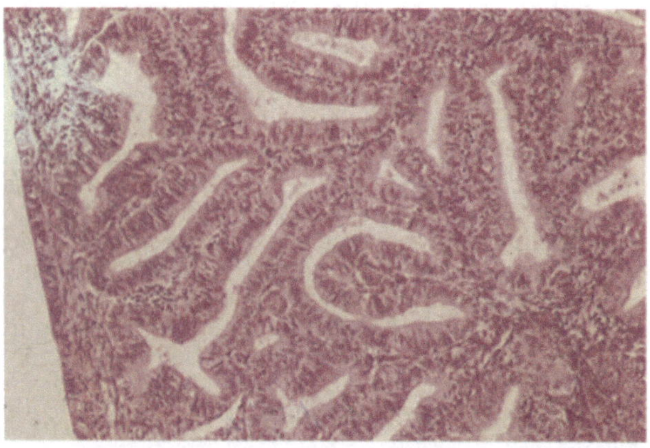

Figure 14.5 Endometrium: glandular hyperplasia with cellular atypia. The glands are crowded, show occasional outpouchings and the stroma is reduced to a wisp between 'back to back' glands. The glandular epithelium maintains its nuclear polarity and the nucleo–cytoplasmic ratio is normal. H & E × 100

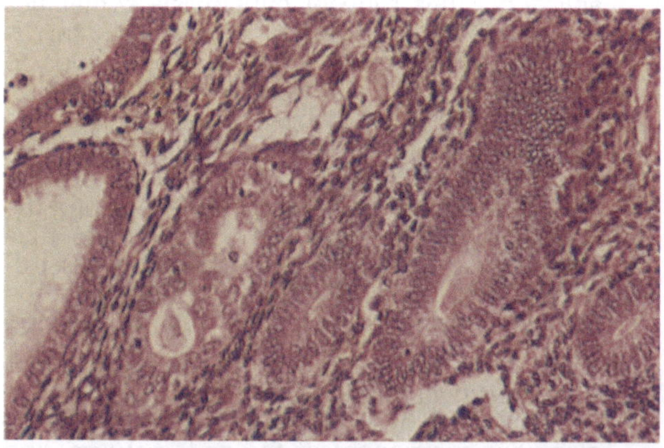

Figure 14.6 Endometrium: glandular hyperplasia with mild cellular atypia. The three glands to the right are lined by columnar epithelium of basal type whilst the gland to their immediate left is lined by atypical epithelium. The cells are pleomorphic, have lost their polarity and show early budding. The biopsy is from a patient with severe cellular atypia elsewhere in the uterus. H & E × 250

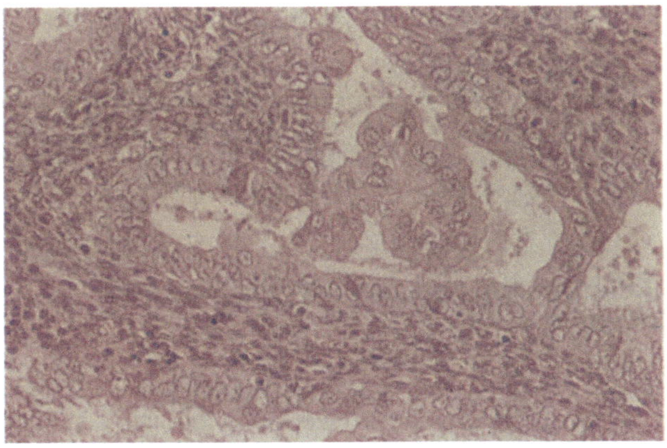

Figure 14.7 Endometrium: glandular hyperplasia with severe cellular atypia. This hyperplastic gland is lined by cells with a higher than normal nucleo–cytoplasmic ratio and rounded nuclei with occasional nucleoli. A bridge of epithelium supported by fine fibrous tissue traverses the gland. H & E × 250

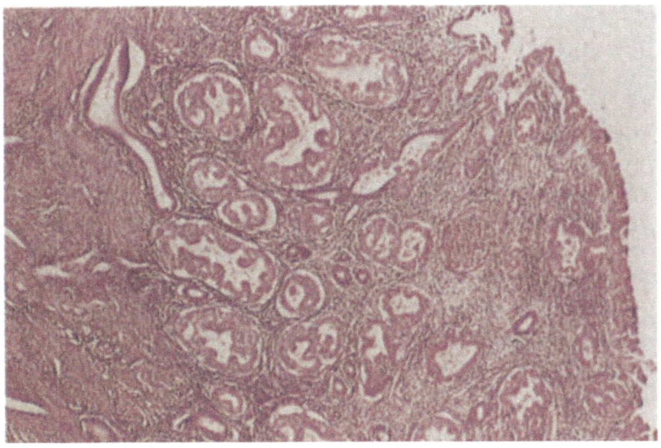

Figure 14.8 Endometrium: intraendometrial adenocarcinoma. The endometrium shows severe glandular architectural and cytological atypia. To the right adenocarcinoma is infiltrating the stroma focally. It is limited to the superficial part of the endometrium and does not invade the basal endometrium or myometrium. To the left, normal myometrium and intact basal endometrial glands are seen. H & E × 40

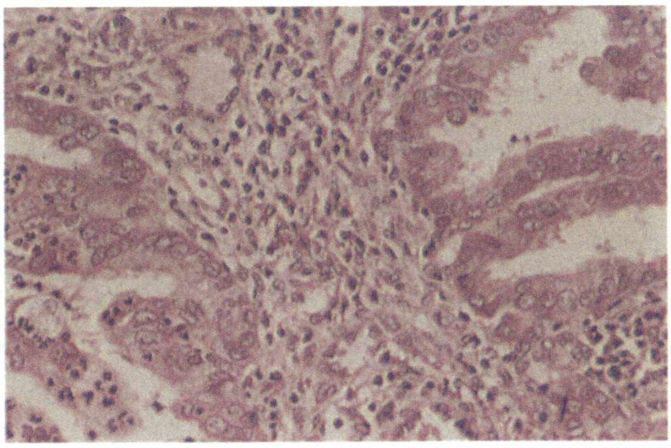

Figure 14.9 Endometrium: intraendometrial adenocarcinoma. The stroma between these two glandular acini is fibrosed and infiltrated by lymphocytes and plasma cells, suggesting stromal invasion. The epithelium in the acinus to the right shows severe cellular atypia whilst in the acinus to the left there are polymorphonuclear leukocytes, a further indication of invasive malignancy (see Figure 14.11). H & E × 250

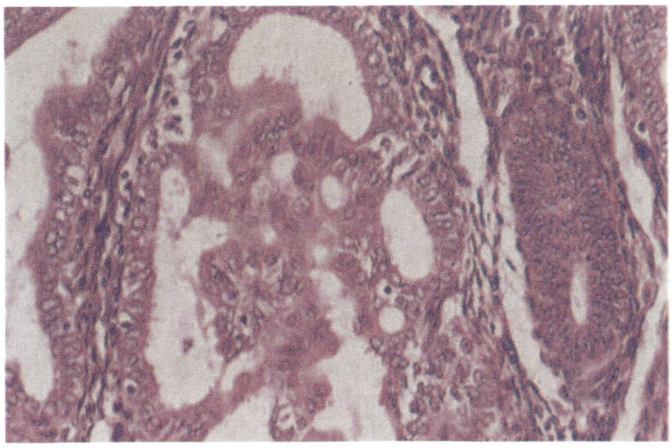

Figure 14.10 Endometrium: intraendometrial adenocarcinoma. In contrast to Figure 14.7 where cells are supported by fibrous tissue as they form bridges across the glandular acini, in this case of carcinoma, the epithelial cells are forming bridges unsupported by fibrous tissue. The individual cells are large, show variable loss of polarity, have large pleomorphic nuclei and nuclear chromatin is abnormally dispersed. Note the mildly hyperplastic epithelium without cellular atypia in the gland to the right. H & E × 250

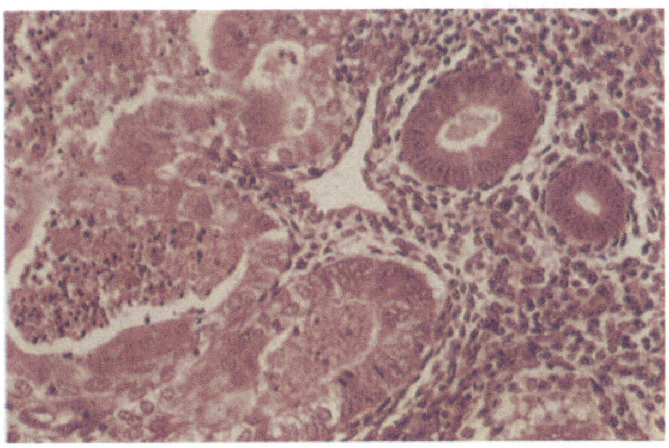

Figure 14.11 Endometrium: intraendometrial adenocarcinoma. The glands to the left of the field are irregular in shape, lined by large pleomorphic cells with atypical nuclei and there are many mitoses. The gland lumena contain polymorphonuclear leukocytes and cellular debris. Note how the cells of this focus of carcinoma contrast with those of the normal glands to the right. H & E × 250

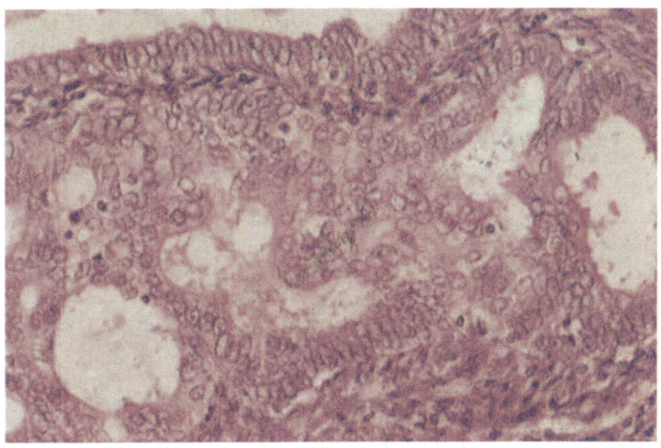

Figure 14.12 Endometrium: intraendometrial adenocarcinoma. The glandular acini in the centre of the field are filled by random masses of cells with rounded, pleomorphic nuclei and eosinophilic cytoplasm: the nucleo–cytoplasmic ratio is high in many cells. The term cellular anarchy is sometimes applied to describe this appearance. H & E × 250

endometrial stroma or one which is not invading the myometrium. It is doubtful, however, if a neoplasm in which there is no invasion of the stroma can be recognized, whilst one which is invading the stroma, though still restricted to the endometrium, is not a true *in situ* tumour in the strict sense of the word. Hence the term 'intraendometrial adenocarcinoma' is preferred to describe an adenocarcinoma which is not invading the myometrium (Figure 14.8).

Histological Distinction between Hyperplasia and Adenocarcinoma

In hysterectomy specimens the task of differentiating between these two lesions is relatively simple for if there is definite myometrial invasion the lesion is, irrespective of histological niceties, an adenocarcinoma: if there is no myometrial invasion there is no practical necessity for differentiating the two conditions as both have the same excellent prognosis and are cured by hysterectomy. Difficulties are, however, encountered in curettage specimens and suggested criteria for indicating that the glands in such a specimen are neoplastic rather than hyperplastic include the formation of intraglandular bridges without a stromal support, the presence of nuclear debris and polymorphonuclear leukocytes within glandular lumens, stratification of cells to form a 'gland within gland' pattern, loss of nuclear polarity, marked nuclear irregularity, rounding of the nuclei, nucleolar prominence, the presence of pale eosinophilic cytoplasm, the finding of numerous mitotic figures, the complete absence of stroma between glands and the piling up of cells into random sheets or masses[2–5]. Features suggesting stromal invasion (Figure 14.9), and therefore implying the malignant nature of the glands, include fibrosis of the interglandular stroma, focal stromal necrosis and a stromal accumulation of inflammatory cells and histiocytes[2].

To a very considerable extent, however, many of these histological features are those which tend to differentiate between a glandular hyperplasia with marked cellular atypia and an intraendometrial adenocarcinoma, and it is of greater importance to attempt to differentiate, in a curettage specimen, between a hyperplasia and the best differentiated adenocarcinoma that is behaving biologically as a carcinoma, i.e. is invading the myometrium. In this respect the most significant indicators of undoubted malignancy are the presence of true intraglandular bridges which are devoid of a stromal support (Figure 14.10), the finding of polymorphonuclear leukocytes within glands (Figure 14.11), the presence of abnormal mitotic figures and the piling up of cells (Figure 14.12) into random sheets and masses[4].

Relationship between Hyperplasia and Neoplasia

Because of variations in nomenclature and of methodological faults in both prospective and retrospective studies it has proved very difficult to establish the relationship between endometrial hyperplasia and the risk of subsequent development of an endometrial adenocarcinoma. Nevertheless, it appears that the only form of endometrial hyperplasia which is associated with any significant risk of evolution into a frank adenocarcinoma is glandular hyperplasia with cellular atypia: the magnitude of this risk remains, however, quite uncertain but it is a reasonable estimate that approximately 10% of women who have a glandular hyperplasia with severe atypia will eventually develop an adenocarcinoma.

To distinguish between a glandular hyperplasia with cellular atypia and an adenocarcinoma is perhaps a false division for there are highly plausible grounds for believing that this type of hyperplasia is, in fact, a form of intraendometrial neoplasia[6]: indeed a good case can be made out for considering glandular hyperplasia with mild atypia as intraendometrial neoplasia Grade I, cases with moderate atypia as intraendometrial neoplasia Grade II, and both those cases with severe atypia and intraendometrial adenocarcinoma as intraendometrial neoplasia Grade III.

References

1. Welch, W.R. and Scully, R.E. (1977). Precancerous lesions of the endometrium. *Hum. Pathol.*, **8**, 503–512
2. Silverberg, S. G. (1977). *Surgical Pathology of the Uterus*, (New York: Wiley)
3. Tavassoli, F. and Kraus, F. T. (1978). Endometrial lesions in uteri resected for atypical endometrial hyperplasia. *Am. J. Clin. Pathol.*, **70**, 776–779
4. Hendrickson, M. R. and Kempson, R. L. (1980). *Surgical Pathology of the Uterine Corpus.* (Philadelphia, London and Toronto: W. B. Saunders)
5. Robertson, W. B. (1981). *The Endometrium*, (London: Butterworths)
6. Fox, H. and Buckley, C. H. (1982). The endometrial hyperplasia and their relationship to neoplasia. *Histopathology*, **6**, 493–510

Endometrium: Epithelial Neoplasms 15

Included within the overall diagnostic term of 'endometrial adenocarcinoma' are a number of tumours which differ histologically from the common conventional adenocarcinoma which occurs at this site: to regard all these as a single entity may conceal possible differences in prognosis between the various tumour types, and it seems reasonable therefore to designate the straightforward adenocarcinoma of the endometrium in some specific manner. The term 'endometrioid adenocarcinoma' has been applied to this tumour and is, in the absence of any obviously better name, used here, albeit with some reluctance.

Endometrioid Adenocarcinoma

These are adenocarcinomata which bear an anarchic resemblance to normal proliferating endometrium. Most are well differentiated (Figure 15.1) and formed of closely packed, irregular, convoluted glandular acini which are lined by columnar cells showing a variable degree of pleomorphism, nuclear hyperchromatism and mitotic activity. The epithelium is often single layered but foci of irregular multilayering, intralumenal tufting and transluminal bridging are common. The stroma is scanty and in many cases absent, the neoplastic glands having a 'back to back' appearance: foci of necrosis, haemorrhage and leukocytic infiltration are common. Foamy, non-mucin containing, histiocytes are seen in the stroma of about 15% of cases but these are not specific to adenocarcinoma and are of no diagnostic or prognostic significance[1]. A minority of endometrioid adenocarcinomata are less well differentiated (Figure 15.2) and consist of a mixture of solid sheets of cells with poorly formed glandular acini, whilst a few consist almost entirely of anaplastic cells (Figure 15.3) with only occasional foci of tentative acinar differentiation.

The differential diagnosis between a well differentiated endometrioid adenocarcinoma and a glandular hyperplasia with severe cellular atypia has been discussed in the previous section but it is worth reiterating here that if, in a hysterectomy specimen, there is no evidence of myometrial invasion, no practical purpose is served in attempting to distinguish between these two conditions, it appearing reasonable to class both as intraendometrial neoplasia Grade III. Conversely, if myometrial invasion is present the lesion is, irrespective of histological niceties, an adenocarcinoma.

The sparse reticulin content of the very poorly differentiated adenocarcinomata serves as a distinguishing feature from the reticulin-rich endometrial stromal sarcoma, whilst the cytological features of such neoplasms differ from those of a malignant lymphoma of the endometrium.

Endometrioid Adenocarcinoma with Squamous Metaplasia

Many, indeed most, endometrioid adenocarcinomata contain easily recognized foci of squamous metaplasia (Figure 15.4), which are usually in an intraglandular site: the metaplastic epithelium has a bland, benign appearance, the squamous cells blend imperceptibly with the epithelial lining of the gland and there is no invasion of the stroma by squamous tissue. Those adenocarcinomata showing prominent or extensive squamous metaplasia are often put into the diagnostic category of 'adenoacanthoma' but the quantitative criteria for this diagnosis are imprecise, ill-defined and highly subjective. Furthermore, it is now clearly established that adenocarcinomata with squamous metaplasia, to even a considerable extent, have exactly the same prognosis as do adenocarcinomata of the same degree of differentiation which lack squamous metaplasia[2]. There is no good reason, therefore, for considering the adenoacanthoma as a discrete or separate entity, and this diagnostic term should be abandoned.

Papillary Adenocarcinoma

Many endometrial adenocarcinomata have a papillary pattern in some areas. Occasionally, however, endometrial neoplasms are wholly, or largely, papillary (Figure 15.5): these closely resemble a tubal carcinoma or a serous ovarian adenocarcinoma and often contain many psammoma bodies. Tumours of this type could develop from foci of endometrial tubal metaplasia, or may arise from uncommitted cells in the endometrium which take one of the possible alternative routes of Müllerian differentiation, i.e. a tubal pathway. These neoplasms are too uncommon for it to be known if their prognosis differs from that of the endometrioid type of adenocarcinoma: they may, however, prompt a suspicion of a metastasis from an ovarian adenocarcinoma, a possibility which can often be eliminated by tracing an origin from, and a transition between, the adjacent endometrium.

Clear Cell Adenocarcinoma

Three forms of clear cell adenocarcinoma of the endometrium can be identified.

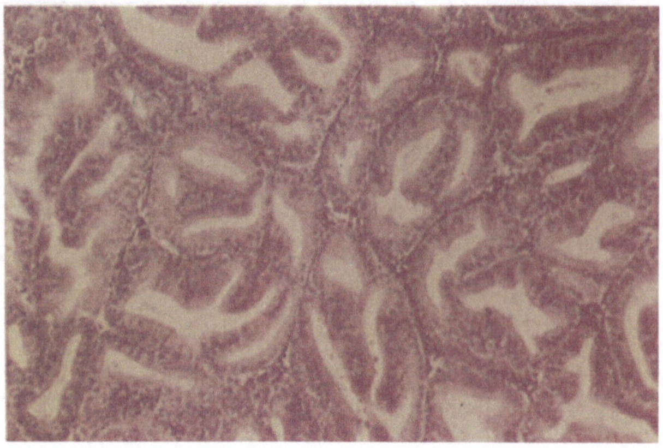

Figure 15.1 Endometrium: well differentiated endometrioid adenocarcinoma (Grade I). The tumour consists of closely packed well-formed glandular acini with irregular infoldings and outpouchings of their epithelium. There is minimal cellular atypia and nuclear pleomorphism and mitoses are infrequent. The neoplasm was however invading the myometrium. H & E x 100

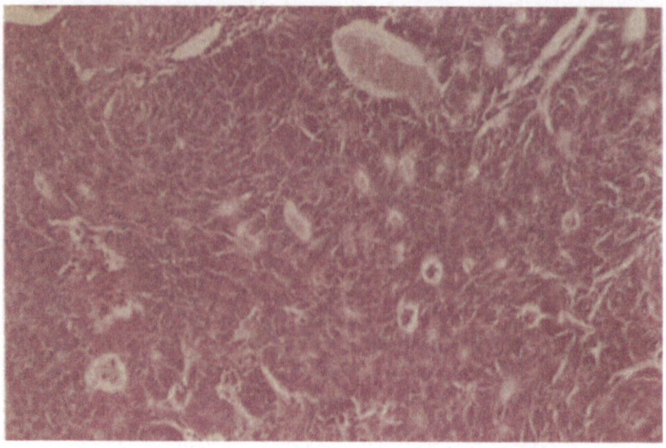

Figure 15.2 Endometrium: moderately well differentiated endometrioid adenocarcinoma (Grade II). The neoplasm is composed of small, ill-formed glandular acini and small sheets of cells showing no acini. Cellular atypia is more marked than in Figure 15.1, the glandular epithelium is multilayered, there is nuclear pleomorphism and mitoses are frequent. H & E x 100

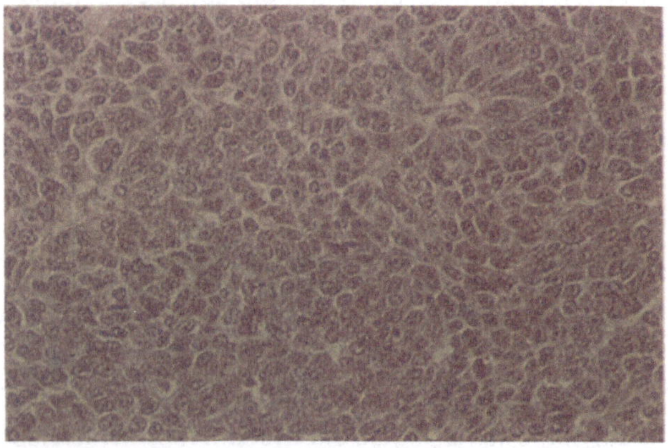

Figure 15.3 Endometrium: undifferentiated carcinoma (Grade III). The tumour consists entirely of sheets of undifferentiated cells with high nucleo–cytoplasmic ratios and showing only poor, abortive gland formation. Such neoplasms may be confused with stromal sarcomata (Figure 16.3). H & E x 250

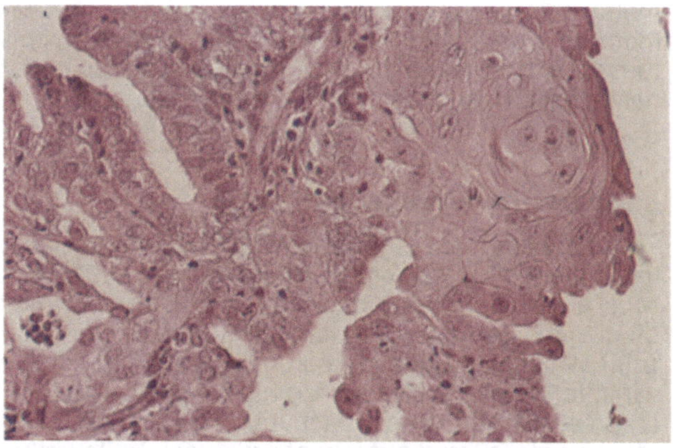

Figure 15.4 Endometrium: endometrioid adenocarcinoma with squamous metaplasia. Well-differentiated adenomatous acini lie to the left and above, and in the upper right of the field is a focus of mature, benign squamous metaplasia. H & E x 250

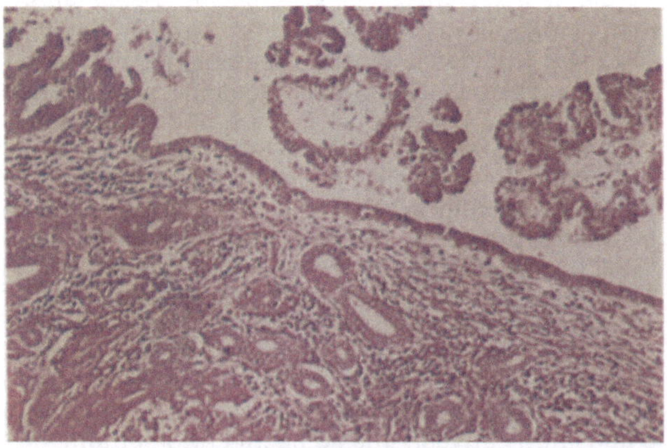

Figure 15.5 Endometrium: papillary adenocarcinoma. A well-differentiated papillary carcinoma can be seen developing at the left, from an atrophic endometrium. Fragments of tumour resembling serous carcinoma of the ovary lie within the uterine cavity. H & E x 100

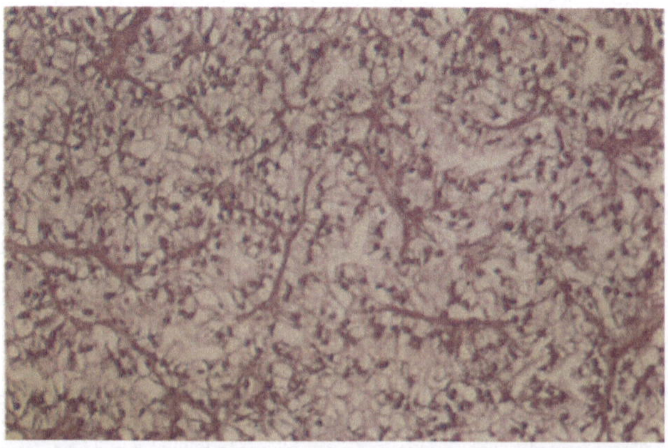

Figure 15.6 Endometrium: clear-celled endometrioid adenocarcinoma. The tumour is composed of large cells with clear cytoplasm, well-defined cell boundaries and large round or ovoid hyperchromatic nuclei with prominent nucleoli. In this example the cells are forming irregular acini. H & E x 100

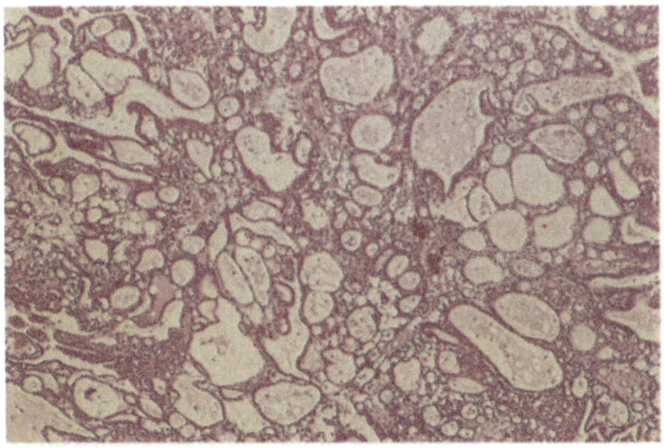

Figure 15.7 Endometrium: clear-celled endometrioid adenocarcinoma. The pattern of this tumour is identical to that seen in mesonephroid carcinoma of the ovary (Figures 27.9–27.11). It is composed of tubules, microcysts, papillae and solid areas. H & E × 40

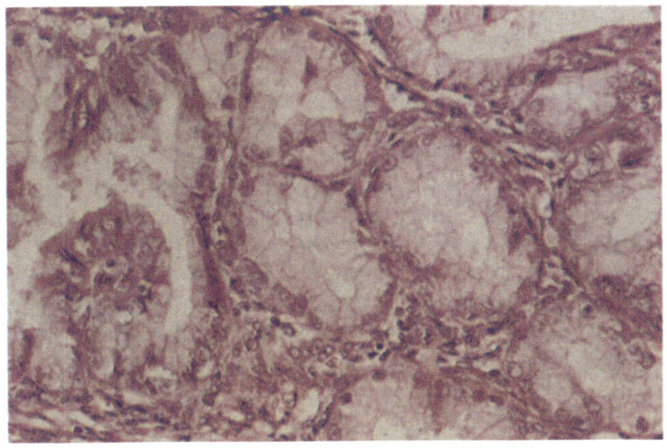

Figure 15.8 Endometrium: mucinous adenocarcinoma. The acini in this well-differentiated infiltrating adenocarcinoma are lined by tall columnar cells with faintly eosinophilic, granular cytoplasm, well-defined cell boundaries and round or oval basal nuclei. Intraendometrial foci such as this may be difficult to distinguish from mucinous metaplasia in hyperplastic endometrium. H & E × 250

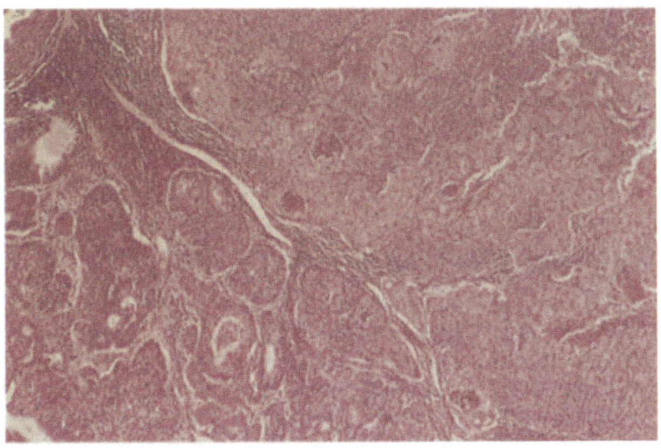

Figure 15.9 Endometrium: adenosquamous carcinoma. The field demonstrates the two distinct components of the tumour. To the lower left it is composed of moderately well-differentiated adenocarcinoma and to the upper right there are sheets of rather poorly differentiated squamous carcinoma. H & E × 40

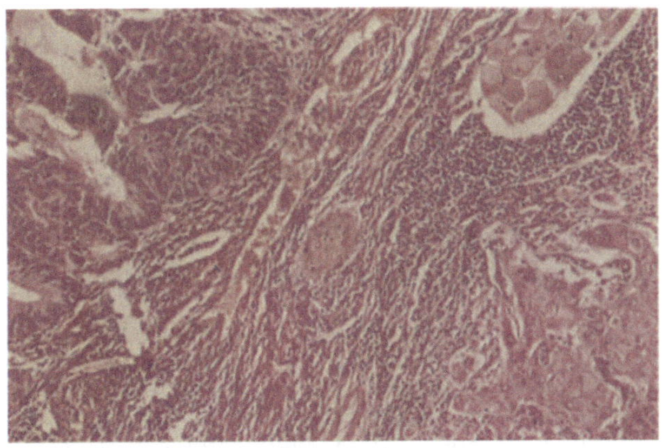

Figure 15.10 Endometrium: adenosquamous carcinoma. This detail from the tumour shown in Figure 15.9 shows the clearly malignant nature of the glandular elements to the upper left and the infiltrating, malignant squamous carcinoma to the right. Note the intense stromal lymphocytic response. H & E × 100

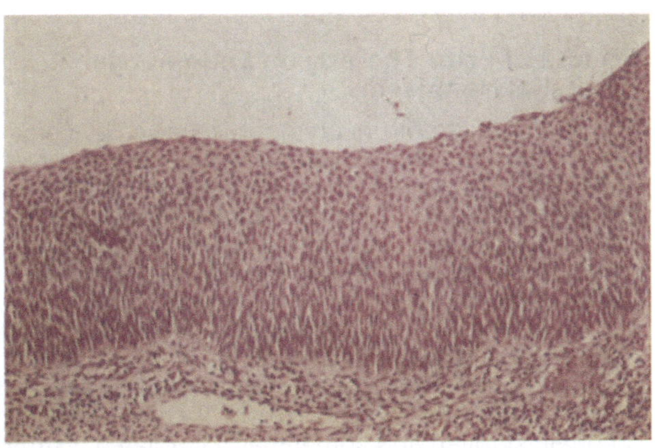

Figure 15.11 Endometrium: squamous intraepithelial neoplasia. The uterus in this unusual case was lined by squamous epithelium showing intraepithelial neoplasia Grade III. The whole depth of the epithelium consists of cells of basaloid type showing a complete absence of maturation. Invasive squamous carcinoma arose from this epithelium elsewhere in the uterus. H & E × 100

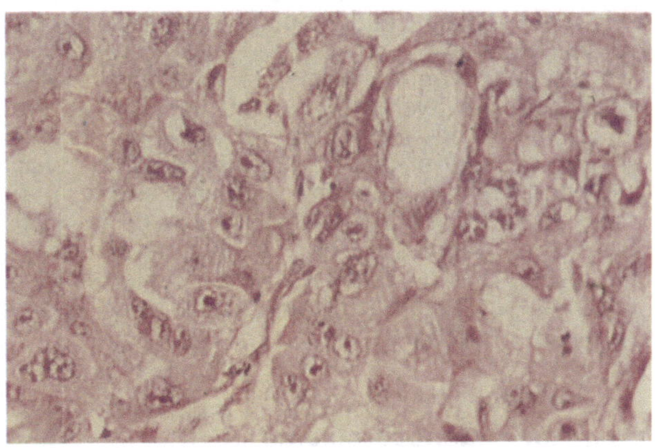

Figure 15.12 Endometrium: adenocarcinoma following irradiation. The tumour consists of large pleomorphic cells with pale granular or clear vacuolated cytoplasm and large pleomorphic nuclei with prominent eosinophilic nucleoi: some cells are multinucleated. These appearances are typical of those seen following irradiation, and there may, in addition, be focal necrosis and a plasmo-lymphocytic infiltrate. Stromal changes include collagen hyalinization, bizarre fibroblasts, a plasma cell infiltrate and vascular sclerosis. H & E × 250

The first is an otherwise conventional endometrioid adenocarcinoma containing a few clear-celled areas: if such foci are relatively inconspicuous, as is usually the case, then the neoplasm should not be classed as a clear cell carcinoma but should retain its status as an endometrioid adenocarcinoma.

A second form is that in which areas of typical endometrioid adenocarcinoma are overshadowed by a prominent clear cell component, the clear cells usually being arranged in sheets or in irregular acini (Figure 15.6): such a neoplasm merits a diagnosis of 'clear celled variant of endometrioid adenocarcinoma'.

A third form, and the one which is usually being referred to when the clear cell adenocarcinoma of the endometrium is discussed[3], is that which mimics exactly the mesonephroid adenocarcinoma of the ovary: it is characterized by the presence of cells with clear or eosinophilic cytoplasm showing a complex permutation of tubules, microcysts, papillae and solid sheets (Figure 15.7). 'Hob-nail' type cells lining the tubules are a typical feature, and elsewhere the nuclei may be angulated and hyperchromatic or round and vesicular. These neoplasms tend to be at a more advanced clinical stage at diagnosis than are endometrioid adenocarcinomata though, at any given stage, their prognosis is the same[4]

Mucinous Adenocarcinoma

This type of endometrial neoplasm occurs in two forms.

One is an endometrial neoplasm which is morphologically very similar to an endocervical adenocarcinoma: endocervical-type epithelium is seen focally in a significant proportion of otherwise unremarkable endometrioid adenocarcinomata; but a wholly, or largely, endocervical type neoplasm, which often has a papillary pattern, may cause considerable diagnostic confusion in a curettage specimen unless fractional curettage has been performed[5]. In a hysterectomy specimen the corporeal site of the neoplasm, its transition from the adjacent endometrium, and its content of endometrial-type stroma usually leaves the diagnosis in little doubt. It is assumed that neoplasms of this type represent Müllerian differentiation of neoplastic endometrial cells along an endocervical pathway.

A second type of mucinous neoplasm closely resembles a very well differentiated mucinous adenocarcinoma of the ovary (Figure 15.8): it is extremely difficult in cases of this type to distinguish between a hyperplasia and an adenocarcinoma and it is, indeed, doubtful whether the term 'mucinous' is strictly applicable to a lesion of this type, mucin stains suggesting strongly that it is a form of hypersecretory endometrioid adenocarcinoma rather than a true mucinous neoplasm.

Secretory Adenocarcinoma

This is not a true entity but represents an endometrioid adenocarcinoma which retains a sufficient sensitivity to hormonal stimuli to undergo secretory change when exposed to progesterone, subnuclear vacuoles being seen in neoplastic glandular acini. In premenopausal women such a change may be due to endogenous hormone activity, whilst in postmenopausal patients it is usually due to the administration of exogenous progestagens.

Adenosquamous Carcinoma

Tumours of this type account for about 5% of all endometrial epithelial neoplasms, contain both malignant glandular and malignant squamous components (Figure 15.9) and have a relatively poor prognosis. The glandular component of these neoplasms does not usually differ from that of a typical endometrioid adenocarcinoma, but the squamous element shows clearly malignant cytological features, infiltrates the stroma in a malignant fashion and although often intimately admixed with the adenocarcinomatous tissue is separate from it and is not seen in an intraglandular site (Figure 15.10). In order to make the diagnosis of an adenosquamous carcinoma it is necessary to exclude the possibility of a cervical origin of the malignant squamous tissue.

An adenosquamous carcinoma must be clearly distinguished from an endometrioid adenocarcinoma with squamous metaplasia, though it has to be borne in mind that the adenocarcinomatous component of the neoplasm may show squamous metaplasia, such metaplastic foci being distinct from the overtly malignant squamous tissue.

Squamous Cell Carcinoma

A primary squamous cell carcinoma of the endometrium is extremely rare. Most cases appear either to complicate a pyometra or to develop in elderly women with ichthyosis uteri: in occasional cases of the latter condition it is sometimes possible to detect an intraepithelial stage of the neoplasm (Figure 15.11). Before diagnosing a primary endometrial squamous cell carcinoma it is necessary to exclude the possibility of its being an adenosquamous carcinoma with a marked predominance of the squamous component, and also to exclude an origin from a cervical neoplasm.

The prognosis of a squamous cell carcinoma in this site is extremely poor.

Effects of Prior Therapy on Endometrial Epithelial Neoplasms

The pathologist not uncommonly receives hysterectomy specimens from patients who have received prior treatment either with progestagens or irradiation for an endometrial adenocarcinoma. Progestagens induce subnuclear vacuolation in the glandular epithelial cells, inhibit mitotic activity and produce a predecidual change in the stromal cells. If the uterus has received prior irradiation the epithelial cells, both neoplastic and non-neoplastic, may show striking nuclear enlargement with marked pleomorphism and hyperchromatism[6] (Figure 15.12); their cytoplasm is granular, swollen and sometimes vacuolated. Within the endometrial stroma irradiation may result in focal hyalinization, the formation of bizarre fibroblasts and sclerosis of the blood vessels.

Because cytological abnormalities are induced in the non-neoplastic tissue there may be difficulty in distinguishing foci of adenomyosis from areas of invasive carcinoma in the irradiated uterus, and similar difficulty may be encountered in excluding neoplastic involvement of the endocervical canal: the fact that irradiation produces cytological, but not architectural, abnormalities in the glands is of considerable aid in making the distinction between tumour invasion and radiation induced changes in non non-neoplastic tissue.

References

1. Dawagne, M. P. and Silverberg, S. G. (1982). Foam cells in endometrial carcinoma: a clinicopathologic study. *Gynecol. Oncol.*, **13**, 67–75
2. Barrowclough, H. and Jaarsma, K. W. (1980). Adenoacanthoma of the endometrium: a separate entity or a histological curiosity? *J. Clin. Pathol.*, **33**, 1064–1067
3. Kurman, R. J. and Scully, R. E. (1976). Clear cell carcinoma of the endometrium: an analysis of 21 cases. *Cancer*, **37**, 1853–1865
4. Crum, C. P. and Fechner, R. E. (1979). Clear cell adenocarcinoma of the endometrium: a clinicopathologic study of 11 cases. *Am. J. Diagn. Gynecol. Obstet.*, **1**, 261–267
5. Czernobilsky, B., Katz, Z., Lancet, M. and Gaton, E. (1980). Endocervical-type epithelium in endometrial carcinoma: a report of 10 cases with emphasis on histochemical methods for differential diagnosis. *Am. J. Surg. Pathol.*, **4**, 481–489
6. Krauss, F. T. (1973). Irradiation changes in the uterus. In Hertig, A. T., Norris, H. J. and Abell, M. R. (eds.). *The Uterus* pp. 457–488. (Baltimore: Williams and Wilkins)

Endometrium: Stromal and Mixed Müllerian Neoplasms

16

Whilst endometrial stromal tumours clearly originate in the endometrium the site of origin of mixed Müllerian tumours of the uterine body is commonly less obvious: most probably develop, however, in the endometrium and they are therefore considered under this topographic heading.

Both these types of tumour can exist in benign or malignant forms and the classification of the malignant varieties (collectively classed as endometrial sarcomata) is complex: all should, however, be considered both in terms of whether they are pure (i.e. contain only one cellular component) or mixed, and in respect of whether they are homologous and contain only cell types normally found in the uterus, or heterologous, i.e. contain cell types normally alien to the uterus[1]. Thus, for instance, an endometrial stromal sarcoma is a pure homologous tumour, whilst oncological exotica such as uterine chondrosarcomata, rhabdomyosarcomata or osteogenic sarcomata are pure heterologous tumours. A uterine carcinosarcoma is a mixed homologous sarcoma whilst a similar neoplasm containing such non-uterine components as striated muscle or cartilage is a mixed heterologous sarcoma.

Endometrial Stromal Tumours

Endometrial Stromal Nodule

This is the only recognized benign tumour of endometrial stromal tissue (Figure 16.1). It presents as a single, well defined, intraendometrial nodule formed of uniform cells which closely resemble those of the normal endometrial stroma during the proliferative phase: they have small dense, ovoid or fusiform nuclei, scanty cytoplasm and ill-defined margins, and are arranged in sheets, interlacing bundles or whorls. The nodules have a well circumscribed, rounded, pushing margin and tend to compress the surrounding tissues: they contain less than 10 mitotic figures per 10 high power fields (usually considerably less) and show no evidence of vascular invasion[2]. It should be noted that these neoplasms can only be distinguished from an endometrial stromal sarcoma of low grade malignancy by thorough examination of their margin, a task usually only possible in a hysterectomy specimen.

Low Grade Endometrial Stromal Sarcoma

This is a neoplasm with infiltrating margins which has a particular tendency to invade vascular channels, and has less than 10 mitotic figures per 10 high power fields[3]: formerly it was variously known as stromal endometriosis, endolymphatic stromal myosis or endometrial stromatosis. The tumour tends to produce a symmetrical uterine enlargement but sometimes presents as a localized mass with ill-defined margins: the neoplastic tissue is characteristically yellowish and, because of its propensity to infiltrate the vascular and lymphatic channels of the myometrium, cords of tumour may protrude from the cut surface of the uterine wall to give a comedo appearance. Histologically, there is extensive infiltration of the myometrium and of its vascular and lymphatic spaces (Figure 16.2); indeed, in some cases the tumour appears to lie solely within these channels with little or no infiltration of the adjacent muscle. The tumour consists of irregular sheets of uniform cells which usually resemble endometrial stromal cells of the proliferative phase (Figure 16.3): occasionally the infiltrating tumour has a richly vascular pattern and may closely resemble a haemangiopericytoma (Figure 16.4). The mitotic count is below 10 per 10 high power fields. The tumour requires to be differentiated from intravenous leiomyomatosis but this distinction is not usually difficult.

About 40% of low grade endometrial stromal sarcomata extend beyond the uterus at the time of diagnosis and recurrence, or metastasis, occurs in about half of the cases. The tumour is, however, of an indolently malignant nature and proves fatal in only 20–25% of cases, usually after an extremely protracted course.

High Grade Endometrial Stromal Sarcoma

Neoplasms of this type (Figure 16.5) tend to present as soft, white, fleshy masses protruding into the uterine cavity. They extensively infiltrate the myometrium, often in a destructive manner, but less commonly invade vascular or lymphatic channels than do their low grade counterparts. The tumour cells still resemble those of proliferative phase endometrial stroma but usually, though not invariably, show a greater degree of nuclear pleomorphism than is found in low grade tumours: they grow in sheets or cords and, by definition, have a mitotic count in excess of 10 per 10 high power fields.

The tumour spreads rapidly to the parametrium and mesentery whilst vaginal and pulmonary metastases are common, the 5 year survival rate being only in the region of 15–25%.

Endometrial Stromal Tumour with Sex Cord Pattern

Some endometrial stromal tumours, of all degrees of malignancy, contain epithelial-like elements arranged in sheets, nests or tubules and occasional neoplasms consist largely, or entirely, of such elements (Figure 16.6) which tend to grow in a pattern reminiscent of that of an ovarian sex cord stromal tumour[4]. Such tumours are too rare for their true nature and natural history to have been fully defined, but it is probably advisable to regard them as being of at least low grade malignancy.

Mixed Müllerian Tumours

These tumours are thought to develop from undifferentiated Müllerian mesenchymal cells which have a capacity for differentiating into a medley of epithelial and mesenchymal tissues. Epithelial differentiation is, however, invariably along Müllerian pathways whilst mesenchymal differentiation may be along homologous or heterologous lines.

Benign Mixed Müllerian Tumour

This neoplasm, also known as a Müllerian adenofibroma[5] usually presents as a large polypoid, papillary mass which commonly fills the uterine cavity and has a spongy or microcystic appearance on section. Histologically (Figure 16.7), it contains epithelial and mesenchymal components which both appear benign. The epithelial element covers broad papillary fronds which project from the surface and into cystic spaces within the neoplasm and forms a lining to glandular acini, clefts and cystic spaces which are set in the mesenchymal component: the epithelial cells are cytologically benign and may be of endometrial, tubal, endocervical, squamous or non-descript cuboidal type and, whilst in most tumours there is a melange of epithelia, in a few only one type is present. The mesenchymal component of the neoplasm consists of spindle-shaped fibroblastic cells which tend to be condensed around or beneath the epithelial component: there are no histological features to suggest malignancy and the mitotic count is less than 4 per 10 high power fields. These tumours are benign but may recur if excision is not complete: therefore, they are probably best treated by hysterectomy.

Mixed Müllerian Tumours of Low Grade Malignancy

These tumours, which occur in almost every age group, also contain both an epithelial and a mesenchymal component, but one of these elements shows the histological features of malignancy. The more common type is the Müllerian adenosarcoma (Figure 16.8) in which there is a benign epithelial component and a malignant sarcomatous component[6]. This tumour resembles, both macroscopically and histologically, the Müllerian adenofibroma and the epithelial component does not differ in any significant manner from that seen in an adenofibroma, though it may show a minor degree of cellular atypia and irregularity. The mesenchymal component, which usually shows a pronounced condensation beneath the surface epithelium and around the contained glandular structures, is formed by round, ovoid or spindle-shaped cells which often bear a close resemblance to those seen in an endometrial stromal sarcoma; their cytoplasm is scanty and their margins are indistinct whilst there is a variable degree of nuclear pleomorphism. There are more than 4 and less than 20 mitotic figures per 10 high power fields and heterologous elements such as rhabdomyoblasts or cartilage may be present. These neoplasms are of low grade malignancy but commonly invade the myometrium: pelvic or vaginal recurrence occurs in about 50% of patients after hysterectomy but distant metastases are distinctly uncommon. Even those women with local recurrence of tumour tend to survive for prolonged periods.

The other form of mixed Müllerian tumour of low grade malignancy is that in which a malignant epithelial component is set in a benign mesenchymal component: these neoplasms, best known as Müllerian carcinofibromata[7], are extremely rare and their prognosis is not yet accurately determined.

Mixed Müllerian Tumours of High Grade Malignancy

These occur predominantly in elderly women and present as a bulky, soft, polypoidal tumour mass which tends to fill the uterine cavity and extend into the endocervical canal, sometimes protruding through the external os to present in the vagina: areas of necrosis and haemorrhage are common. Histologically, there is an intimate admixture of carcinomatous and sarcomatous elements, with the latter usually predominating. The carcinomatous component is often identical with an endometrioid type of endometrial adenocarcinoma but sometimes resembles a tubal, clear cell or endocervical adenocarcinoma: in occasional instances it is predominantly or wholly of squamous type. The sarcomatous element may be largely undifferentiated or may resemble an endometrial stromal sarcoma, and if no heterologous tissues are present the neoplasm is classed as a carcinosarcoma (Figure 16.9). If heterologous mesenchymal tissues are present the neoplasm is commonly known as a mixed mesenchymal sarcoma (Figure 16.10): the alien tissues most commonly noted are malignant striated muscle, cartilage or bone (Figure 16.11). Rhabdomyoblasts with cross striations are often present whilst large plump eosinophilic cells with granular cytoplasm, but lacking obvious cross striations, are commonly seen (Figure 16.12), it being disputed as to whether these are primitive rhabdomyoblasts or not. It is usual to encounter a mixture of heterologous elements but sometimes a rhabdomyosarcomatous component predominates and this is occasionally the sole sarcomatous tissue present. Marked cellular pleomorphism is the rule in malignant mixed Müllerian tumours with the formation of bizarre tumour giant cells and the presence of markedly aberrant mitotic figures.

These neoplasms are highly malignant and most have spread outside the uterus into the pelvic tissues and to the local lymph nodes at the time of initial diagnosis: metastases may be purely carcinomatous, entirely sarcomatous or contain a mixture of both malignant elements and occur in the lungs, liver and bone. Death is almost invariable, and rapid, if there is extrauterine spread and remains the rule if the tumour, though still confined to the uterus, has invaded the myometrium to a depth greater than 50% of its thickness[8]. The histological features of the neoplasm offer no guide to prognosis.

References

1. Ober, W. B. (1959). Uterine sarcomas: histogenesis and taxonomy. *Ann. N. Y. Acad. Sci.*, **75**, 568–585

2. Tavassoli, F. N. and Norris, H. J. (1981). Mesenchymal tumours of the uterus VII. A clinicopathological study of 60 endometrial stromal nodules. *Histopathology*, **5**, 1–10

3. Hendrickson, M. R. and Kempson, R. L. (1980). *Surgical Pathology of the Uterine Corpus*. (Philadelphia, London, Toronto: W. B. Saunders)

4. Clement, P. B. and Scully, R. E. (1976). Uterine tumors resembling ovarian sex cord tumors: a clinicopathologic analysis of 14 cases. *Am. J. Clin. Pathol.*, **66**, 512–525

5. Vellios, F., Ng, A. B. P. and Reagan, J. W. (1973). Papillary adenofibroma of the uterus: a benign mesodermal mixed tumor of Müllerian origin. *Am. J. Clin. Pathol.*, **60**, 543–551

6. Clement, P. B. and Scully, R. E. (1974). Müllerian adenosarcoma of the uterus: a clinicopathologic analysis of ten cases of a distinctive type of Müllerian mixed tumor. *Cancer*, **34**, 1138–1149

7. Östör, A. G., and Fortune, D. W. (1980). Benign and low grade variants of mixed Müllerian tumours of the uterus. *Histopathology*, **4**, 369–382

8. Barwick, K. W. and LiVolsi, V. A. (1979). Malignant mixed Müllerian tumors of the uterus. *Am. J. Surg. Pathol.*, **3**, 125–135

Figures 16.1–16.2 will be found overleaf.

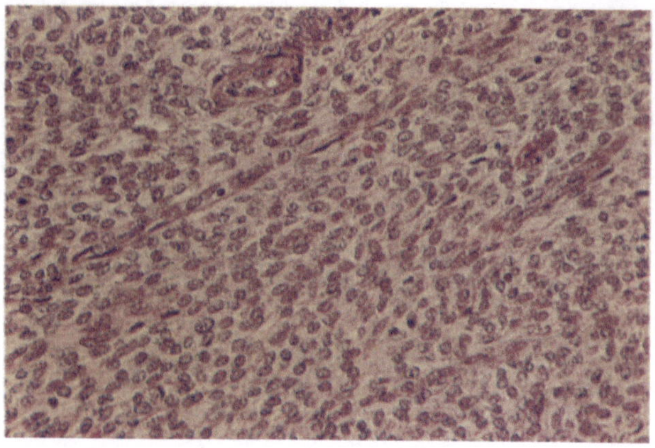

Figure 16.1 Endometrium: benign stromal nodule. The lesion is composed of sheets and bundles of uniform ovoid cells with scanty cytoplasm and ill-defined cell boundaries. The cells closely resemble those of the normal proliferative phase endometrium. The margins of the lesion are clearly defined and non-infiltrative. H & E x 250

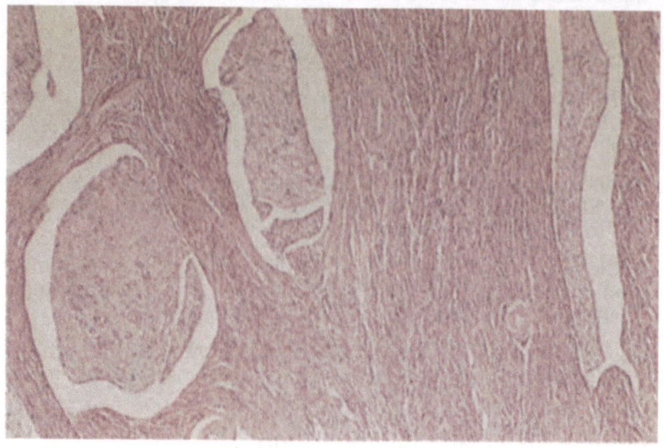

Figure 16.2 Myometrium: low grade stromal sarcoma. The vascular spaces in the myometrium are distended by well-differentiated, stromal sarcoma. There is no infiltration of the muscle in this field. H & E x 40

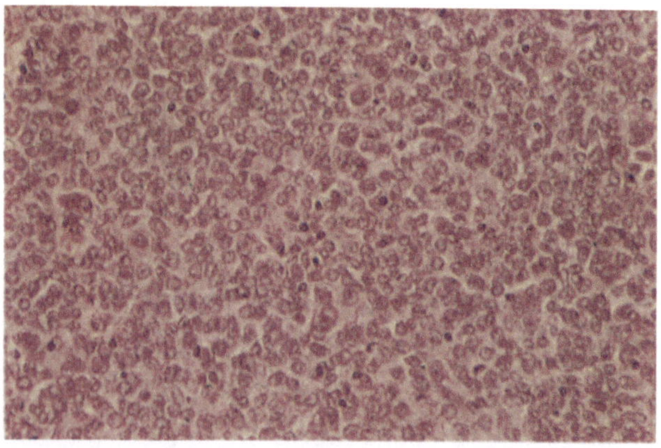

Figure 16.3 Endometrium: low grade stromal sarcoma. The tumour is composed of sheets reminiscent of the stromal cells of follicular phase, but showing more nuclear atypia, higher nucleo–cytoplasmic ratios and occasional multinucleation. There are less than 10 mitoses per 10 high-power fields. Compare the cellular detail with those of the neoplasm's benign counterpart in Figure 16.1. H & E x 250

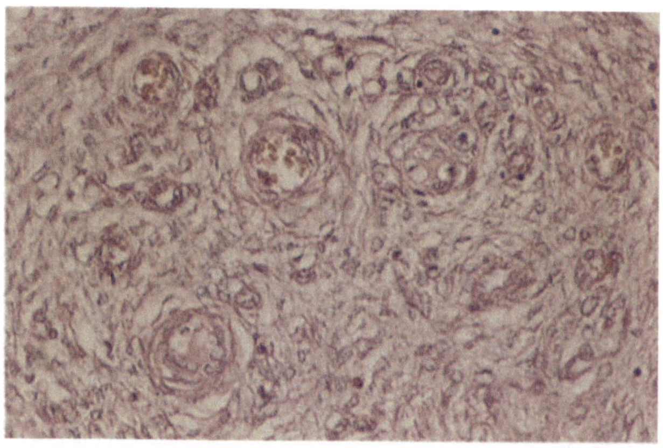

Figure 16.4 Endometrium: stromal sarcoma with haemangiopericytic pattern. This low grade stromal sarcoma (shown in Figure 16.2) is extremely vascular. The tumour cells are arranged around small well-formed blood vessels and there is a resemblance to haemangioperocytoma (Figure 10.11). H & E x 250

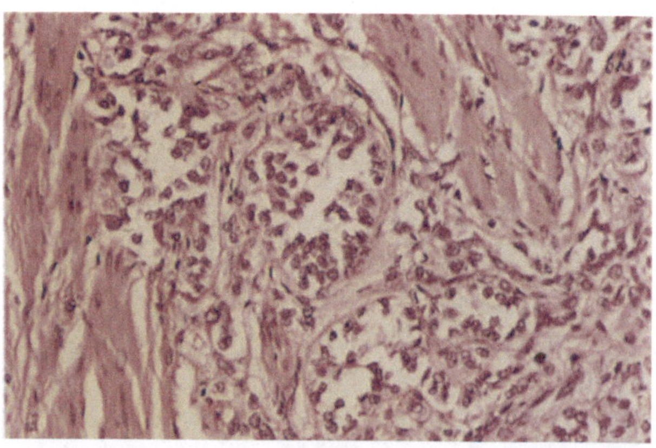

Figure 16.5 Endometrium: high grade stromal sarcoma. The tumour, which is composed of small pleomorphic cells, similar to those of the stroma in the proliferative phase, is infiltrating the myometrium. This infiltrative growth pattern is characteristic of the high grade stromal sarcoma; the low grade tumour generally has a non-infiltrative convex expanding margin. H & E x 250

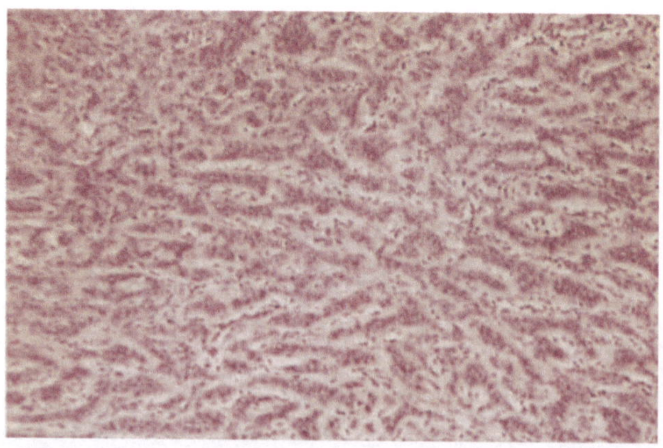

Figure 16.6 Endometrium: stromal tumour with sex cord pattern. The stromal sarcomatous cells are forming cords which ramify through the tissue in a pattern reminiscent of that of an ovarian sex cord tumour. H & E x 100

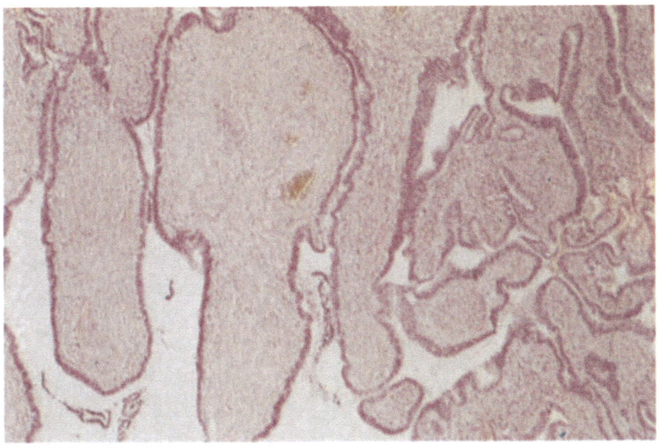

Figure 16.7 Endometrium: Müllerian adenofibroma. This polypoidal tumour is composed of cystic spaces into which blunt, broad papillae project (to the left) and small cysts and clefts (to the right). The epithelium is cubo–columnar and of endometrial type: the mesenchyme is a mixture of fibrous tissue and endometrial-like stroma; both components are benign and show only minimal cellular atypia. There are fewer than 4 stromal mitoses per 10 high power fields. H & E × 40

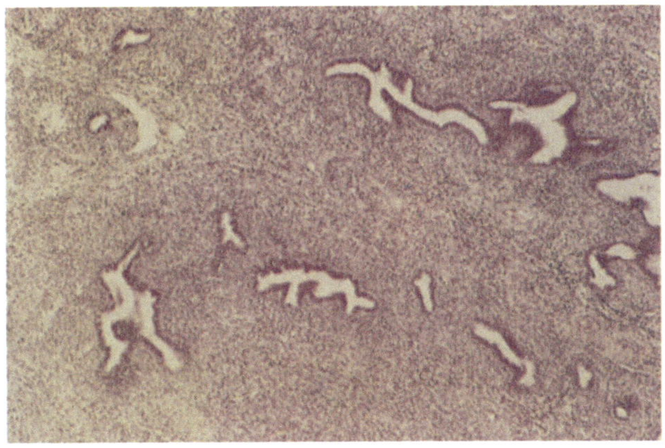

Figure 16.8 Endometrium: Müllerian adenosarcoma. Irregular glands lined by epithelium of endometrial and endocervical type lie in a pleomorphic cellular stroma which is condensed around the glands to form a cambium layer. H & E × 40

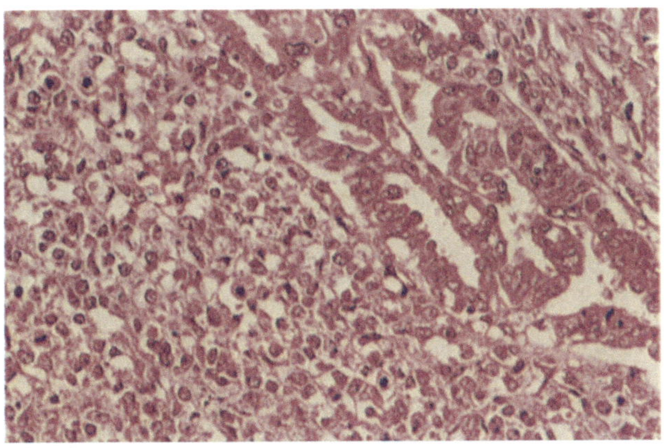

Figure 16.9 Endometrium: mixed Müllerian tumour of high grade malignancy (carcinosarcoma). This tumour, which contains no heterologous elements, is composed of moderately well-differentiated adenocarcinoma (to the upper right) and stroma with the pattern of high grade stromal sarcoma. H & E × 250

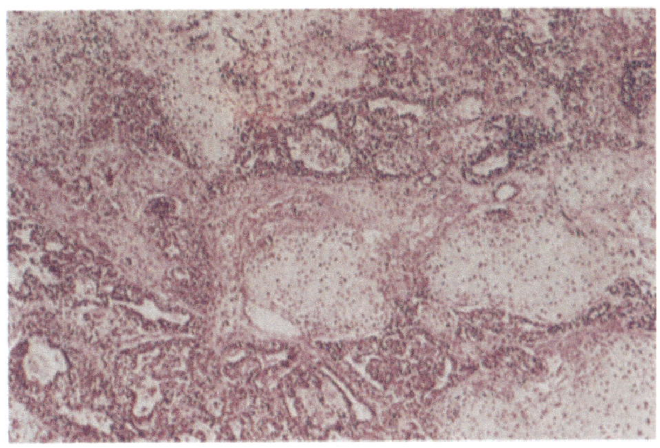

Figure 16.10 Endometrium: mixed Müllerian tumour of high grade malignancy. The general morphology of one of these neoplasms showing the highly cellular sarcomatous stroma with foci of atypical cartilage and poorly differentiated, irregular foci of adenocarcinoma. H & E × 40

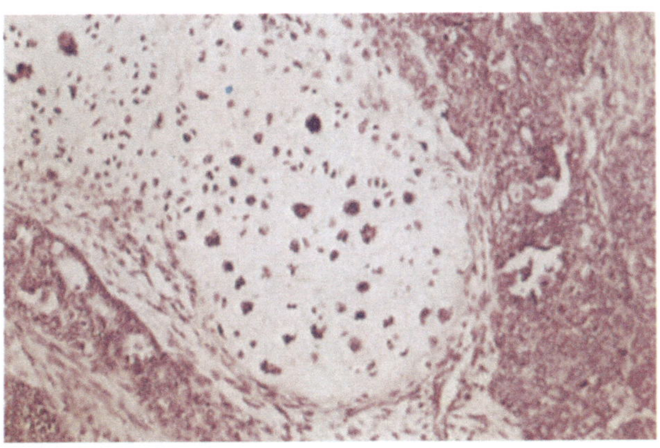

Figure 16.11 Endometrium: mixed Müllerian tumour of high grade malignancy with heterologous elements. The tumour is composed of undifferentiated carcinoma and poorly differentiated adenocarcinoma, to the sides of the field, and chondro-sarcoma, centrally. H & E × 100

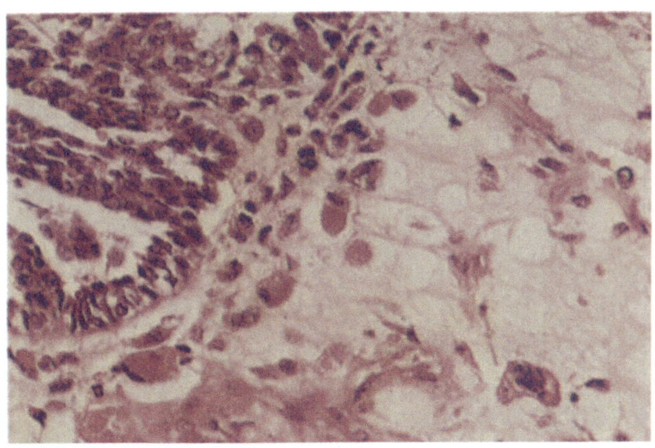

Figure 16.12 Endometrium: mixed Müllerian tumour of high grade malignancy. To the upper left there is a focus of moderately well-differentiated adenocarcinoma and in the underlying stroma there are several large cells with granular, eosinophilic cytoplasm and eccentric hyperchromatic nuclei: these are rhabdomyoblasts. H & E × 250

Myometrium: Non-Neoplastic Conditions and Miscellaneous Neoplasms 17

Non-neoplastic Conditions

Adenomyosis

This is a disease principally of parous women in the later years of their reproductive life, and is characterized by the presence of endometrial tissue deep within the myometrium (Figure 17.1): there is almost invariably an associated hypertrophy of smooth muscle fibres around the islands of ectopic endometrium. When considering this condition it has always to be borne in mind that the interface between the normal endometrium and the myometrium is often very irregular, and that tangential cutting of the basal endometrium may produce apparently isolated islands of endometrial tissue surrounded by myometrium. It is for this reason that the word 'deep' is insisted upon in the definition of adenomyosis though there has been considerable dispute as to its interpretation. Very often it has been suggested that to justify a diagnosis of adenomyosis the ectopic endometrium should be one high power microscopic field, or a proportion of a low power microscopic field, below the base of the endometrium; but these are poorly defined criteria which take no account of variations in myometrial thickness, and the defining criterion that the intramyometrial glands must be at a distance of more than one quarter of the full thickness of the uterine wall below the endometrial–myometrial junction is to be preferred[1].

The nodules of adenomyosis may be distributed diffusely throughout the myometrium, in which case the uterus shows a roughly symmetrical enlargement which is usually due as much, or indeed more, to the associated muscular hypertrophy than to the ectopic endometrium: the cut surface has a trabeculated firm appearance with focally depressed areas corresponding to the islands of endometrial tissue. Less commonly, adenomyosis occurs focally and presents as a poorly demarcated, tumour-like, asymmetrical thickening of the myometrium: this localized form is often known as an 'adenomyoma', but this is a poor term because of its implication of neoplasia.

Histologically, foci of adenomyosis consist of both endometrial glands and stroma (Figure 17.2): the stromal element usually resembles normal endometrial stroma of the proliferative phase whilst the glands are commonly of the basal type and do not therefore show cyclical activity. Occasionally the glands are of the immature type and whilst sensitive to oestrogens are unresponsive to progesterone, thus tending to undergo simple hyperplasia (cystic glandular hyperplasia) and, occasionally, glandular hyperplasia with either architectural or cytological atypia. It is theoretically possible for this to progress to an adenocarcinoma but if such a change does occur it must be of the greatest rarity. True cyclical change in adenomyosis is very uncommon but secretory transformation of the glands, and decidualization of the stromal element, is sometimes seen during pregnancy and in women receiving progestational agents (Figure 17.3).

Adenomyosis is due to a downgrowth of the basal layer of the endometrium into the myometrium, and serial sectioning will invariably demonstrate a continuity between the basal endometrium and the apparently isolated underlying foci of endometrium. The aetiology of the condition is, however, obscure and although trauma, in the form of curettage, and oestrogenic stimulation have been suggested as causal factors there is no real proof that either play a significant aetiological role.

Myometritis (*Figure 17.4*)

This may complicate a severe puerperal or postabortal endometritis, and is sometimes seen in women wearing an IUCD but is distinctly uncommon. An eosinophilic infiltration of the myometrium is occasionally encountered: this usually follows minor uterine surgery, such as cone biopsy or curettage, and appears to represent an idiosyncratic response to trauma.

Myometrial Hypertrophy

This term is applied to describe a symmetrically enlarged, unduly heavy uterus which is free of any other pathological abnormality. The weight of the uterus varies with both age and parity, and the upper limits of normality have been defined as 130 g for the nulliparous uterus, 210 g for uteri from women who have had 1–3 pregnancies and 250 g for those of a parity of 4 or more[2]. Histologically, the hypertrophied myometrium is characterized by hyperplasia and hypertrophy of the smooth muscle fibres, and there is a variable increase in fibrous and elastic tissue. Occasionally, there is a mild perivascular lymphocytic infiltrate. The aetiology and pathogenesis of this condition are not known.

Miscellaneous Tumours

Adenomatoid Tumours

These are relatively common in the myometrium and, if sought for, can be found in approximately 1% of uteri[3]. They occur most commonly on the posterior surface of the uterus, near the cornua, and although

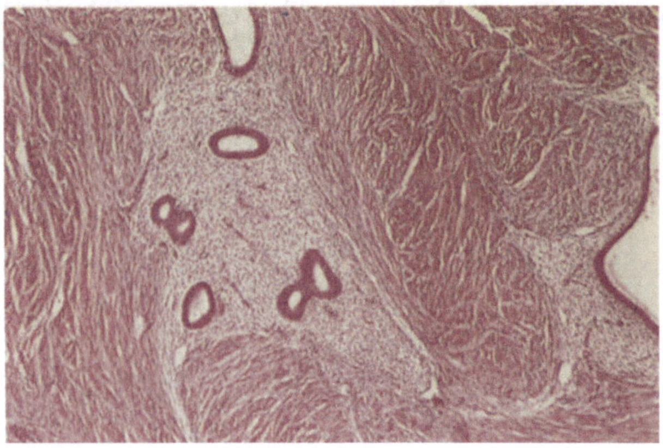

Figure 17.1 Myometrium: adenomyosis. Foci of endometrial tissue with non-secretory glands of proliferative type in a cellular stroma are seen in mildly hypertrophied myometrium. H & E × 40

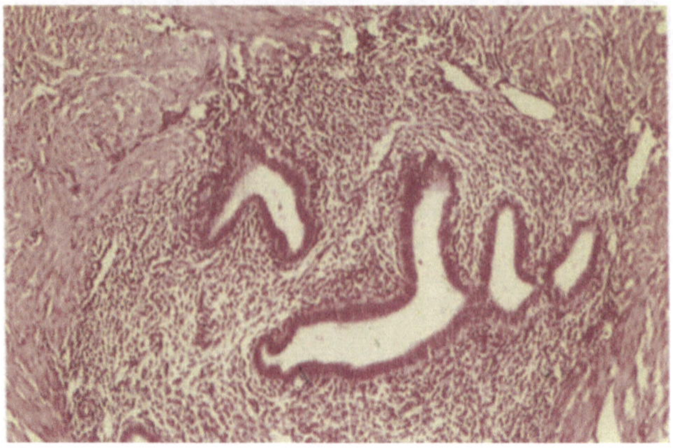

Figure 17.2 Myometrium: adenomyosis. The stroma in this example is of proliferative type and the glands are lined by epithelium of basal type, showing neither secretory nor proliferative activity. H & E × 100

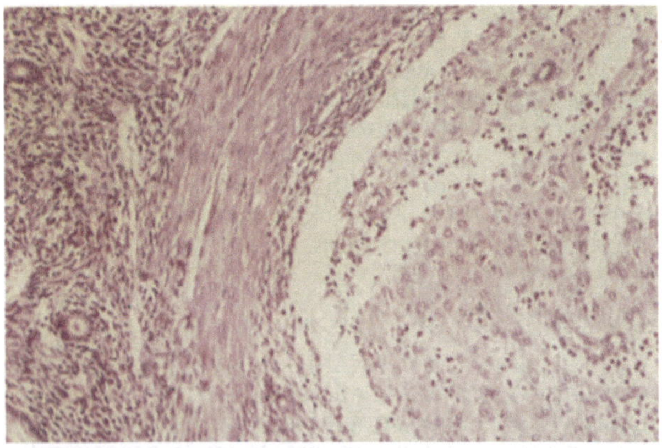

Figure 17.3 Myometrium: adenomyosis. This patient, who had extensive endometriosis, had been treated with progestagens. The stroma of the adenomyotic focus to the right shows marked stromal pseudodecidualization and the glands are small and inactive. The focus to the left remains hormonally unresponsive. H & E × 100

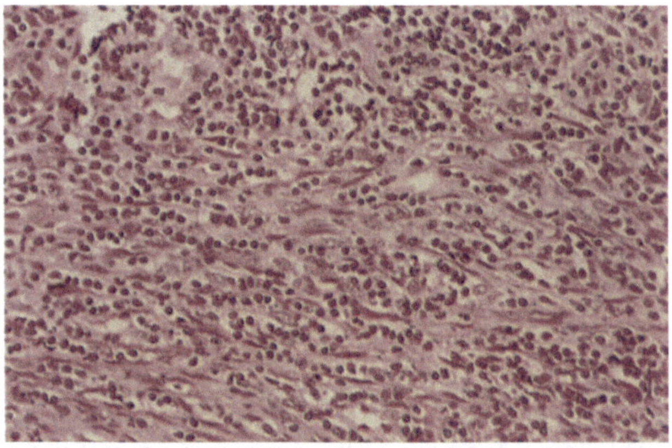

Figure 17.4 Myometrium: myometritis. The myometrium is heavily infiltrated by plasma cells and lymphocytes. The specimen is from a patient who had been wearing an inert intrauterine contraceptive device for many years and eventually developed pelvic sepsis. H & E × 250

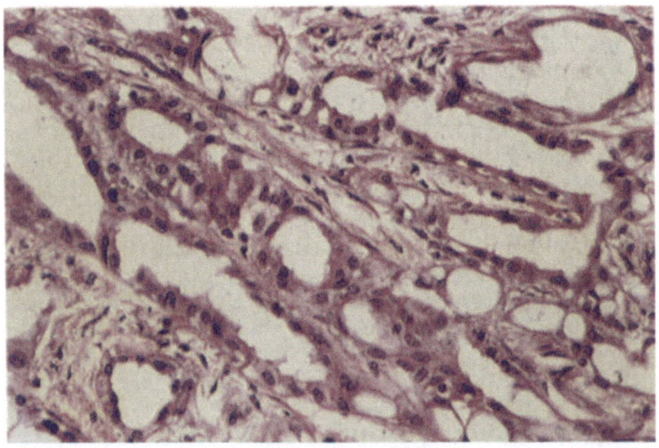

Figure 17.5 Myometrium: adenomatoid tumour. The tumour is composed of narrow tubules lined by cuboidal and flattened cuboidal cells lying in a fine fibrous stroma. H & E × 250

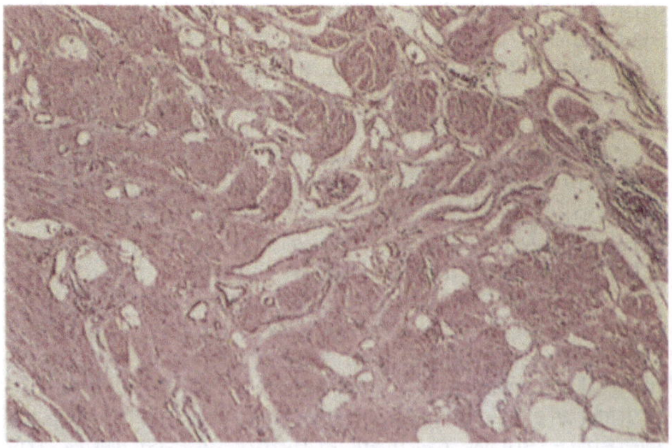

Figure 17.6 Myometrium: adenomatoid tumour. In this angiomatoid form of the tumour, cystic spaces lined by flattened epithelium form a honeycomb which replaces much of the outer third of the myometrium. Superficially the lesion resembles an angioma but the presence of mucin within the spaces distinguishes these conditions. H & E × 40

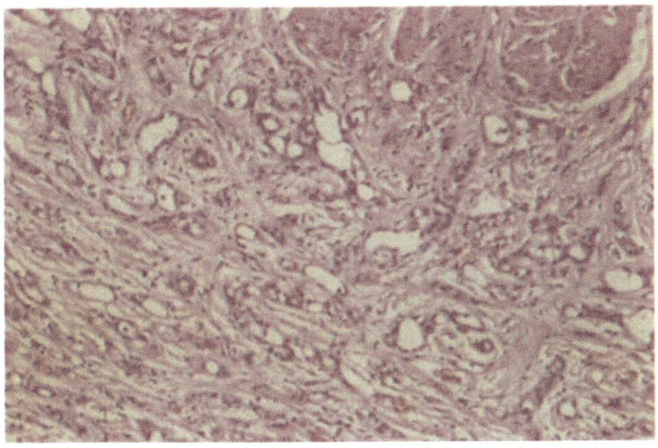

Figure 17.7 Myometrium: adenomatoid tumour. In this area a mixed tubular (to the upper right) and solid trabecular pattern (to the lower left) is apparent. H & E × 100

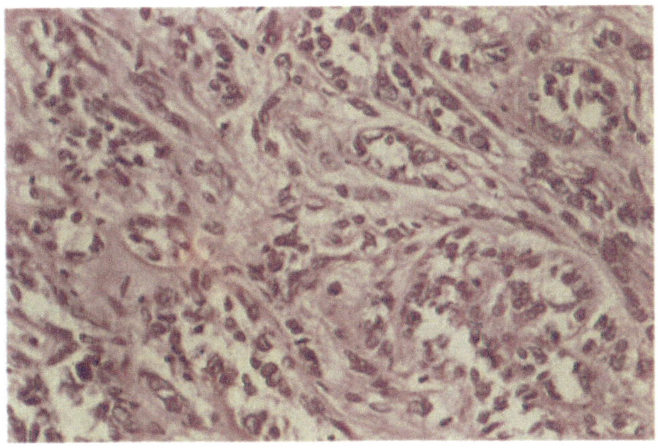

Figure 17.8 Myometrium: malignant mesothelioma. The tumour is composed of pleomorphic cells with hyperchromatic pleomorphic nuclei. Mitoses are present. There is biphasic differentiation, the tumour having stromal and 'glandular' components. This neoplasm metastasized widely and the patient died. H & E × 25

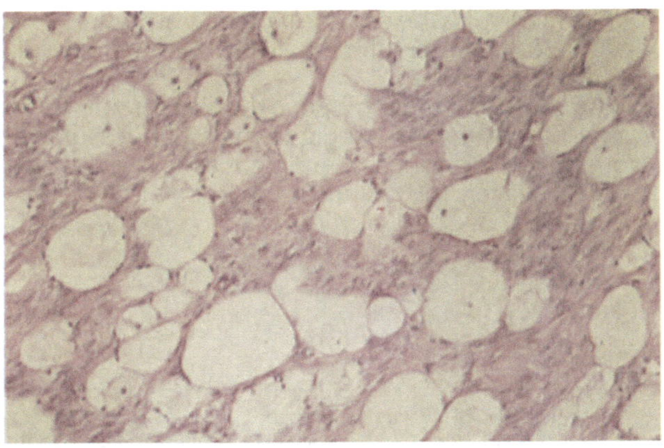

Figure 17.9 Myometrium: lymphangiocystic fibroma. This whole neoplasm is well represented by this field in which spaces, partly lined by flattened cells, form a mesh. The intervening cells are a mixture of smooth muscle cells, with their typical rectangular nuclei, and fibrous tissue with fusiform nuclei. H & E × 100

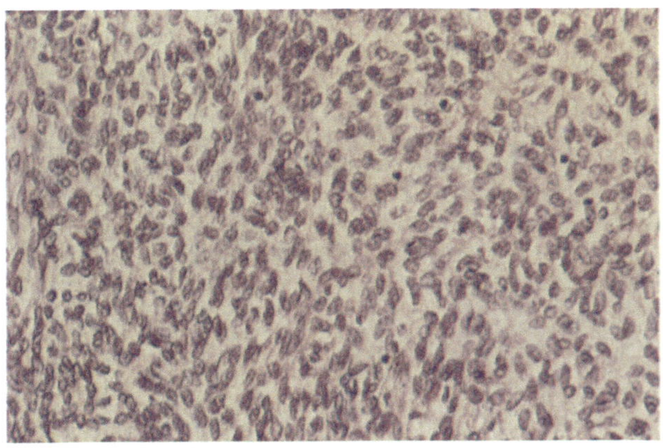

Figure 17.10 Myometrium: haemangiopericytoma. In this field the appearances are those of undifferentiated mesenchyme. The cells are uniform and have round or ovoid nuclei. H & E × 250

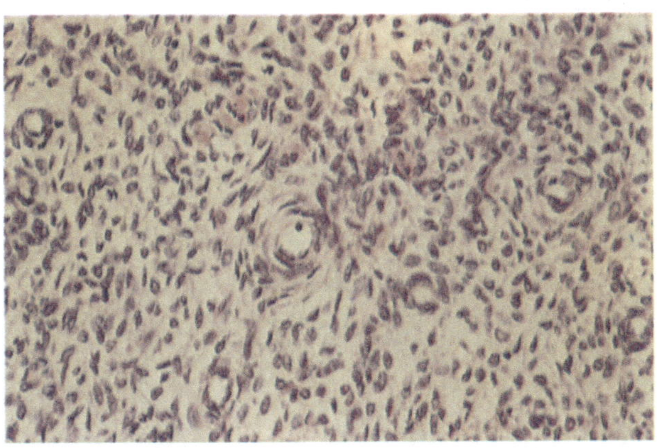

Figure 17.11 Myometrium: haemangiopericytoma. This is an example of a more overtly vascular area. Several small vessels surrounded by circumferentially orientated tumour cells can be seen amidst undifferentiated mesenchyme. H & E × 250

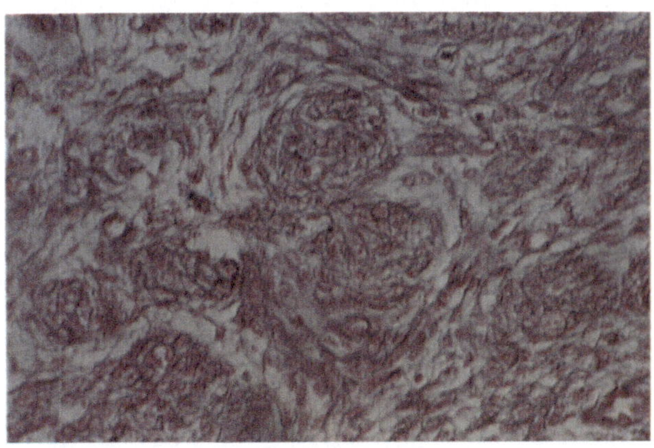

Figure 17.12 Myometrium: haemangiopericytoma. The vascular nature of the neoplasm is more clearly seen in this section stained to show the reticulin pattern. Reticulin stain × 250

most are subserosal a proportion appear to be intramural. They are small, usually measuring 0.5–2 cm in diameter, poorly delineated and greyish-tan or slightly yellow. Histologically, a variety of patterns can be recognized and although, in any given tumour, a particular histological form tends to predominate it is usual to find a mixture of patterns[4]. In the adenoid, or tubular, pattern (Figure 17.5) there are [illegible] multiple, complex, gland-like spaces which are lined by cuboidal cells, whilst in the angiomatoid, or canalicular, form (Figure 17.6) there are relatively large rounded spaces which are lined by flattened cells and resemble lymphatic channels. Less commonly encountered are the solid, or plexiform pattern where there are solid cords or columns of cells with abundant eosinophilic cytoplasm and the cystic pattern (Figure 17.7) which is characterized by the presence of many large cyst-like spaces which are subdivided by thin septa to give a honeycomb appearance. The neoplasm grows in an infiltrative manner with tumour cells interspersed between muscle cells, fibrous tissue and elastic fibres: nevertheless, the cytological appearances are bland and mitotic figures are rarely seen. Alcian-blue positive material is present within the glands or tubules, and the tumour content of this material is markedly diminished by prior treatment with hyalurodinase: this feature, together with ultrastructural studies[5,6] has led to the firm identification of the adenomatoid tumour as a benign mesothelioma which originates from the serosa. They are invariably asymptomatic incidental findings.

Malignant Mesothelioma

Although adenomatoid tumours are always benign a malignant counterpart, a true malignant mesothelioma, of the myometrium is occasionally encountered, albeit with the greatest rarity. Such neoplasms differ from the adenomatoid tumour by their marked cellular atypia and appear to behave in a highly malignant manner (Figure 17.8).

Lymphangiocystic Fibroma (Figure 17.9)

This has been described as a tumour consisting of numerous lymphatic channels set in a matrix of fibrous connective tissue[7]. Whether such neoplasms are a true entity or whether they simply represent marked lymphangiectasia in a leiomyoma is a debatable, and currently unresolved, point but they appear to behave in a benign fashion.

Haemangiopericytoma

The diagnosis of a haemangiopericytoma of the myometrium has tended of late to fall into disrepute, largely because many examples described as such were in fact either highly vascular leiomyomata or low grade endometrial stromal sarcomata. Nevertheless, haemangiopericytomata do occur in this site[8,9], and appear either as a single spherical intramural mass, measuring up to 20 cm in diameter, or as a polypoid lesion projecting into the uterine cavity. Their margins are not sharply defined and their cut surface is grey or yellowish and lacks the whorled appearance of a leiomyoma. Histologically, these tumours are composed of mesenchymal cells having an undifferentiated appearance (Figure 17.10). They have a single, round or ovoid, nucleus with a fine chromatin pattern and a well marked nuclear membrane and scanty eosinophilic cytoplasm. Numerous vessels are present but these are frequently collapsed and only revealed by a reticulin stain: sometimes, however, there is a more overtly vascular pattern (Figure 17.11), the vessels being of variable calibre, with walls of differing thickness. Pericytic cells form a circumferential mantle around the blood vessels, and reticulin stains show a fine mesh of reticulin fibres surrounding individual cells (Figure 17.12). Some haemangiopericytomata are broken up into lobules by connective tissue septa which may surround small or large aggregates of cells. Mitotic figures are uncommon.

The uterine haemangiopericytomata should be regarded as being of low grade malignancy but with a quite high incidence of recurrence: it is not uncommon, however, for recurrent tumour not to become manifest for 5, or more, years after the removal of the initial neoplasm.

References

1. Hendrickson, M. R. and Kempson, R. L. (1980). *Surgical Pathology of the Uterine Corpus*, (Philadelphia, London, Toronto: W. B. Saunders)
2. Langlois, P. L. (1970). The size of the normal uterus. *J. Reprod. Med.*, **4**, 220–228
3. Tiltman, A. J. (1980). Adenomatoid tumours of the uterus. *Histopathology*, **4**, 437–443
4. Quigley, J. C. and Hart, W. R. (1981). Adenomatoid tumors of the uterus. *Am. J. Clin. Pathol.*, **76**, 627–635
5. Ferenczy, A., Fenoglio, J. and Richart, R. M. (1972). Observations on benign mesothelioma of the genital tract (adenomatoid tumor): a comparative ultrastructural study. *Cancer*, **30**, 244–260
6. Salazar, H., Kanbour, A. and Burgess, F. (1972). Ultrastructure and observations on the histiogenesis of mesotheliomata 'adenomatoid tumors' of the female genital tract. *Cancer*, **29**, 141–152
7. Langley, F. A. (1973). The pathology of the myometrium. In Fox, H. and Langley, F. A. (eds.). *Postgraduate Obstetrical and Gynaecological Pathology*. pp. 147– 175. (Oxford: Pergamon Press)
8. Silverberg, S. G., Willson, M. A. and Board, J. A. (1971). Hemangiopericytoma of the uterus: an ultrastructural study. *Am. J. Obstet. Gynecol.*, **110**, 397–404
9. Langley, F. A. (1976). Malignant tumours of the uterine mesenchyme. *Clin. Obstet. Gynaecol.*, **3**, 425–457

Myometrium: Smooth Muscle Neoplasms

18

Leiomyomata

These tumours are so ubiquitous and well known that their general features require little comment. Histologically, they consist of fusiform smooth muscle cells with abundant eosinophilic cytoplasm and elongated, blunt-ended or tapering, nuclei which are arranged in bundles and whorls (Figure 18.1), the bundles often intersecting at right angles to each other and usually being separated from each other by a variable amount of fibrous tissue. Some of the bundles will, of course, be cut in cross-section and the neoplastic cells will then appear to be rounded with central circular or polygonal nuclei. Leiomyomata are cytologically bland and, by definition, have less than 2 mitotic figures per 10 high power microscopic fields.

Although the typical uterine leiomyoma hardly poses a diagnostic problem difficulties may arise if the histological appearances are markedly altered by degenerative changes, if one of the uncommon histological variants of these neoplasms is encountered or if a histologically typical leiomyoma appears to be growing in a manner more characteristic of a malignant neoplasm.

Degenerative Changes

Hyaline change, of a variable extent, is present in most leiomyomata (Figure 18.2) and the hyalinized areas may undergo liquefactive necrosis to produce the picture of cystic degeneration: calcification, oedema, myxoid change (Figure 18.3), mucous change and fatty change are all moderately common and can alter the normally orderly appearance of a leiomyoma. Infarction of a leiomyoma sometimes occurs and a specific form of necrosis which occurs particularly, but not only, in pregnancy is 'red degeneration' which is characterized macroscopically by a dull beefy red appearance of the neoplasm, and is probably due to haemorrhagic infarction of an extensively hyalinized tumour. More common is focal necrosis which occurs most frequently during pregnancy and in women on oral contraceptives: this is often associated with focal cellular atypia and mitotic activity, but the localized nature of these abnormalities, and their relationship to the area of necrosis, allows for a clear distinction to be drawn from malignant change. In this respect it should also be borne in mind that very few leiomyosarcomata appear to arise from a previously benign leiomyoma.

Histological Variants

Many leiomyomata are focally hypercellular, but the term 'cellular leiomyoma' is reserved for those tumours in which this pattern predominates (Figure 18.4). In such neoplasms the elongated muscle cells are closely packed and their long, blunt-ended nuclei approximated. Cellular atypia is either absent or minimal and there are less than 2 mitotic figures per 10 high power fields. Distinction from an endometrial stromal sarcoma can be made on the basis of the spindly nature of the cells and the pattern of distribution of reticulin fibres, which parallel cellular bundles rather than surround individual cells.

The term 'epithelioid leiomyoma' is used to describe smooth muscle neoplasms formed of rounded or polygonal cells which are arranged in nests, cords or sheets. There are, however, several forms of this particular type of tumour. The 'leiomyoblastomatous' form of epithelioid leiomyoma is composed of rounded or polygonal cells with central, round or angulated, nuclei and eosinophilic or partially cleared cytoplasm: any cytoplasmic clearing is most marked at the cellular periphery and the nucleus with its surrounding rim of eosinophilic cytoplasm is then sometimes likened to a fried egg. The 'clear cell' variant of this tumour is formed of cells with completely cleared cytoplasm (Figure 18.5), and in this type of neoplasm the nucleus may be pushed to one side to give a signet ring appearance, a change sometimes seen in the leiomyoblastomatous form but with lesser frequency. The plexiform type of epithelioid leiomyoma[1], also known as a 'plexiform tumourlet' (Figure 18.6), is formed of cells with scanty eosinophilic cytoplasm and bland 'crumpled' nuclei which are arranged in long cords separated by hyalinized collagen. The criteria for a diagnosis of malignancy are somewhat less well defined for epithelioid leiomyomata than in the more conventional smooth muscle tumours, though those with less than 2 mitotic figures per 10 high power fields can still safely be regarded as benign: it is thought, however, that those with a mitotic count of 5 or more mitoses per 10 high power fields should be considered as malignant[2] whilst those with 3 or 4 mitotic figures per 10 high per fields should fall into the category of smooth muscle tumour of uncertain malignant potential (*vide infra*).

The bizarre leiomyomata, also known as 'symplastic' or 'atypical' leiomyomata, are characterized by the presence of multinucleated giant cells and cells with irregular nuclei of bizarre shape (Figure 18.7). This cellular atypia should not be taken as evidence of malignancy for, as with all uterine smooth muscle tumours, the diagnosis of malignancy is determined principally by the mitotic count and no matter how atypical and abnormal the cells in a leiomyoma may appear the neoplasms should not be considered as malignant if there are less than 2 mitotic figures per 10 high power fields. Using this criterion most bizarre leiomyomata are totally benign despite their initially disconcerting histological appearance.

Some leiomyomata show marked nuclear palisading and hence tend to resemble a neurolemmoma

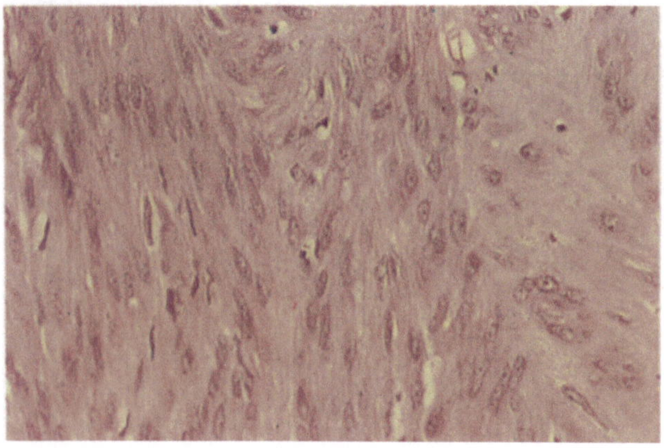

Figure 18.1 Myometrium: leiomyoma. The tumour is formed by interlacing bundles of smooth muscle cells with elongated, oblong or fusiform nuclei and pale eosinophilic cytoplasm. To the right, there is early hyalinization, a very common finding. H & E × 250

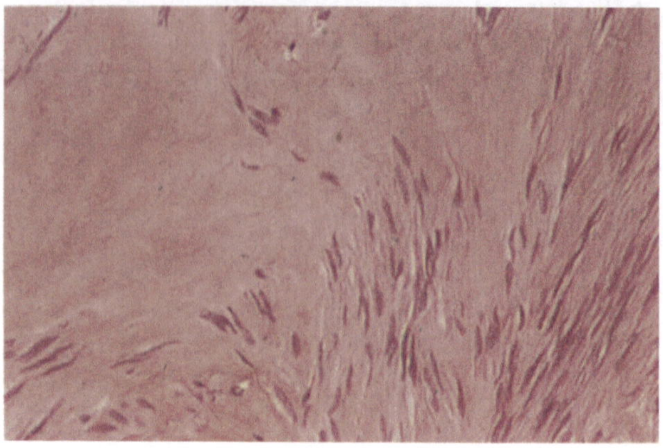

Figure 18.2 Myometrium: leiomyoma, hyaline degeneration. This leiomyoma shows extensive hyalinization. The smooth muscle cells have elongated, somewhat compressed nuclei. H & E × 250

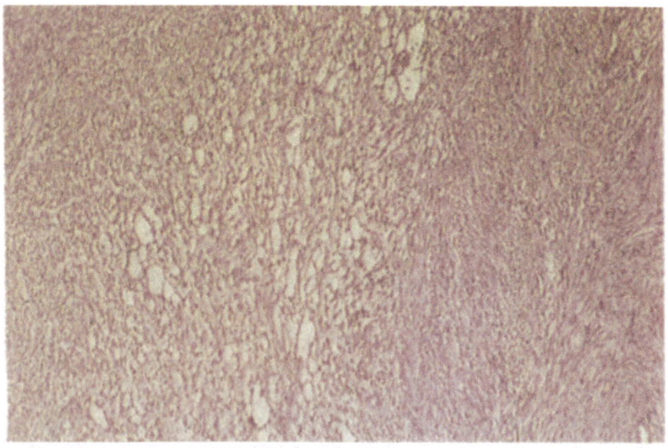

Figure 18.3 Myometrium: leiomyoma, myxoid change. The leiomyoma is of conventional form at the right of the field but centrally shows myxoid degeneration, small irregular unlined spaces containing mucopolysaccharides replacing the more solid structure. H & E × 40

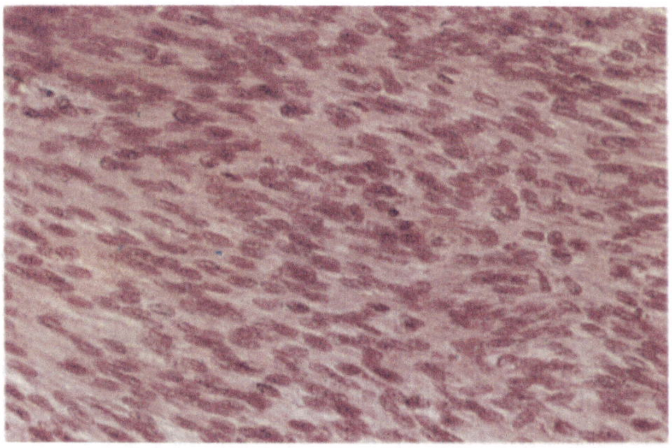

Figure 18.4 Myometrium: cellular leiomyoma. The whole neoplasm is composed of closely packed smooth muscle cells with rather plump, rounded nuclei and relatively high nucleo-cytoplasmic ratios. There are however no mitoses and the tumour is completely benign. H & E × 250

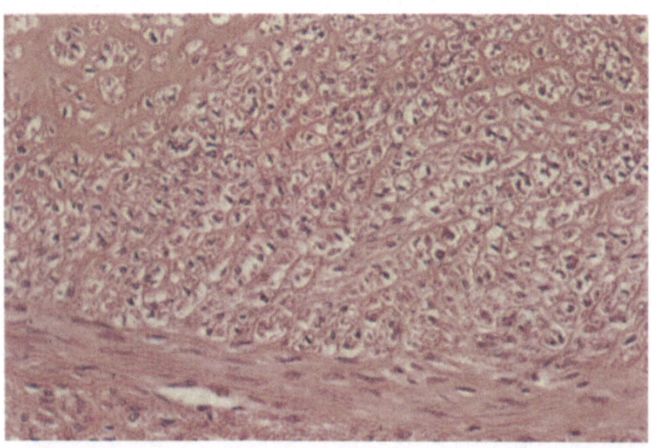

Figure 18.5 Myometrium: epithelioid, clear cell leiomyoma. The tumour is composed of large cells with central or slightly eccentric nuclei and clear cytoplasm arranged in cords and clusters. At the lower margin of the section is a band of leiomyoma of typical appearance. H & E × 250

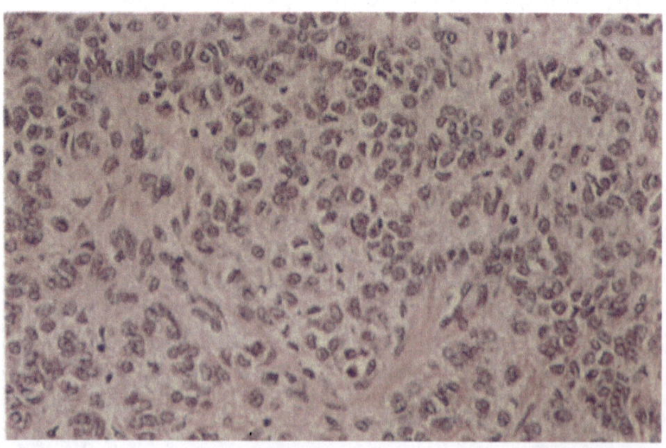

Figure 18.6 Myometrium: plexiform tumourlet. The small round cells with bland, 'crumpled' nuclei and scanty cytoplasm are arranged in nests and cords which are separated by hyalinized collagen. There are no mitoses. H & E × 250

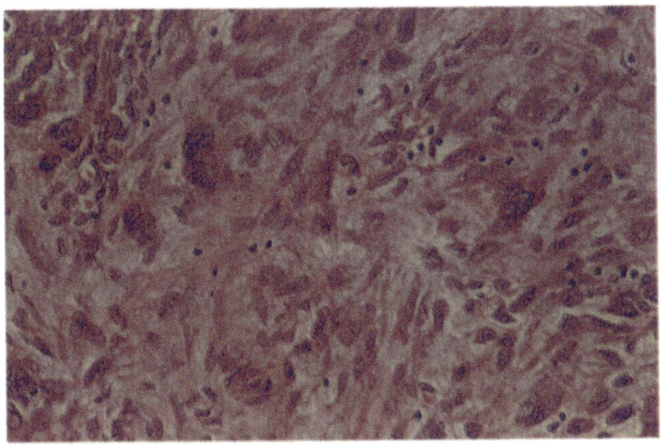

Figure 18.7 Myometrium: bizarre leiomyoma. This field shows several multinucleated smooth muscle cells; the nuclei are pleomorphic and hyperchromatic. The surrounding tumour cells show varying degrees of nuclear atypia and pleomorphism. Despite the bizarre appearances, the tumour is benign, there are no mitoses: the appearance is often associated with degenerative changes. H & E × 250

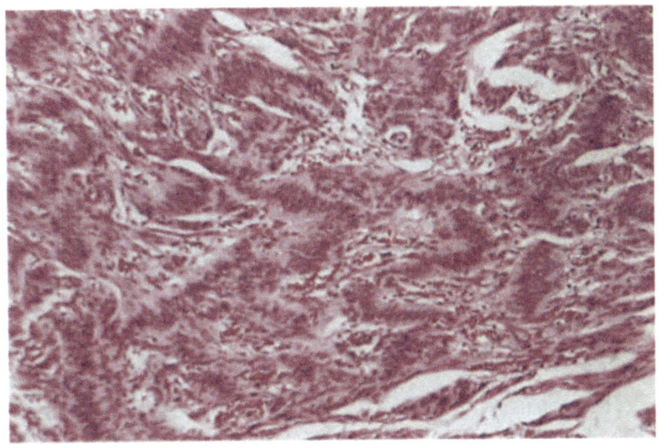

Figure 18.8 Myometrium: leiomyoma, neurolemmomatous pattern. The palisading of the smooth muscle nuclei creates an appearance similar to that seen in neurolemmomata of Antoni A pattern. H & E × 100

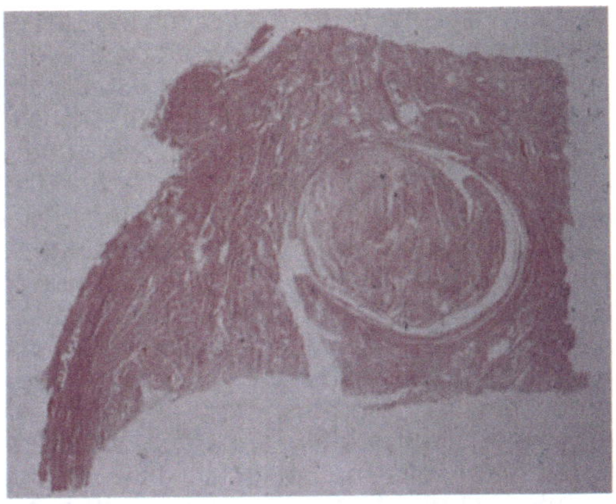

Figure 18.9 Myometrium: intravenous leiomyoma. The centre of the field is occupied by a small round tumour which is growing along and distending a vein. Elastic stains will usually reveal the true nature of the wall of such an intramyometrial space. The neoplasm in this example shows extensive hyalinization and occasional bizarre cells but no mitotic activity. H & E × 2.4

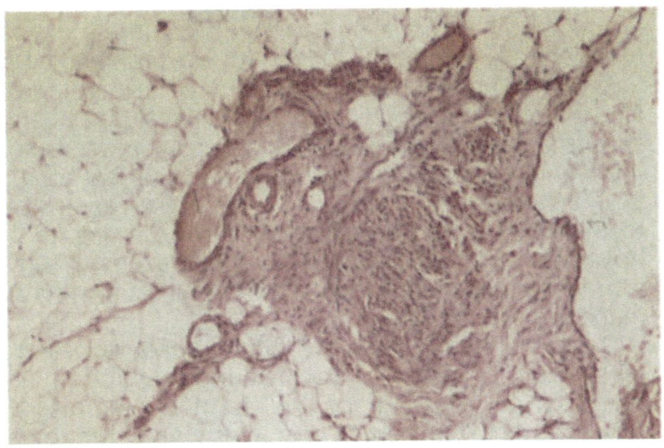

Figure 18.10 Omentum: leiomyomatosis peritonealis disseminata. A nodule of submesothelial smooth muscle cells in the centre of the field is forming a leiomyoma-like nodule. There is a little perinodular fibrosis around which the normal omental adipose tissue is seen. H & E × 100

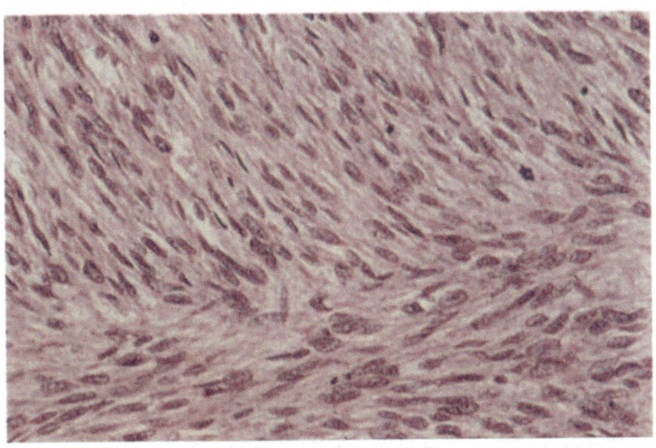

Figure 18.11 Myometrium: low grade leiomyosarcoma. The tumour is composed of bundles of plump, well-differentiated smooth muscle cells with elongated ovoid nuclei and copious cytoplasm. Mitoses are frequent and several are seen in this field. H & E × 250

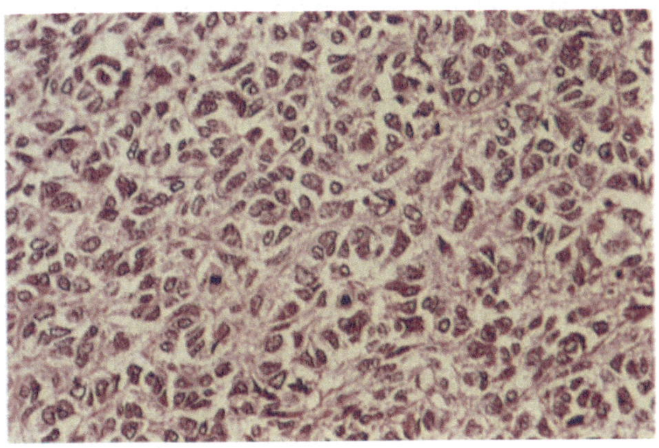

Figure 18.12 Myometrium: high grade leiomyosarcoma. The tumour is composed of pleomorphic cells with nuclear hyperchromatism, frequent mitoses (four in this field alone), fairly abundant eosinophilic cytoplasm and ill-defined cell boundaries. There were less anaplastic, more typical leiomyosarcomatous elements elsewhere in the tumour. H & E × 250

(Figure 18.8): despite this pattern they are of smooth muscle origin and, indeed, it is doubtful if neurolemmomata ever develop in the uterus.

In some leiomyomata there is an admixture with fat cells, these latter sometimes forming nodules within the tumour: these neoplasms should be classed as lipoleiomyomata and their histological appearance is their only unusual feature.

Unusual Growth Patterns of Leiomyomata

A few leiomyomata show apparent invasion of vascular channels within the neoplasm but the term 'intravenous leiomyomatosis' is restricted to those rare tumours in which there is either macroscopically visible extension of tumour into vascular spaces, or histological evidence of growth into vessels beyond the confines of a leiomyoma[3]. Whether in fact this condition is truly due to invasion of blood vessels by an extravascular leiomyoma or whether these are neoplasms arising from the smooth muscle of the vessel walls is uncertain but the histological diagnosis is dependent upon the finding of leiomyomatous tissue within venous or lymphatic channels in the uterine wall (Figure 18.9): the intravascular tumour tissue often has a lobulated appearance, is histologically bland, frequently extensively hyalinized and shows a paucity of mitotic figures. In most cases intravenous leiomyomatosis is limited to the uterus and hysterectomy is curative: extrauterine extension to the veins of the broad ligament or the vagina is, however, not uncommon whilst, exceptionally, tumour can extend into the inferior vena cava and may reach the right atrium.

Some apparently benign leiomyomata appear to give rise to metastases in the lungs or abdominal lymph nodes. In many of the reported examples of this syndrome of 'benign metastasizing leiomyoma' the uterine tumour has been inadequately examined, and it is possible that a diagnosis of leiomyosarcoma has been missed: in other cases the syndrome may well have been due to the synchronous occurrence of independent uterine and pulmonary leiomyomata. In a few instances, however, surgical trauma to the uterus does appear to have caused dissemination of a benign leiomyoma.

The condition of 'leiomyomatosis peritonealis disseminata' is characterized by multiple leiomyoma-like nodules in the submesothelial connective tissue of the abdomen, the most common sites of involvement being the omentum, bowel serosa, mesentery and the surface of the uterus. The nodules usually measure less than 1 cm in diameter but may attain a size of 10 cm. Histologically, the appearances are those of a small leiomyoma (Figure 18.10) and there are usually few mitotic figures. This condition usually arises during pregnancy, in patients with a granulosa cell tumour or in women using oral steroid contraceptives, and may therefore be hormone-dependent: it probably represents a multicentric metaplastic change in the submesothelial connective tissue[4].

Smooth Muscle Tumours of Uncertain Malignant Potential

This term recognizes the fact that there is a grey area between the clearly benign and the overtly malignant smooth muscle tumours of the uterus: it would clearly be unduly rigid to insist that a tumour with 9 mitotic figures per 10 high power fields was benign whilst one with a mitotic count of 10 was malignant. Hence, those smooth muscle tumours with a mitotic count of 5–9 per 10 high power fields but which appear cytologically bland are put into this perhaps somewhat unsatisfactory category of tumours of uncertain malignant potential, as also are those with mitotic counts of 2–4 per 10 high power fields in which there is some cellular atypia[5]. No neoplasm falling into this category has yet been shown to metastasize, but the treatment of choice is, in the absence of pregnancy which increases the mitotic count in benign leiomyomata, a hysterectomy.

Leiomyosarcoma (Figures 18.11 and 18.12)

All uterine smooth muscle tumours with 10 or more mitotic figures per 10 high power fields are, irrespective of other histological features, classed as leiomyosarcomata: neoplasms with 5–9 mitotic figures per 10 high power fields also fall into this category if they show any cellular atypia. Although these carefully defined criteria must be insisted upon for the diagnosis of a leiomyosarcoma the fact is that, in reality, most uterine leiomyosarcomata are obviously malignant. These neoplasms usually present as intramural masses which lack the clearly circumscribed margin of a leiomyoma and cannot be easily shelled out from the myometrium: on section they are usually soft and fleshy, sometimes being described as 'brain-like' or 'fish-like', and their characteristically greyish appearance is altered by the presence of foci of necrosis and haemorrhage. Histologically, the typical leiomyosarcoma is formed of spindle cells with relatively abundant eosinophilic cytoplasm: nuclear atypia, cellular pleomorphism and abundant mitotic activity are usually readily apparent, whilst multinucleated giant cells and osteoclast-like cells may be seen: abnormal mitotic figures occur with some frequency. The range of appearances in a leiomyosarcoma is, however, wide ranging from a tumour differing from a leiomyoma only by its high mitotic count to a virtually anaplastic sarcoma.

The overall 5 year survival rate for women with a uterine leiomyosarcoma is only about 20%[6]: there is pelvic and intra-abdominal spread, whilst blood borne metastases occur in the lungs, pleura, kidneys and liver. Features indicative of a particularly poor prognosis include extrauterine spread at the time of initial diagnosis, a very high mitotic count and cellular anaplasia.

References

1. Nunez-Alonso, C. and Battifora, H. A. (1979). Plexiform tumors of the uterus: ultrastructural study. *Cancer*, **44**, 1707–1714
2. Kurman, R. J. and Norris, H. J. (1976). Mesenchymal tumors of the uterus. VI. Epithelioid smooth muscle tumors including leiomyoblastoma and clear cell leiomyoma. *Cancer*, **37**, 1853–1865
3. Norris, H.J. and Parmley, T. (1975). Mesenchymal tumours of the uterus. V. Intravenous leiomyomatosis: a clinical and pathological study of 14 cases. *Cancer*, **36**, 2164–2178
4. Tavassoli, F. A. and Norris, H. J. (1982). Peritoneal Leiomyomatosis (Leiomyomatosis peritonealis disseminata): a clinicopathologic study of 20 cases with ultrastructural observations. *Intern. J. Gynecol. Pathol.*, **1**, 59–74
5. Hendrickson, M. R. and Kempson, R. L. (1980). *Surgical Pathology of the Uterine Corpus*. (Philadelphia, London, Toronto: W. B. Saunders)
6. Christopherson, W. M. and Richardson, M. (1981). Uterine mesenchymal tumors. *Pathol. Ann.*, **16**, 215

Fallopian Tube and Broad Ligament: Non-Neoplastic Conditions I

19

The Normal Fallopian Tube

The Fallopian tube extends from the ostium laterally to the uterine cornu medially and comprises four sections, the infundibulum, into which the ostium opens, the ampulla, which is the longest section, the isthmus and the interstitial part which lies within the uterine musculature. The wall is formed by an inner mucosa, an intermediate muscular layer and a serosal covering. The mucosa is thrown into a series of folds or plicae which are simple and few in the medial portion of the tube, but more complex and numerous laterally. The muscular wall comprises a well-defined inner, circular layer and a filamentous, ill-defined, outer longitudinal layer. A second longitudinal layer lies deep to the circular muscle in the interstitial and proximal parts of the tube where its filaments extend into the mucosal folds. The tubal ostium is surrounded by a series of finger-like projections, the fimbria, and it is not unusual to see vestigial, non-communicating accessory ostia adjacent to the definitive ostium. Walthard's rests, which appear as sago-like granules on the tubal serosa, are so common as to be regarded as normal.

The mucosa comprises a scanty lamina propria covered by an epithelial monolayer in which three cell types are recognized (Figure 19.1), the ciliated, secretory and intercalary or peg cells; intraepithelial lymphocytes are usually also present. The mucosa in each section of the tube contains different proportions of each cell type, ciliated cells being most numerous on the fimbria and in the ampulla and scanty in the isthmus and interstitial segments.

The tall, columnar, ciliated cells have round or oval nuclei with finely granular chromatin and prominent nucleoli, the longitudinal axis of the nuclei lying at right angles to or parallel to the basement membrane; the cytoplasm is pale and the lumenal surface bears cilia. The narrow, more dense and darkly staining nuclei of the secretory cells vary in position, at some stages of the cycle coming to lie above the lumenal surface of the ciliated cells giving an impression that the epithelium is multilayered; their apical cytoplasm may be vacuolated. The intercalary cells are narrow columnar cells with thin, darkly staining nuclei and are probably a variant of the secretory cell. Mitoses are rarely seen in the epithelium of the normal tube.

Cyclical Changes and the Effects of Hormones

Before puberty both secretory and ciliated cells are shallow and cilia are few in number. After the menarche, a regular cyclical change occurs. During the follicular phase of the menstrual cycle, ciliated cells, which are shallow postmenstrually, increase in height and width to reach their maximum at the time of ovulation and then diminish in the luteal phase whilst secretory cells, which also increase in height in the follicular phase, remain tall throughout the luteal phase, their nuclei sometimes lying above the lumenal surface of the adjacent ciliated cells. During menstruation it is not uncommon to see fragments of endometrium within the tubal lumen and these may be associated with macrophages: a similar appearance may be seen postpartum (Figure 19.2).

In pregnancy both secretory and ciliated cells are shallow and intercalary cells increase in number. Focal, patchy, mucosal stromal decidualization occurs quite frequently, and occasionally an Arias-Stella-like change is seen in the epithelium. A mild, acute, non-specific (so-called 'physiological') salpingitis is not uncommon postpartum, this almost certainly being a reaction to the tissue breakdown products from the uterine cavity.

After the menopause, the epithelial cells may remain tall and columnar for many years but gradually they become more shallow, the plicae blunted and the lamina propria fibrosed (Figure 19.3): cilia are inconspicuous. Hormone replacement therapy may, of course, reverse these atrophic changes.

In patients with excessive oestrogenic stimulation, such as that seen with a granulosa cell tumour, the epithelium may become tall and multilayered, these changes being remarkably focal and localized (Figure 19.4).

Epithelial Metaplasia

Metaplastic change is uncommon in the Fallopian tube. Occasionally, however, the epithelium is replaced by foci of mucus-secreting cells of endocervical type[1] or by stratified squamous epithelium (Figure 19.5): intraepithelial neoplasia has been described in the latter case. Foci of metaplastic oncocytes with copious eosinophilic cytoplasm can be differentiated from neoplastic cells by the absence of nuclear atypia and mitoses.

The Fallopian Tube after Sterilization

Occlusion of the tube by a plastic clip placed at right angles to the longitudinal axis of the lumen, elicits a local, active, non-specific chronic inflammatory cell infiltrate which is often dense and consists mainly of lymphocytes and histiocytes (Figure 19.6). The tube is compressed, serosa grows over the clips, the lumen tapers to the point of occlusion on both sides of the device and there is focal mural and serosal fibrosis.

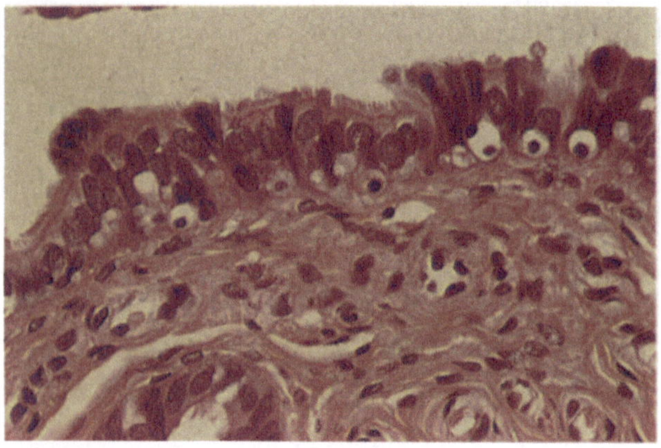

Figure 19.1 Fallopian tube: normal epithelium in the early luteal phase. The ciliated cells are shorter than the secretory cells, bear uniform cilia on their free margins and have round or ovoid nuclei with finely granular chromatin. The nuclei of the secretory cells are more deeply staining, elongated and lie above the free surface of the ciliated cells; there are subnuclear vacuoles in the cytoplasm of some of these cells. H & E × 400

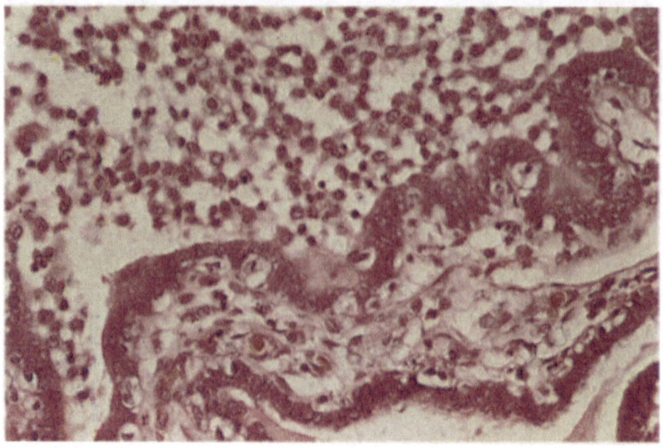

Figure 19.2 Fallopian tube: postpartum. The tubal lumen contains macrophages and endometrial stromal fragments. Note the absence of inflammation in the plica to the lower right: this is not an inflammatory phenomenon. H & E × 250

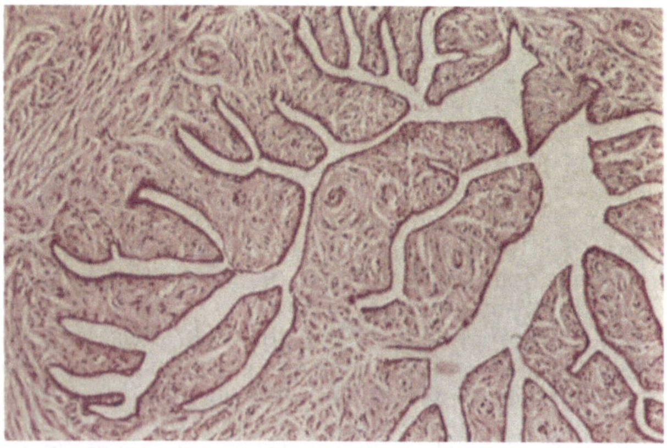

Figure 19.3 Fallopian tube: postmenopausal. The plicae are short and blunt and their stroma is fibrous. The covering epithelium is atrophic, its constituent cells are flattened or cubo-columnar; cilia are not visible. H & E × 100

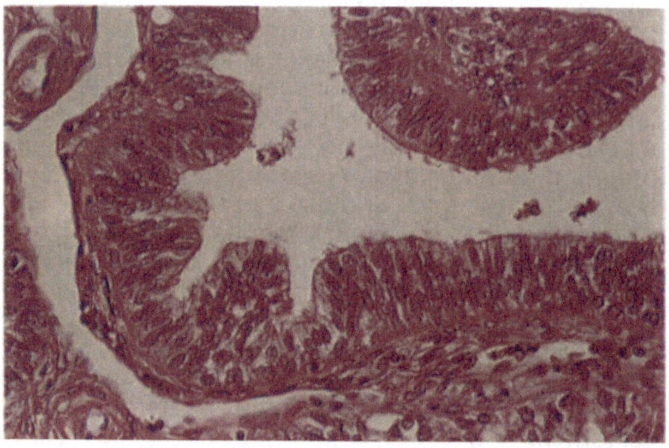

Figure 19.4 Fallopian tube: excess oestrogenic stimulation. The tubal epithelium is multilayered, the cells comprising a mixture of ciliated and secretory cells. Compare with the normal epithelium shown in Figure 19.1. H & E × 250

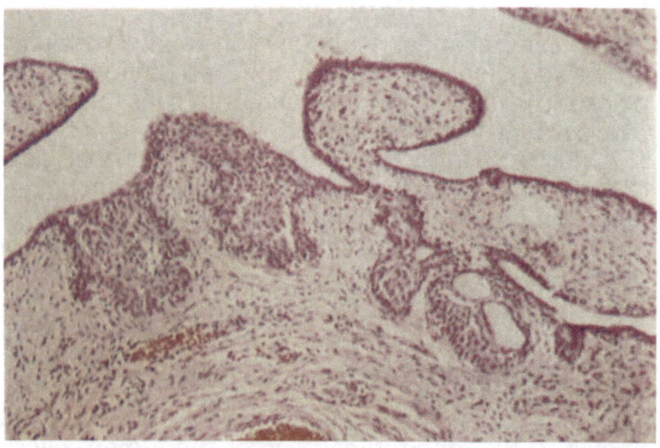

Figure 19.5 Fallopian tube: squamous metaplasia. Foci of immature, metaplastic squamous epithelium and reserve cell hyperplasia (Figures 7.5 and 7.6) are seen in this tube from a postmenopausal patient. H & E × 100

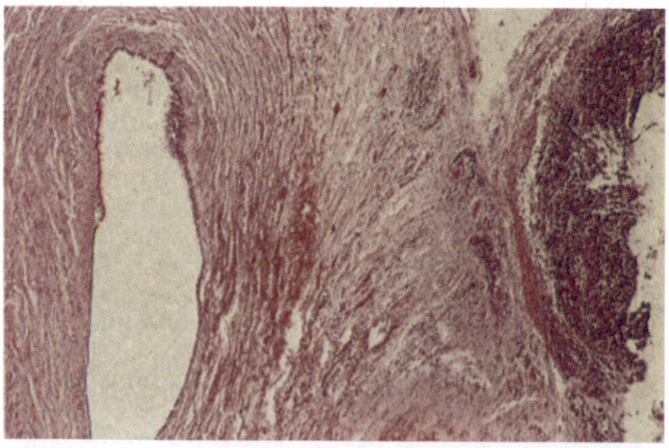

Figure 19.6 Fallopian tube: post-sterilization. The tubal lumen lies to the left; it is rather distended. At the extreme right can be seen the dense lymphocytic infiltrate which surrounded the clip which was used to occlude the tube. A scanty, focal lymphocytic infiltrate is present in the muscular wall. H & E × 40

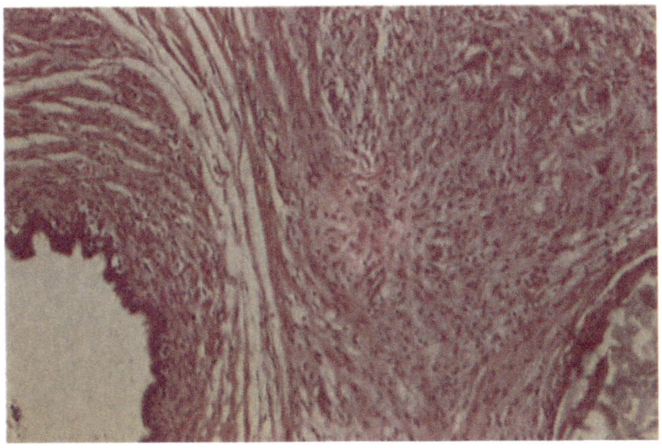

Figure 19.7 Fallopian tube: post-sterilization. The tubal lumen, to the left, is mildly dilated and within the wall to the lower right there is suture material. To the upper right there are macrophages and foreign body giant cells. There is a scattering of lymphocytes in all layers of the wall. H & E × 100

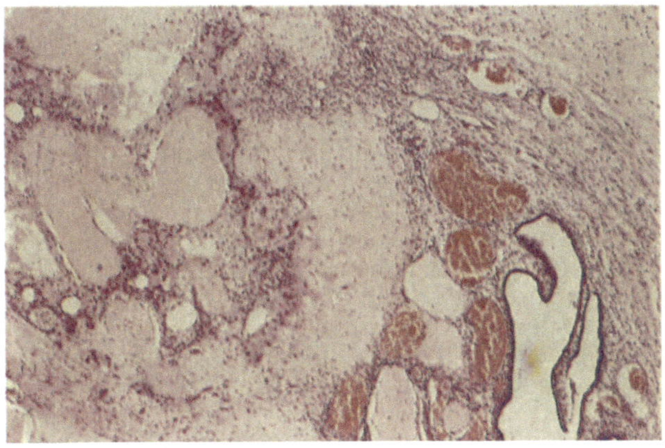

Figure 19.8 Fallopian tube: ectopic gestation. The residual tubal lumen lies to the lower right whilst in the wall to the upper left can be seen ghost-like placental villi, apparently viable trophoblast and decidual cells. The tube was removed from a woman of 34 years who had requested sterilization. H & E × 40

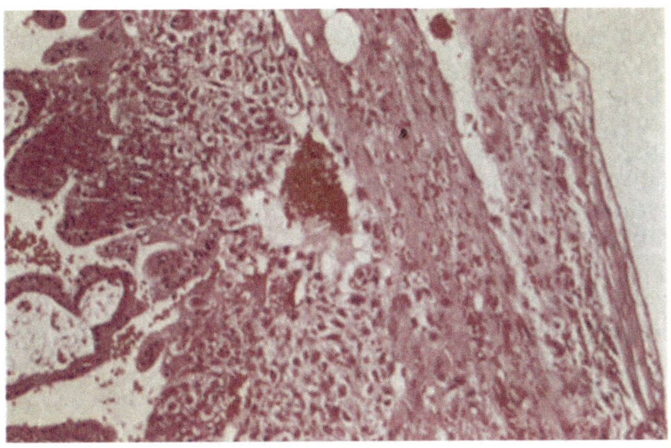

Figure 19.9 Fallopian tube: ectopic gestation. The tubal lumen, to the left, contains first trimester placental villi. Extravillous trophoblast is growing out to infiltrate the wall to the right. Note the absence of a decidua and the proximity of the penetrating trophoblast to the serosal surface at the right. H & E × 100

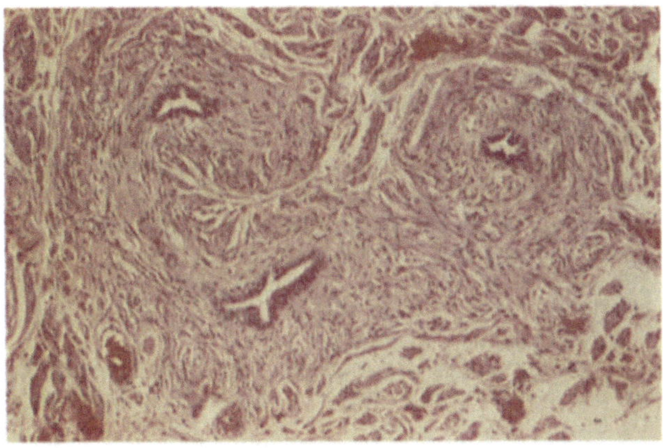

Figure 19.10 Broad ligament: mesonephric remnants. These tubules with muscular walls and a cubo–columnar epithelial lining are typical of mesonephric ductules. H & E × 100

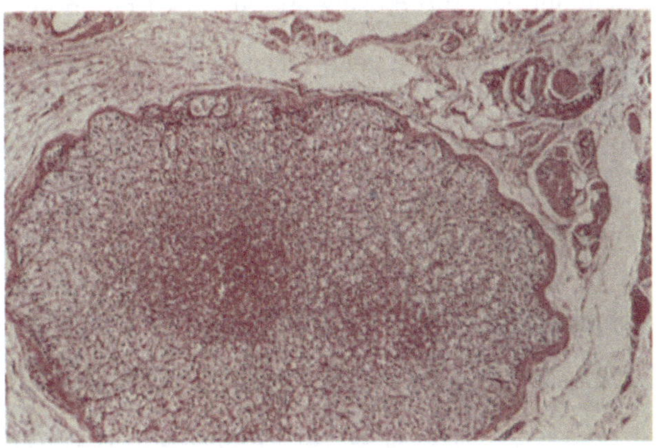

Figure 19.11 Broad ligament: adrenal cortical rest. A well-circumscribed, encapsulated nodule of adrenal tissue is seen. It contains a larger outer zona glomerulosa and an inner zona fasciculata. H & E × 40

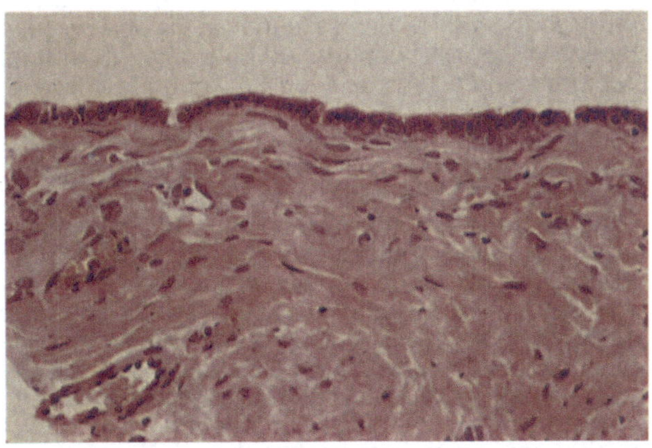

Figure 19.12 Broad ligament: paraovarian cyst. The cyst is lined by cubo–columnar epithelium of tubal type and the wall is muscular. The cyst is of Müllerian origin. H & E × 250

A similar appearance is seen following simple tubal ligation without excision.

If complete occlusion is not obtained, the usual tapering of the lumen is not seen: a lumen may be traced alongside the device due to a failure to enclose the complete lumen at the time of application or on rare occasions, a lumen may be seen weaving between the teeth of an apparently adequately positioned device.

Damage to the tube remote from the clamped segment is unusual with either simple ligation or clipping[2], only minimal dilatation occurring, whereas following tubal resection, a hydrosalpinx is common in the residual tube: the mucosal folds are shallow, the cells cuboidal and there is loss of cilia, whilst microscopic polyps may form[3]. A brisk, active chronic inflammatory process in the wall and serosa is often associated with foreign body granulomata around suture material (Figure 19.7).

Ectopic Pregnancy

Ectopic gestation occurs in approximately 1 in 200 pregnancies, most commonly in the Fallopian tube. In almost half these patients careful histological examination reveals an underlying pathological lesion, usually evidence of previous inflammation or, less commonly, salpingitis isthmica nodosa[4]. When interpreting inflammatory changes in the tube in an ectopic pregnancy it must be remembered that inflammation is usually a concomitant of the haemorrhage associated with the pregnancy and may not indicate underlying disease.

The majority of pregnancies (80%) implant in the ampulla and almost all terminate early in gestation by spontaneous abortion or tubal rupture. That not all tubal pregnancies end as clinical emergencies is shown by the occasional incidental finding of hyalinized or calcified products of conception in supposedly normal tubes (Figure 19.8).

In tubal abortion, the fetus and sac may have been passed into the abdominal cavity, the tubal lumen may be blood-filled and the serosa and fimbria show little or no abnormality, whereas in complete or partial tubal rupture, the rupture site is usually clearly visible, blood clot and placental tissue often protruding through the defect. Serosal surfaces may be covered by thrombus or fibrinous exudate and, if rupture occurred some time previously, by granulation or fibrous tissue.

Implantation undoubtedly occurs primarily in the mucosa but the thin wall of the tube and the mucosa are ill adapted for pregnancy and in some cases rapid penetration of the thin musculature by trophoblast results in the development of the gestational sac in the subserosal tissue: rupture of such a pregnancy may result in a histological picture which suggests a serosal implantation, but careful examination of the remainder of the tube usually discloses the continuity between the intralumenal and subserosal space.

Histologically, the tubal implantation site is similar to that seen in the uterus, but there is a paucity of decidua and the trophoblast commonly penetrates the vasculature in all layers of the wall including the serosa (Figure 19.9).

The appearance of the resected tube in ectopic gestation depends upon the duration of the pregnancy, the mode of its termination and the time which has elapsed since the demise of the fetus. Thus, at one extreme, the tube may contain an apparently viable gestational sac complete with fetus and there may be a clearly identifiable implantation site whilst, at the other, there may be only non-specific granulation tissue and a complete absence of trophoblast. In the majority of cases, the tube contains a mixture of blood clot and placental villi which show a variety of postmortem changes.

Embryonic Remnants

Mesonephric and paramesonephric remnants are often seen on histological examination of the broad ligament. Both occur as small tubules which have a muscular wall (Figure 19.10): the paramesonephric remnants are lined by an epithelium of tubal type, whilst the mesonephric variety are lined by a cuboidal or low columnar epithelium.

Adrenal Cortical Rests

Well defined adrenocortical rests are not uncommon in the broad ligament and are usually found just below the peritoneum, adjacent to the ovarian vein: they are rarely visible macroscopically. Histologically, the rests tend to be rounded, often with an apparent capsule, and they contain all three layers of the normal adrenal cortex (Figure 19.11): medullary tissue is absent.

Cysts

Paraovarian Cysts

These are of two types. The majority are of paramesonephric (Müllerian) origin and are often considered to develop from blind accessory tubal lumena. Such cysts are usually 5–15 cm in diameter, but can occasionally attain huge dimensions: they lie within the ligament with the tube stretched over their upper surface and, if very large, can compress or flatten the ovary. The cysts are freely movable within the ligament and easily enucleated: they are unilocular, contain clear fluid, have a wall formed by connective tissue and smooth muscle and are lined by an epithelium of tubal type (Figure 19.12). The less common variety of paraovarian cyst is of mesonephric origin and is usually smaller than a paramesonephric cyst: these cysts tend to lie away from the tube, which is not stretched over them, and cannot be enucleated from the ligament. Histologically, this type of cyst has a rather thick fibromuscular wall and is lined by a single layer of non-ciliated cuboidal cells.

References

1. Pauerstein, C. J. (1974). *The Fallopian Tube: A Reappraisal.* (Philadelphia: Lea and Febiger)
2. Bernhardt-Huth, D., Frantzen, Ch. and Schlösser, H. W. (1979). Morphological alterations of rabbit oviducts following ligature of the tubal isthmus. *Virch. Arch. Pathol. Anat. Histol.*, **384**, 195–211
3. Vasquez, G., Winston, R. M. L., Boeckx, W. and Brosens, I. (1980). Tubal lesions subsequent to sterilisation and their relation to fertility after attempts at reversal. *Am. J. Obstet. Gynecol.*, **138**, 86–92
4. Honoré, L. H. (1978). Salpingitis isthmica nodosa in female infertility and ectopic pregnancy. *Fertil. Steril.*, **29**, 164–168

Fallopian Tube and Broad Ligament: Non-Neoplastic Conditions II

20

Acute Inflammation

Infection may reach the Fallopian tube along the lumen from the uterus (endosalpingitis), via the vasculature or lymphatics from the uterus (interstitial salpingitis), from distant sites by haematogenous spread or directly from adjacent organs.

Endosalpingitis

Infection in the uterus or the presence of an IUCD predispose to the development of an acute endosalpingitis. In the past, it was assumed that the majority of infections were due to *N. gonorrhoea*, but it has become clear that many infections are due to anaerobic organisms (particularly *Bacteroides*), *Chlamydiae* and possibly *Mycoplasma*, the role which *N. gonorrhoea* plays having been perhaps overstated.

Inflammation commences in the mucosa and spreads through the tube wall producing a local peritonitis and frequently, because of the close proximity of the ovary, an acute peri-oophoritis or tubo-ovarian abscess. Initially, the Fallopian tube is swollen, congested and inflamed, the serosa becomes dull, hyperaemic and its surface covered by fibrinous exudate. Early in the disease the tube is not distended but as the inflammation proceeds, the lumen fills with pus which may spill into the abdominal cavity to produce a pelvic peritonitis: later, inflammation of the fimbriae leads to their agglutination with consequent ostial obstruction.

Histologically, the mucosa is initially swollen, hyperaemic, focally haemorrhagic and infiltrated by neutrophil polymorphonuclear leukocytes; an acute inflammatory exudate accumulates in the lumen (Figure 20.1). At the same time there is progressive desquamation, necrosis and ulceration of the tubal epithelium and the damage may be extensive. The individual epithelial cells at this stage may show marked reactive atypia, their nuclei being enlarged and both cells and nuclei showing pleomorphism: mitoses may be seen where there is repair or less severe damage (Figure 20.2). Ultimately the tubal lumen becomes filled with cellular debris and pus. Neutrophil polymorphs are seen in all layers of the wall and the serosa where there is a fibrous exudate.

Interstitial Salpingitis

Interstitial salpingitis is the result of infection which reaches the tube via the uterine lymphatics or veins: streptococcal infections typically behave in this manner. In these cases, the infection centres upon the tubal wall with relative sparing of the mucosa (Figure 20.3). Histologically, an acute inflammatory infiltrate can be seen in the tube wall, between the fibres of the musculature, and there may be interstitial oedema, vascular congestion and even microabscess formation (Figure 20.4). The mucosa usually shows a relatively scanty neutrophil polymorph infiltrate and the lumen may be free of exudate. The absence of mucosal damage in these cases is important, for, with the resolution of infection, tubal patency, and hence fertility, is little impaired.

Chronic Inflammation

The sequelae of acute endosalpingitis are variable. In mild, or adequately treated, cases the disorder may resolve leaving minimal or no residual disease. In other cases, occlusion of the tubal ostium and the accumulation of pus within the tube leads to the formation of a pyosalpinx (Figure 20.5). A pyosalpinx is lined by non-specific granulation and fibrous tissue and contains an acute inflammatory exudate and, later, macrophages, some of which contain haemosiderin. A tubo-ovarian or pelvic abscess may also result. In other cases the clinical picture of chronic salpingitis is in fact due to reinfection, a condition to which these patients are prone. Infertility is a common and important complication, the risk of infertility increasing with each successive attack of infection. In the unlikely event of pregnancy occurring, ectopic tubal gestation is common.

Hydrosalpinx Follicularis (*Follicular Salpingitis*)

Following the damage consequent upon acute endosalpingitis, plical fusion may occur during the healing process, with strands of mucosa forming a mesh across the tubal lumen (Figure 20.6). The resultant damage is associated with a high incidence of infertility and ectopic gestation. The tubal epithelium is often flattened, and cilia may be difficult to identify but inflammatory cells are often few and there may be only a scattering of lymphocytes in the lamina propria.

Hydrosalpinx

This is a Fallopian tube in which the wall is thinned and attenuated, the lumen being distended and containing clear serous fluid. Usually the tubal ostium is occluded and the fimbria invaginated; the ampullary and infundibular segments are thin-walled and distended, sometimes almost translucent, and the tube assumes a retort-like shape. However, the isthmus is of normal calibre and communicates with the dis-

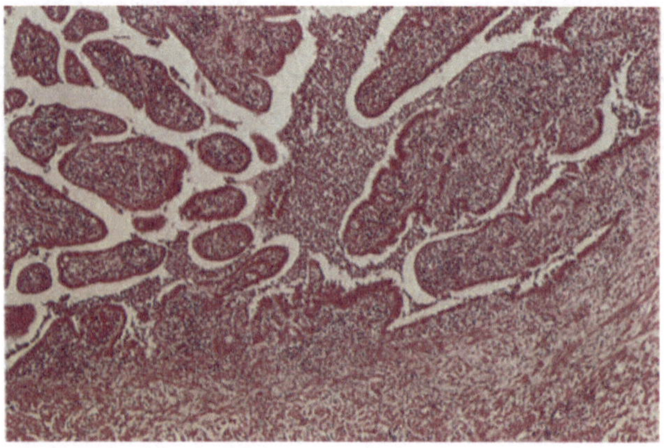

Figure 20.1 Fallopian tube: acute endosalpingitis. The tubal lumen contains an exudate of polymorphonuclear leukocytes and fibrin. The plicae are swollen and are heavily infiltrated by acute inflammatory cells. The wall, at the lower margin of the field, is infiltrated by polymorphonuclear leukocytes and there is early, focal, mucosal ulceration. H & E × 40

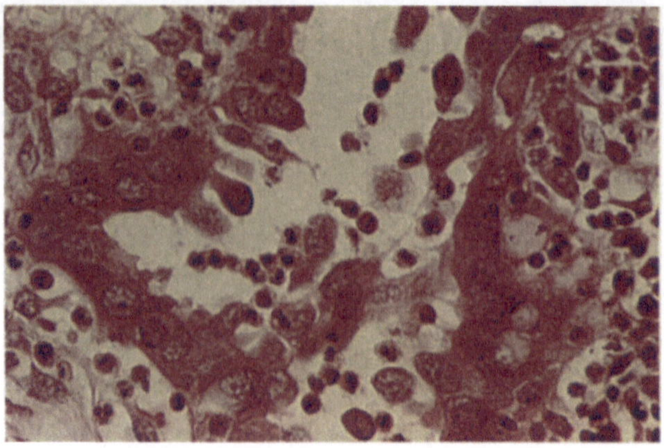

Figure 20.2 Fallopian tube: reactive cellular atypia in endosalpingitis. The epithelial cells are pleomorphic, and show loss of polarity and budding. In some cells there is a high nucleo–cytoplasmic ratio and nucleoli are seen. H & E × 400

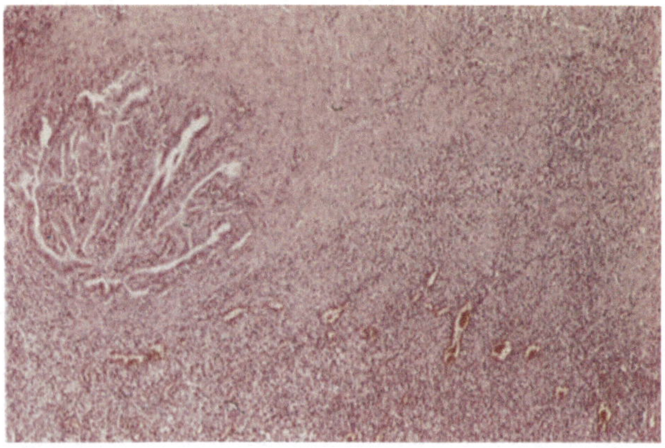

Figure 20.3 Fallopian tube: interstitial salpingitis. The tubal lumen which lies to the left is patent; the mucosa contains only a scanty intrastromal inflammatory infiltrate. Within the wall below and to the right there is a dense active non-specific chronic inflammatory cell infiltrate consisting of neutrophil polymorphonuclear leukocytes, plasma cells, histiocytes and occasional lymphocytes; vascular dilatation is conspicuous. H & E × 40

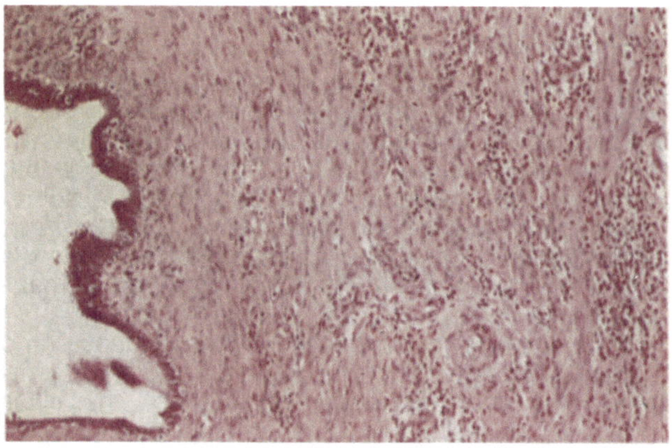

Figure 20.4 Fallopian tube: interstitial salpingitis. The contrast between the normal isthmic mucosa, to the left, and the inflamed musculature to the right is clearly seen. Note the truly interstitial nature of the inflammatory infiltrate. H & E × 100

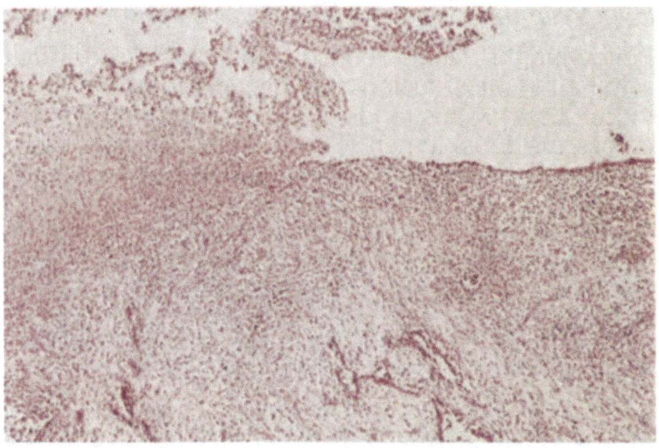

Figure 20.5 Fallopian tube: pyosalpinx. The mucosa is flattened and largely replaced by non-specific granulation tissue. To the left of the field it is ulcerated. H & E × 40

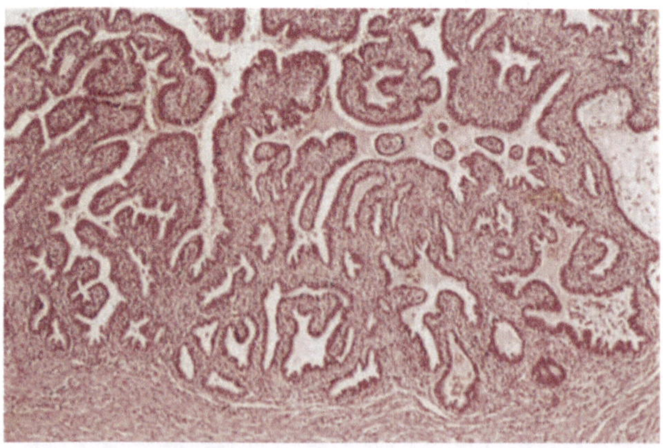

Figure 20.6 Fallopian tube: salpingitis follicularis. In this portion of tube the mucosal plicae are irregularly fused to form a mesh across the lumen. The stroma contains a scanty infiltrate of lymphocytes and the epithelium is focally flattened. There are fibrous scars in the muscular wall. H & E × 40

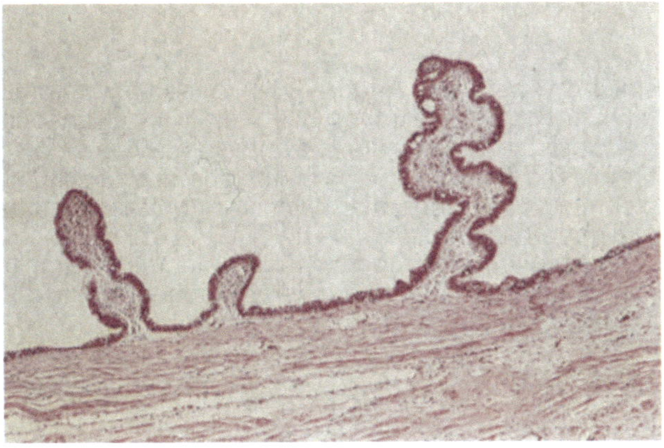

Figure 20.7 Fallopian tube: hydrosalpinx. This is part of a hydrosalpinx. The muscular wall is thinned and the mucosa flattened but shortened individual plicae are present at intervals around the lumen. The epithelium is of fairly normal structure and there is no active inflammation. H & E × 40

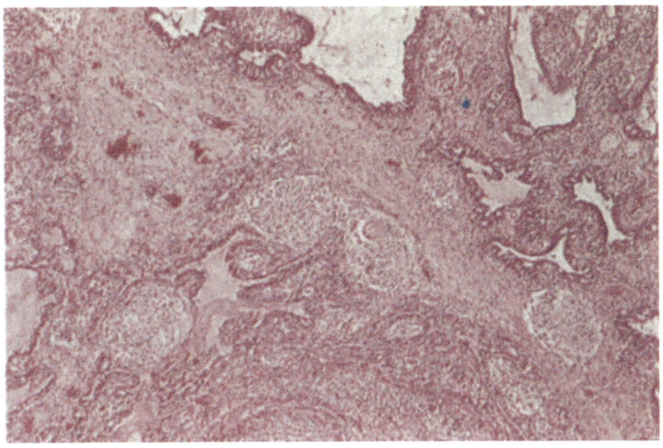

Figure 20.8 Fallopian tube: tuberculosis. The plicae are swollen and several non-caseating granulomata are seen. In addition there is a diffuse plasma cell and lymphocytic infiltrate. H & E × 40

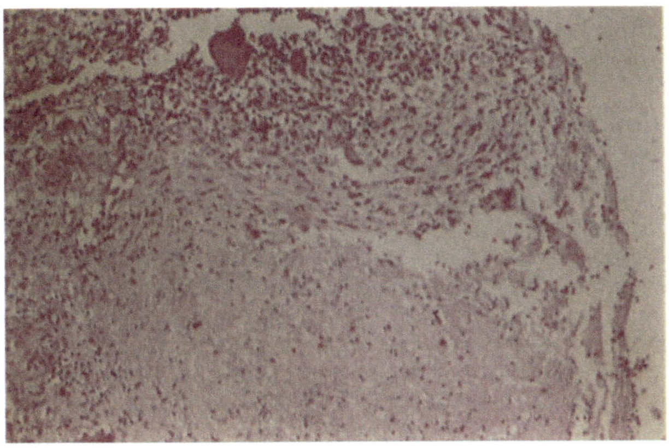

Figure 20.9 Fallopian tube: tuberculosis. The lumen of this tube is lined by fibro-caseous tuberculous granulation tissue. Epithelioid granulomata and Langhans giant cells are seen at the top of the field. The sample is from the wall of a tuberculous pyosalpinx. H & E × 100

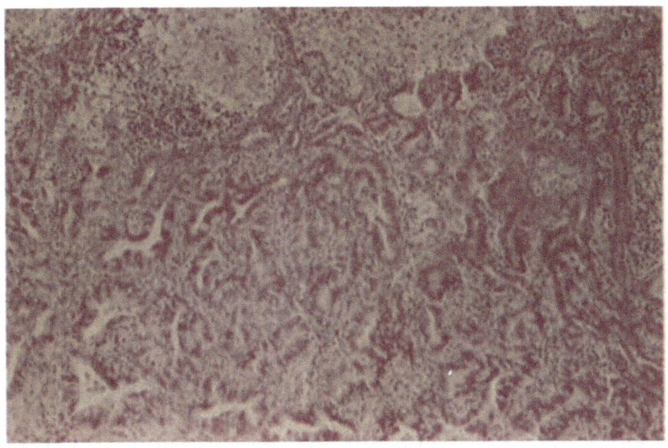

Figure 20.10 Fallopian tube: tuberculosis. In the mucosa, tuberculous granulomata are present at the top of the field. Below, there is a marked degree of mucosal hyperplasia. The resulting picture of complex branching glandular spaces and acini mimics that of well-differentiated carcinoma. However, whilst the epithelium may show reactive changes there is no nuclear hyperchromatism or abnormal mitotic activity. H & E × 100

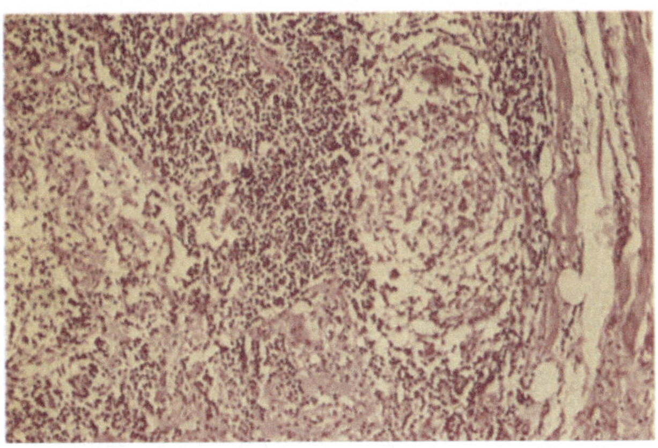

Figure 20.11 Fallopian tube: Crohn's disease. Several well-formed non-caseating sarcoid-like granulomata are present in the tubal musculature and mucosa. They consist of epithelioid cells and macrophage giant cells with a cuff of lymphocytes. H & E × 100

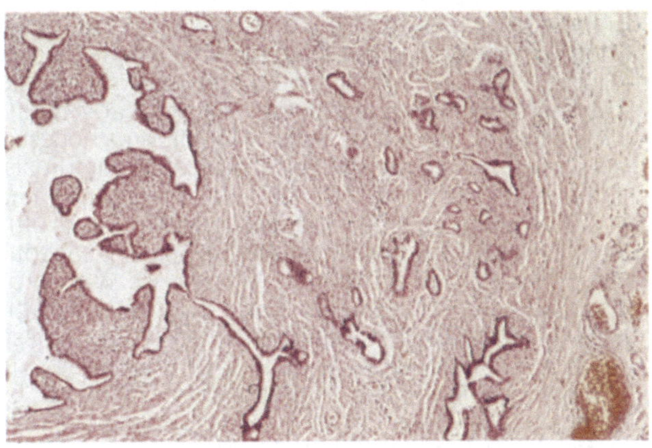

Figure 20.12 Fallopian tube: salpingitis isthmica nodosa. In the lower left of the field a diverticulum can be seen leading from the tubal lumen into the wall where there are numerous similar gland-like structures. The diverticula are lined by epithelium of tubal type and there is hypertrophy of the surrounding muscle particularly in relation to the more deeply situated elements. H & E × 40

tended segment. Histologically, the mucosa is rarely completely flattened for isolated, shortened plicae can usually be identified even in the grossly distended tube (Figure 20.7). Sometimes the plicae contain collections of foamy macrophages and, very occasionally, a scattering of lymphocytes but there is rarely any evidence of active inflammation. The epithelium is usually shallow and cuboidal and cilia are scanty or absent. The muscle is flattened, thinned and in many cases partly or completely replaced by fibrous tissue. The presence of a communicating grossly distended tubal segment and the persistence of occasional plicae has led to the suggestion that the distension is not the consequence simply of the accumulation of fluid but results from underlying destruction of the integrity of the tube wall and the sphincter-like action of the tubal isthmus.

Granulomatous Salpingitis

Chronic granulomatous salpingitis has many causes, but without doubt the most common throughout the world is tuberculosis. Tuberculosis has an incidence ranging from 1% in infertile women in USA and Great Britain to 10% in India. It is found in 20% of women dying of tuberculosis. Infection reaches the tube via the blood stream from a primary site elsewhere in the body, usually the lung. It may also spread via the lymphatics from the intestinal tract or directly from the intestines or bladder. The serosal surface may be directly affected when there is tuberculous peritonitis and the lumen may be initially spared. The disease is almost invariably bilateral.

Characteristically the tube is thickened, fibrosed and covered by dense adhesions. Surprisingly, in the presence of such extensive disease, the ostium may be patent and this finding in a severely abnormal tube should always suggest the possibility of tuberculosis. In other patients the tube is converted into a distended retort-shaped sac filled with caseous material. In both forms of the disease, the serosal surfaces often bears tubercles.

Histologically, the disease is usually first manifest in the mucosa where granulomata, composed of clusters of epithelioid cells cuffed by lymphocytes and associated with Langhans' giant cells, develop. In the adhesive form of the disease, granulomata are often non-caseating and contain Schaumann bodies (Figure 20.8). The histological similarity to sarcoid may therefore be acute and the finding of any tuberculoid granulomata in biopsies from this area necessitates the microbiological exclusion of tuberculosis. In the exudative form of the disease, the granulomata in the mucosa enlarge, undergo caseation and ultimately rupture into the tubal lumen where the caseous material elicits an inflammatory response with progressive mucosal damage, plical fusion and, ultimately, obliteration of the tubal lumen. The wall also contains granulomata although they may be few in number; gradually the wall becomes replaced by fibrous tissue and in the longstanding case there may be focal calcification (Figure 20.9).

In a proportion of cases the tubal mucosa shows striking hyperplasia (Figure 20.10) and misinterpretation of this appearance has led to an erroneous diagnosis of carcinoma[1]. The appearance can be distinguished from carcinoma by the absence of cellular pleomorphism, abnormal nuclear chromatin pattern and abnormal mitoses.

The outcome of tuberculous salpingitis is almost inevitable infertility and should pregnancy occur ectopic gestation is likely.

Other Forms of Infective Granulomatous Salpingitis

In countries where the disease is endemic bilharzial infection of the Fallopian tubes is found in 20% of women at postmortem and is thought to be an important cause of infertility. The presence of ova within the tube wall elicits a marked fibroblastic response.

Tubal actinomycosis has assumed greater importance in recent years as it has been shown to be a rare though serious complication of the use of the IUCD (See Chapter 34).

Pin worm infection is a rare cause of granulomatous salpingitis whilst foreign bodies, often surgical or introduced at the time of surgery, are not an infrequent cause.

Crohn's Disease

The Fallopian tube may be involved secondarily to intestinal disease in two ways. There may, on rare occasions, be an intestino–tubal fistula or, more commonly, a salpingo-oophoritis with non-caseating tuberculoid granulomata in the tubal musculature and mucosa[2] (Figure 20.11). Severe epithelial atypia has been recorded in some of these patients and may lead to an unwarranted diagnosis of carcinoma *in situ*[3].

Salpingitis Isthmica Nodosa

Salpingitis isthmica nodosa has often, and quite incorrectly, been regarded as an inflammatory process. It is, in fact, a diverticular disease of the isthmic portion of the tube, analagous to adenomyosis, and is an important factor in ectopic gestation.

Externally the isthmus bears nodular swellings, up to 1 or 2 cm in diameter, and the wall is thickened. Histologically, a transverse section of the tube shows a normal, narrow, or even occluded lumen and the musculature contains multiple small cyst-like spaces lined by tubal epithelium (Figure 20.12). The muscle around the epithelial elements is hypertrophied, this contributing to the nodularity of the tube.

References

1. Puflett, D. (1972). Tuberculous salpingitis resembling adenocarcinoma. *Med. J. Aust.*, **2**, 149–151
2. Brooks, J. J. and Wheeler, J. E. (1977). Granulomatous salpingitis secondary to Crohn's disease. *Obstet. Gynecol.*, **49** (No. 1 Suppl.), 315–335
3. Wheeler, J. E. (1982). Pathology of the Fallopian tube. In Blaustein, A. (ed.). *Pathology of the Female Genital Tract.* (New York: Springer-Verlag)

Fallopian Tube and Broad Ligament: Neoplasms

21

FALLOPIAN TUBE

Benign Neoplasms

Tubal neoplasms of this type are all very rare, the least uncommon being the adenomatoid tumour which is usually small (1–2 cm across) and occurs in a subserosal site, compressing the muscularis into the tubal lumen (Figure 21.1): histologically and histogenetically this is identical to its myometrial counterpart (see Chapter 17). Benign epithelial neoplasms are exceptional and it is probable that virtually all reported papillomata or adenomata of the tube have been of either an inflammatory or hyperplastic nature: very occasionally a genuine adenofibroma (Figure 21.2) is, however, encountered. Mature cystic teratoma can occur in the tube, these presumably developing from germ cells which have become arrested during their passage through the lumen.

Intraepithelial Neoplasia

Premalignant abnormalities of the tubal epithelium are poorly documented and it has not yet been possible to define, with any degree of confidence, a condition of tubal intraepithelial neoplasia (or 'adeno 'adenocarcinoma *in situ*'). Minor degrees of atypical epithelial proliferation with nuclear crowding, some loss of nuclear polarity, a minor degree of stratification and some nuclear atypia, are relatively common in the tube (Figure 21.3): atypical proliferation of this type is found most frequently in association with a salpingitis, being seen most markedly in cases of tubal tuberculosis, but has also been noted in 14% of otherwise normal surgically removed tubes[1]. There is no evidence that relatively minor proliferative lesions of this type, which are usually focal, ever progress to an adenocarcinoma but a more florid papillary pattern, with marked cellular atypia, translumenal epithelial bridging and mitotic figures, is occasionally seen and should be regarded as a precursor of frank malignancy: how often such a lesion progresses to an invasive adenocarcinoma is, however, unknown.

Malignant Neoplasms

Adenocarcinoma

This is by far the commonest malignant tumour of the tube but nevertheless accounts for only 0.3% of cases of gynaecological cancer[2]: it occurs most commonly in the fifth and sixth decades, the mean age of women with this neoplasm being about 55 years.

Macroscopically, the involved tube may appear externally normal or only slightly swollen but more commonly it resembles a pyo- or hydrosalpinx: perforation of the wall by tumour is relatively uncommon but in advanced cases there may be a large neoplastic mass enveloping the ovary. On opening the tube it is usually seen to be largely filled with friable, crumbling, grey tumour which often shows areas of necrosis: fluid is also often present. The tumour is bilateral in 20% of cases, but it is not yet established whether this is due to the simultaneous development of two primary tumours or to metastasis in one tube from a primary neoplasm in the contralateral tube.

Histologically, the tumour is usually a well differentiated papillary adenocarcinoma (Figure 21.4) and tends to resemble closely a serous adenocarcinoma of the ovary. Less well differentiated neoplasms have a mixed papillary–alveolar pattern whilst the uncommon poorly differentiated adenocarcinomata tend to grow in a solid (or 'medullary') fashion (Figure 21.5). Histological variants of this basic pattern are unusual but rare examples of endometrioid, adenosquamous and transitional cell carcinomata have been described.

The histological diagnosis of tubal adenocarcinoma is often straightforward, but difficulty is sometimes encountered in distinguishing between this neoplasm and the adenomatous hyperplasia which is frequently associated with tubal tuberculosis, a difficulty compounded by the fact that tuberculosis and an undoubted adenocarcinoma sometimes coexist in the same tube (Figure 21.6). Attention to such features as the degree of cellular atypia and the presence of abnormal mitotic figures, nuclear pleomorphism and hyperchromatism usually help in resolving this dilemma whilst invasion of the wall is, of course, a clear indication of frank malignancy.

Because of the rich lymphatic drainage of the tube an adenocarcinoma tends to spread to lymph nodes at a relatively early stage, those most commonly involved being the para-aortic, internal iliac and inguinal nodes. Implantation of tumour via the abdominal ostium on to the peritoneum and ovary and via the uterine cornu into the uterus is also an important route of dissemination whilst direct spread through the tubal wall will involve adjacent structures. Staging of the tumour depends on the extent of spread at the time of diagnosis:

Stage I	Tumour limited to the tube and not penetrating the serosal surface
Stage II	Tumour extending through the serosa with invasion of surrounding organs or with metastases to pelvic organs
Stage III	Metastases to sites outside the pelvis but within the abdomen
Stage IV	Metastases outside the abdomen

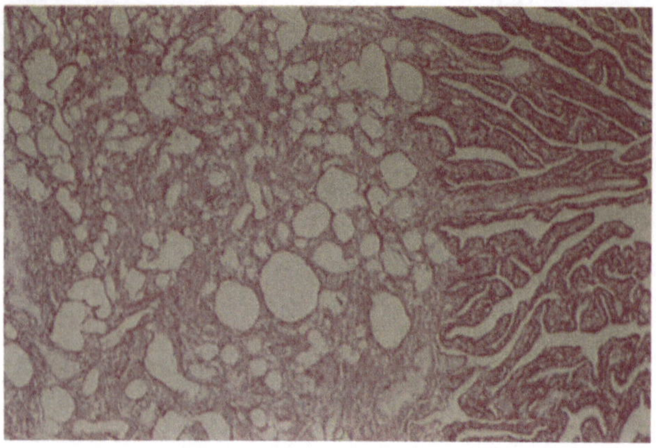

Figure 21.1 Fallopian tube: adenomatoid tumour. The tube wall is eccentrically expanded by a typical adenomatoid tumour (see Figures 17.5, 17.6 and 17.7). The lumen was partly obstructed by the neoplasm which was found unexpectedly in a tube removed at sterilization. H & E × 40

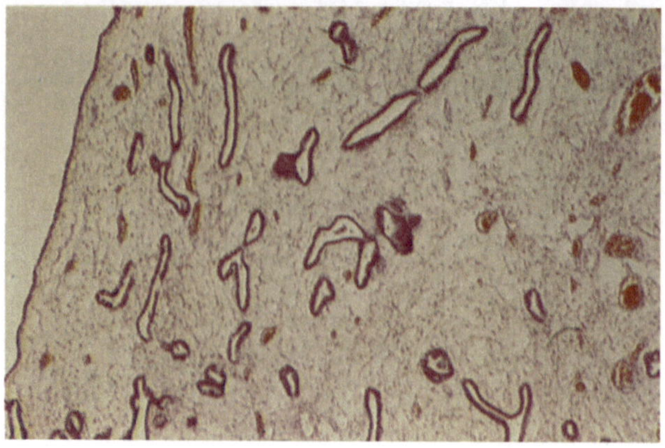

Figure 21.2 Fallopian tube: adenofibroma. The tumour consists of narrow tubules and small acini lined by epithelium of tubal type and by rather flattened cuboidal cells set in a fine fibrous cellular stroma. H & E × 40

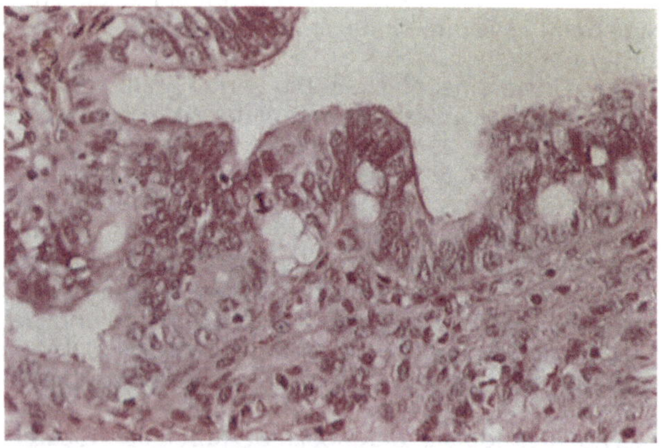

Figure 21.3 Fallopian tube: epithelial atypia. One of many atypical epithelial foci in a Fallopian tube removed at sterilization. The cells show nuclear enlargement and loss of polarity: some epithelial multilayering is present and to the left of centre there is a mitosis of normal configuration. H & E × 250

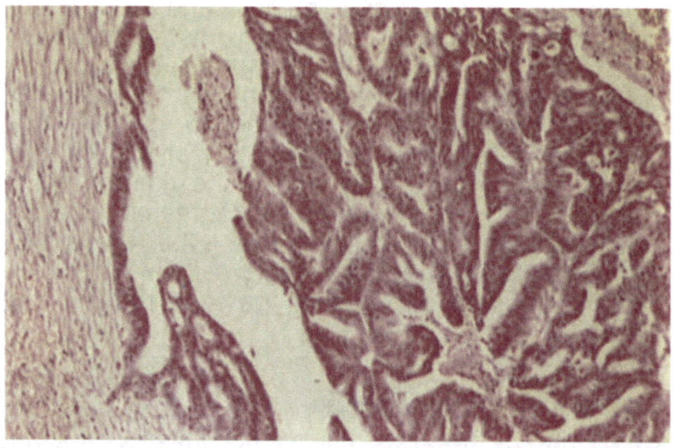

Figure 21.4 Fallopian tube: well-differentiated adenocarcinoma. To the left, the tubal lumen is lined by epithelium showing intraepithelial neoplasia and below there is an abrupt transition to papillary carcinoma which lines the tube and fills the lumen. In this neoplasm, the fine fibro-vascular papillary fronds are covered by atypical epithelium but of recognizable tubal type. The presence of an intraepithelial component distinguishes the lesion from metastatic papillary serous adenocarcinoma of the ovary. H & E × 100

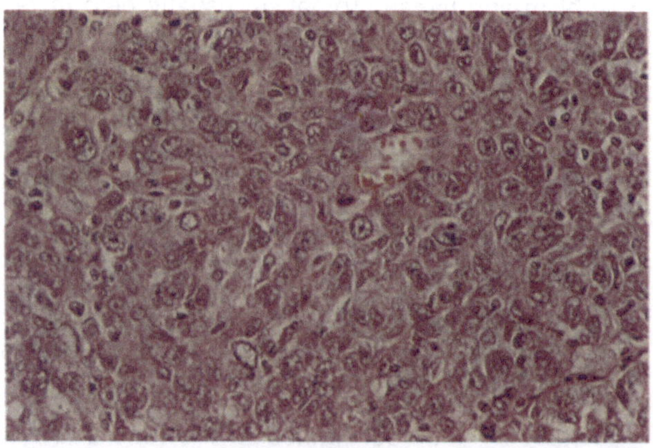

Figure 21.5 Fallopian tube: undifferentiated carcinoma. The tumour grows in sheets of large cells with pleomorphic nuclei, many of which contain nucleoli. Lymphocytes are scattered amongst the neoplastic cells. H & E × 250

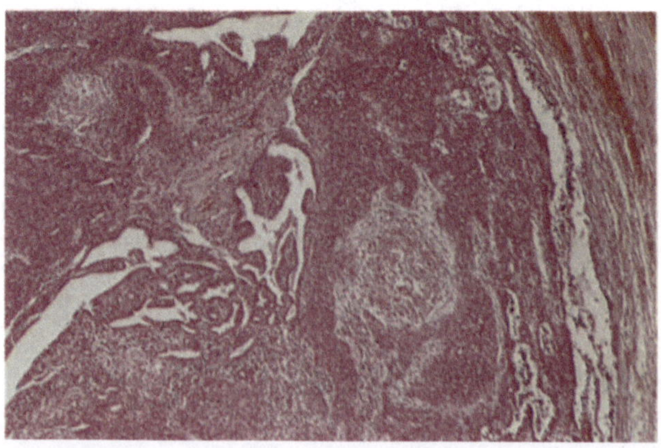

Figure 21.6 Fallopian tube: tuberculosis and poorly differentiated adenocarcinoma. The tubal lumen is filled by carcinoma which in this field is forming undifferentiated sheets and infiltrating cords. Caseating epithelioid granulomata can be seen between the tumour masses. Microbiological studies confirmed the presence of *M. tuberculosis*. H & E × 40

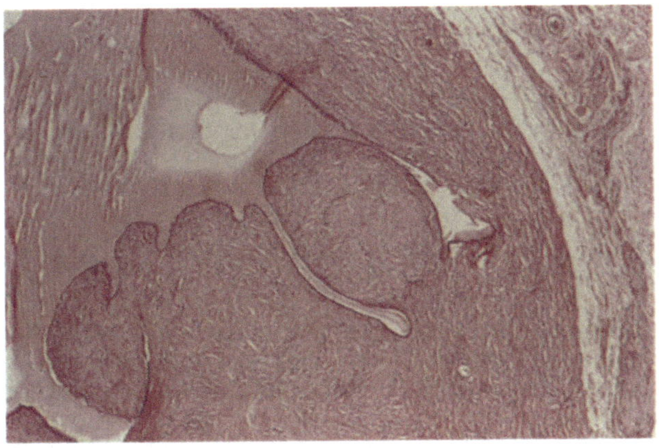

Figure 21.7 Broad ligament: serous papillary cystadenoma arising in a paraovarian cyst. The cyst has a fibrous wall, and is lined by a single layer of flattened, cuboidal epithelium. Below and to the right short, blunt papillary ingrowths protrude into the lumen. H & E × 40

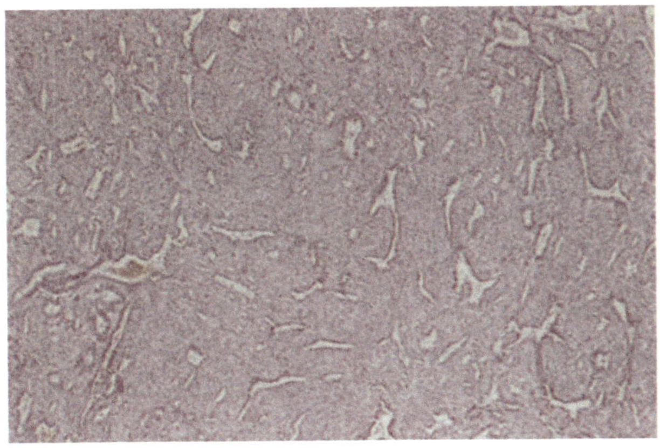

Figure 21.8 Broad ligament: adnexal tumour of Wolffian origin. The tumour has a pattern of narrow, irregular clefts in a cellular stroma. H & E × 40

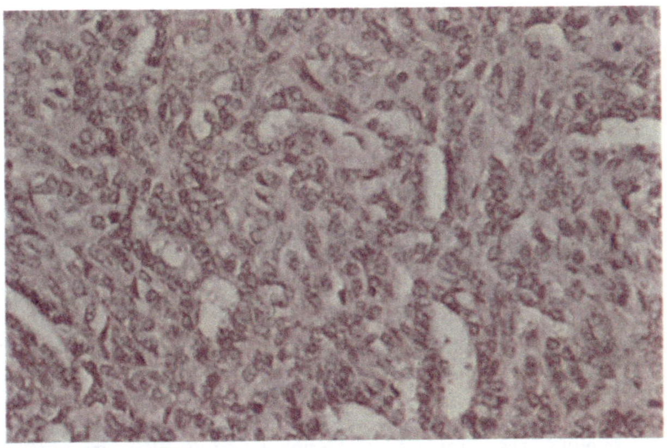

Figure 21.9 Broad ligament: adnexal tumour of Wolffian origin. The tumour in this field is predominantly solid with small unlined clefts and tubules. The cells lining the tubules and forming the stroma are similar. They have round or oval nuclei, rather scanty eosinophilic cytoplasm and ill-defined cell margins; there are no mitoses and nuclear atypia is absent. H & E × 250

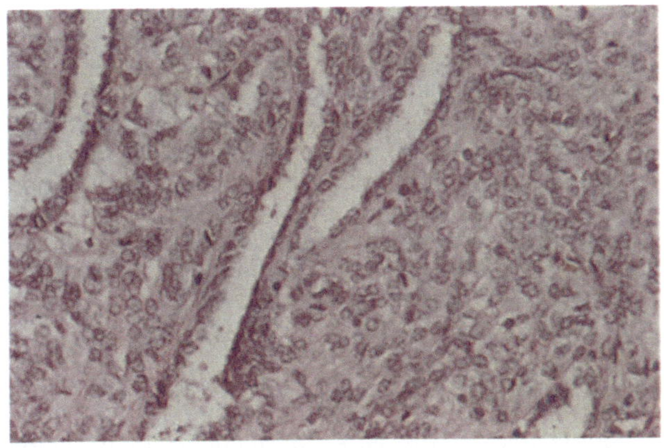

Figure 21.10 Broad ligament: adnexal tumour of Wolffian origin. The pattern in this field is of well-formed tubules lined by a distinct layer of small, regular cuboidal cells with scanty cytoplasm and round nuclei. The cells in the stroma are forming trabeculae and have larger, more vesicular nuclei than do those lining the tubules. H & E × 25

The overall 5-year survival for women with a tubal adenocarcinoma is 27% but that for those with Stage I tumours is 60%, this figure declining to 30% for Stage II cases and falling to below 10% for those with Stage III or IV disease: unfortunately, histological grading of the tumour appears to be of little prognostic value[2].

Choriocarcinoma

These rare neoplasms of the tube probably result from an ectopic pregnancy and present as a large haemorrhagic fleshy mass which may largely destroy the tube: histologically, they are identical to a uterine choriocarcinoma (see Chapter 32).

BROAD LIGAMENT

A variety of tumours can occur in the broad ligament but most of these have their origin elsewhere. Thus, the only reasonably common broad ligament neoplasm, the leiomyoma, is usually a pedunculated or detached subserous uterine leiomyoma which has extended into the ligament, whilst most of the ovarian ovarian-type tumours which have been described within the ligament have probably arisen in the ovary and have become secondarily incarcerated within the ligament. However, primary leiomyomata can arise from the sparse smooth muscle fibres of the ligament, whilst occasional tumours of ovarian type can develop from intraligamentous accessory or supernumary ovarian tissue: an endometrioid adenocarcinoma of the ligament may develop in, and from, a focus of endometriosis.

Serous Papillary Cystadenoma

Neoplasms of this type, identical to their ovarian counterparts, occur in the broad ligament in the absence of accessory ovarian tissue: whilst it is possible that some develop from foci of endosalpingiosis it is probable that the vast majority arise in para-ovarian cysts of paramesonephric type for the development of papillary serous neoplasms within such cysts has been well documented[3]. The occurrence of such a tumour in a para-ovarian cyst may be apparent to the naked eye as a coating of closely packed clusters of verrucous ingrowths on the inner surface of the cyst but is sometimes less obvious, appearing only as a focal thickening of the wall. Histologically, fibrous or oedematous papillary ingrowths are covered by tubal type epithelium which is in continuity with that lining the cyst (Figure 21.7).

Adnexal Tumour of Wolffian Origin (Figures 21.8–21.10

This rare, but distinctive neoplasm[4,5] arises either within the leaves of the ligament or is attached to the tube by a pedicle. The tumour is solid, lobulated and apparently encapsulated: on section the neoplasm may appear rubbery or friable and small cysts or foci of calcification may be apparent. Histologically, there is a complex and variable pattern made up of various permutations of hollow or solid tubules, solid masses of epithelial cells, sieve-like spaces, cellular trabeculae and areas which bear some resemblance to an adenomatoid tumour. The original identification of these tumours as being of Wolffian origin was based largely upon their site but has, to some extent, been confirmed by electron microscopic observations[6]. These neoplasms usually appear to behave in a benign fashion but one has been described which gave rise to hepatic metastases[7].

References

1. Moore, S.W. and Enterline, H.T. (1975). Significance of proliferative epithelial lesions of the uterine tube. *Obstet. Gynecol.*, **45**, 385–390
2. Benedet, J. L. and White, G. W. (1981). Malignant tumors of the Fallopian tube. In Coppleson, M. (ed.). *Gynecologic Oncology*, pp. 621–629. (Edinburgh, London, Melbourne and New York: Churchill-Livingstone)
3. Honoré, L. H. and O'Hara, K. E. (1980). Serous papillary neoplasms arising in paramesonephric parovarian cysts: a report of eight cases. *Acta Obstet. Gynecol. Scand.*, **59**, 525–528
4. Kariminejad, M. H. and Scully, R. E. (1973). Female adnexal tumor of probable Wolffian origin: a distinctive pathologic entity. *Cancer*, **31**, 671–677
5. Sivathondan, Y., Salm, R., Hughesdon, P. E. and Faccini, J. M. (1979). Female adnexal tumour of probable Wolffian origin. *J. Clin. Pathol.*, **32**, 616–624
6. Demopoulos, R. I., Sitelman, A., Flotte, T. and Bigelow, B. (1980). Ultra-structural study of a female adnexal tumor of probable Wolffian origin. *Cancer*, **46**, 2273–2280
7. Taxy, J. B. and Battifora, H. (1976). Female adnexal tumor of probable Wolffian origin: evidence for a low grade malignancy. *Cancer*, **37**, 2349–2354

Ovary: Normal Appearances and Cyclical Changes

22

Pathologists are often required to examine normal ovaries. The wide range of structures in the normal ovary sometimes gives rise to diagnostic difficulties, and it is by no means uncommon for physiological cyclical changes to be interpreted as being of a pathological nature. It is, therefore, necessary for the histopathologist to appreciate the spectrum of morphological features that may be found in the normal ovary.

The normal ovary[1,2] is covered by a single layer of surface epithelium which is in continuity with the peritoneum. Between the surface epithelium and the cortex is a narrow, eosinophilic band of basement membrane material, the tunica albuginea. The cortex, in which germinal cells and follicles in varying stages of development and regression are seen, comprises a superficial, densely spindle-celled fibrous zone rich in reticulin and a less compact deep component. The medulla contains islands of stromal cells, blood vessels, lymphatic channels and autonomic nerves which enter the ovary at the hilum where hilar (Leydig) cells and the rete ovarii, a series of small irregular tubules of Wolffian duct origin, are sited.

Surface Epithelium

This (Figure 22.1) is composed of a single layer of cubo-columnar or flattened cells which may become focally multilayered or show metaplasia (Figure 22.2) to tubal endocervical-like mucinous epithelium or, in association with cortical metaplasia to endometrial-like stroma, to endometrial-type epithelium.

Follicular Development

The Pre-ovulatory Follicle

During the reproductive years the ovarian cortex contains numerous primordial follicles which are single germ cells each surrounded by a layer of flattened granulosa cells (Figure 22.3). Following stimulation by FSH, the granulosa cell layer becomes first cuboidal and ultimately multilayered, this being the primary follicular stage (Figure 22.4), and the zona pellucida, an eosinophilic band of homogenous mucopolysaccharide, forms between the granulosa cells and the germ cell: the stromal cells which immediately surround the follicle form an inner and outer layer, the theca interna and theca externa respectively. The theca interna cells are recognized by their rounded shape and variable lipid content, whilst the cells of the theca externa have large oval to spindle-shaped nuclei and are usually less clearly demarcated from the surrounding stroma.

As follicular maturation proceeds, the granulosa cells increase in number, mitoses are numerous, pseudoglandular structures, Call–Exner bodies, form where a ring of granulosa cells surrounds a small collection of acellular, hyaline, follicular fluid, and a larger cleft in the granulosa cell layer, in which follicular fluid (liquor folliculi) accumulates, forms the cavity or antrum of the Graafian follicle (Figure 22.5). The ovum enlarges and, surrounded by granulosa cells the inner layer of which is stratified to form the corona radiata, protrudes into the antrum forming the cumulus ovaricus. The granulosa cells at this stage are small, regular or minimally irregular cells with ill-defined, rather granular cytoplasm and darkly staining nuclei. No blood vessels penetrate this layer during this phase of development.

The Postovulatory Follicle

Ovulation is followed by collapse of the follicle. The granulosa cells proliferate, and under the influence of LH, become luteinized (Figure 22.6), their scanty cytoplasm becomes more voluminous, markedly eosinophilic and their cell margins more distinct. The thin-walled blood vessels of the theca interna penetrate the granulosa cell layer and the follicle fills with blood, a layer of fibrin and, later, fibrous tissue lines the follicle. The continuous layer of thecal cells becomes discontinuous, pyramidal clusters of luteinized thecal cells remain at the site of the vascular penetration between the lobules of granulosa cells, whilst elsewhere the theca becomes fibrous and indistinguishable from adjacent stromal cells.

The mature corpus luteum, which measures 1–2 cm in diameter, appears variably haemorrhagic and its wall pale to dark yellow. The central cavity contains fibrin and immature fibrous tissue, the inner wall is composed of luteinized granulosa cells arranged in festoons and there is an outer discontinuous layer of luteinized thecal cells (Figure 22.7). Clusters of stromal luteinized, hormone-secreting cells, remote and separate from the follicular structures, also occur throughout the reproductive years and persist in some women after the menopause.

If conception does not occur, the corpus luteum involutes; vacuoles appear in the cytoplasm of the luteal cells, their nuclei become pyknotic and gradually the cells become hyalinized and contracted to form the dense, eosinophilic, convoluted scar, the corpus albicans (Figure 22.8) which is gradually resorbed.

The Corpus Luteum in Pregnancy

If pregnancy ensues, the corpus luteum becomes larger and the cells derived from the theca interna, the

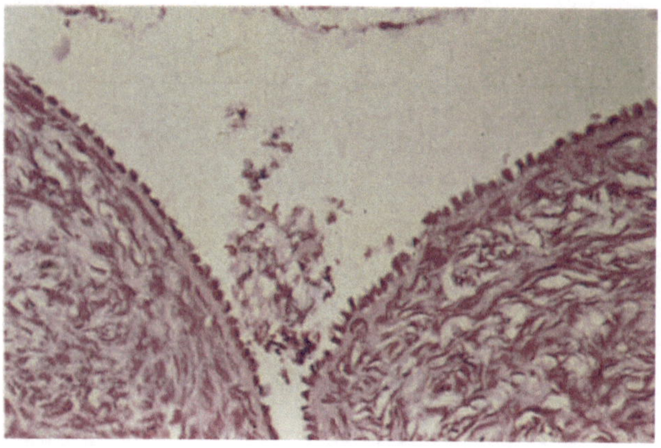

Figure 22.1 Ovary: normal surface epithelium. The surface epithelium is composed of small, regular, flattened cuboidal cells beneath which there is a narrow, pink-staining, homogenous tunica albuginea. The underlying stroma is normal. H & E × 250

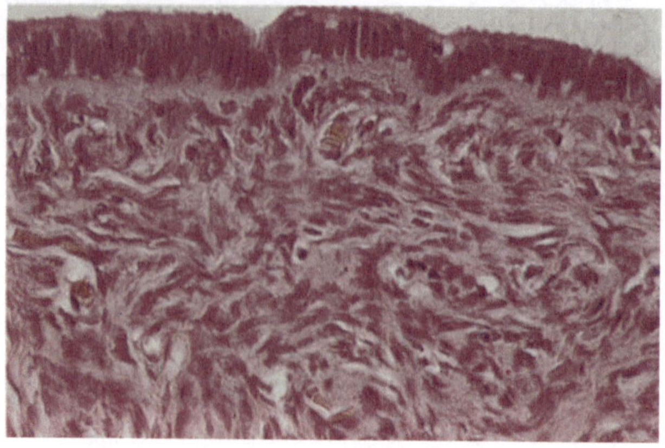

Figure 22.2 Ovary: metaplasia in surface epithelium. The surface epithelium is composed of tall columnar cells of endometrial type with elongated nuclei which lie at right angles to the basement membrane. In some places there is epithelial multilayering and occasional cells show vacuolation of the infranuclear cytoplasm. H & E × 250

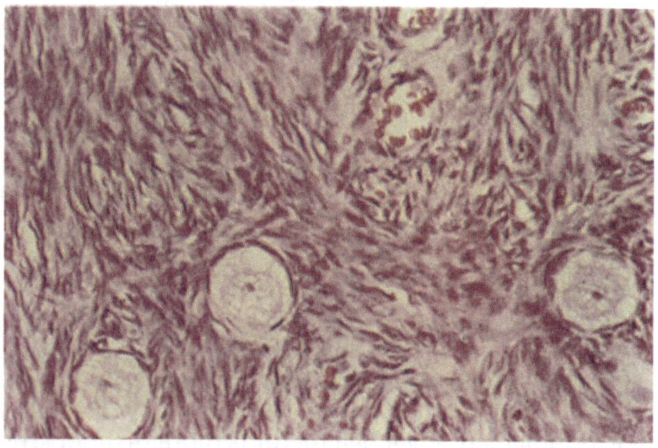

Figure 22.3 Ovary: primordial follicles. Three primordial follicles are present in the field. They have large, pale-staining central germ cells surrounded by a single layer of flattened darkly-staining granulosa cells. H & E × 250

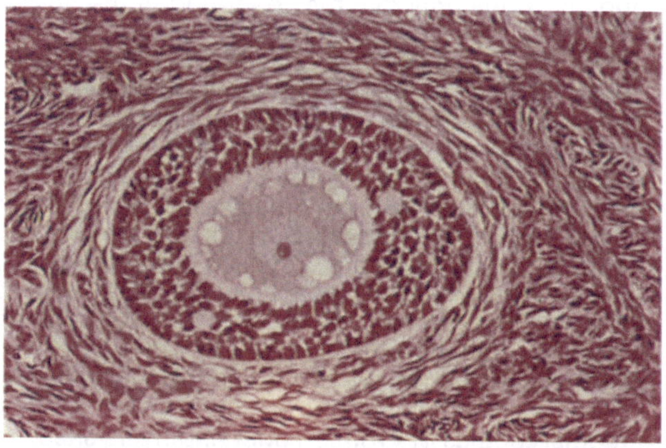

Figure 22.4 Ovary: primary follicle. The central germ cell, with a large pale nucleus, prominent eosinophilic nucleolus and pale cytoplasm, is separated from the granulosa cells by a narrow homogenous pink layer of mucopolysaccharide, the zona pellucida. The granulosa cells are plump and more numerous than in the primordial follicle and are forming pseudo-glandular structures, Call–Exner bodies. Within the bodies there is follicular fluid which appears as pink hyaline droplets. The stroma surrounding the follicle shows early differentiation into theca interna and externa, the cells can be distinguished from the surrounding stroma by their pallor and circumferential orientation. H & E × 250

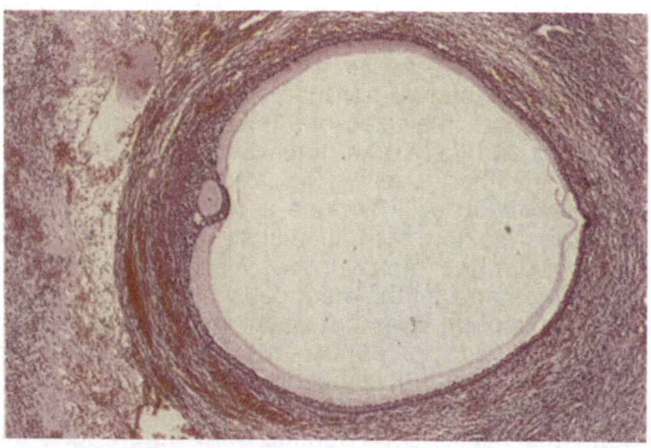

Figure 22.5 Ovary: Graafian follicle (antral follicle). The ovum, surrounded by the darkly-staining granulosa cells of the cumulus ovaricus, lies to the left of and protrudes into the antrum. An attenuated layer of granulosa cells surrounds the antrum outside which the thecal cells form a pale, spindle-celled outer layer, theca externa and a more darkly-staining round-celled inner layer, theca interna. The surrounding stroma is congested. H & E × 40

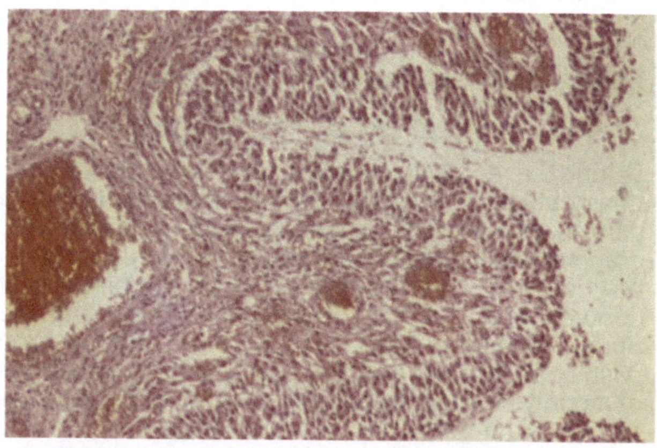

Figure 22.6 Ovary: early post-ovulatory follicle. The follicle, to the right, is lined by granulosa cells which stain less darkly than in the pre-ovulatory follicle. This is due to luteinization which is seen as an increase in eosinophilic cytoplasm and a reduction in nucleo–cytoplasmic ratio. The cells of the theca interna show a similar change. H & E × 100

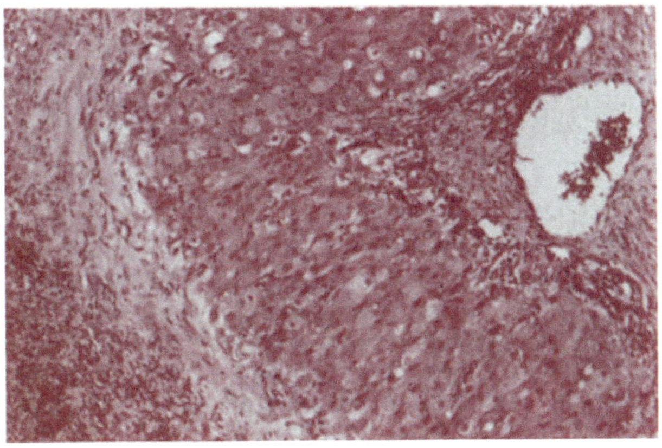

Figure 22.7 Ovary: corpus luteum. The central cavity of the corpus lies to the left and is filled by blood and immature fibrous tissue. The granulosa cells, forming the inner layer of the wall, are large, have small central nuclei and dense, copious eosinophilic luteinized cytoplasm. The smaller, luteinized thecal cells form an irregular, discontinuous outer layer and stain more darkly in this section. H & E x 100

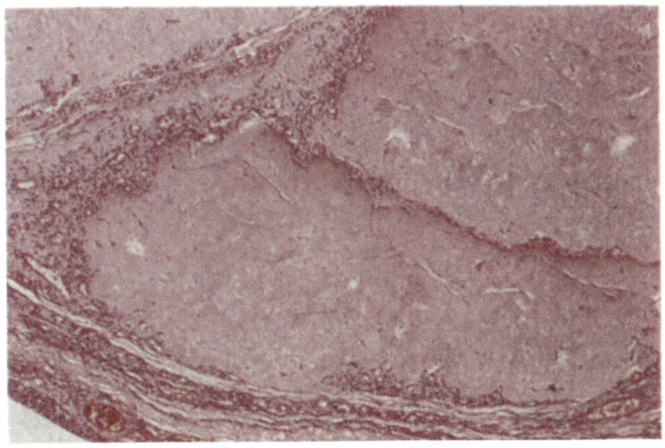

Figure 22.8 Ovary: corpus albicans. The centre of the field is occupied by two adjacent corpora albicantia. They are composed of hyalinized fibrous tissue and still have the somewhat scalloped outline of the corpora lutea from which they develop. H & E x 40

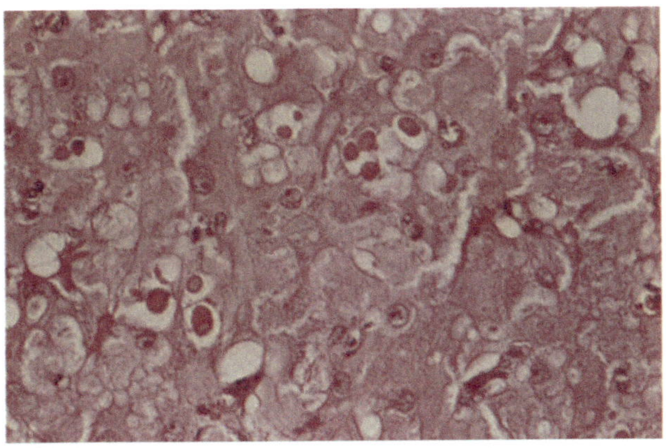

Figure 22.9 Ovary: corpus luteum of pregnancy. The granulosa cells are heavily luteinized, have copious eosinophilic cytoplasm and large nuclei with prominent nucleoli. Pink hyalinized colloid bodies or droplets can be seen lying between the granulosa cells. H & E x 250

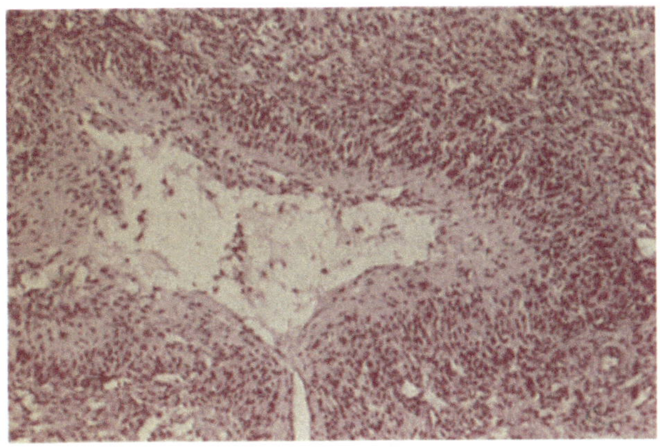

Figure 22.10 Ovary: atretic follicle. Atresia occurred in this follicle after the development of the antrum. The wall is formed by a rather ill-defined layer of small, regular, darkly-staining granulosa cells and the lumen has collapsed leaving a stellate cavity which is partly filled by young granulation tissue. In time this will shrink further leaving a corpus fibrosa. H & E x 100

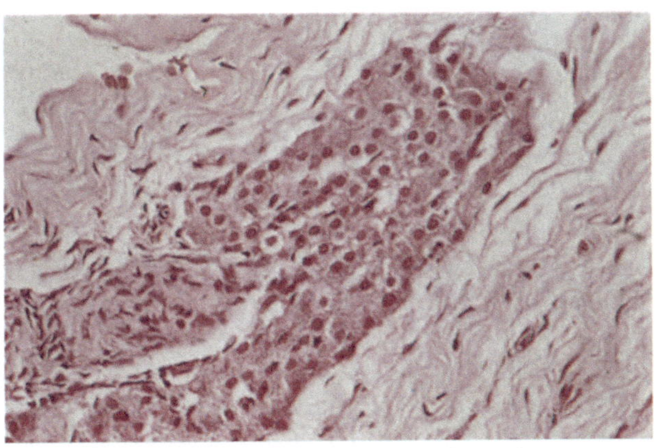

Figure 22.11 Ovary: hilar cells. A cluster of large round hilus cells with central round or ovoid nuclei and copious eosinophilic cytoplasm lie adjacent to a nerve in the ovarian hilum. Several small clusters of cells may be present. H & E x 250

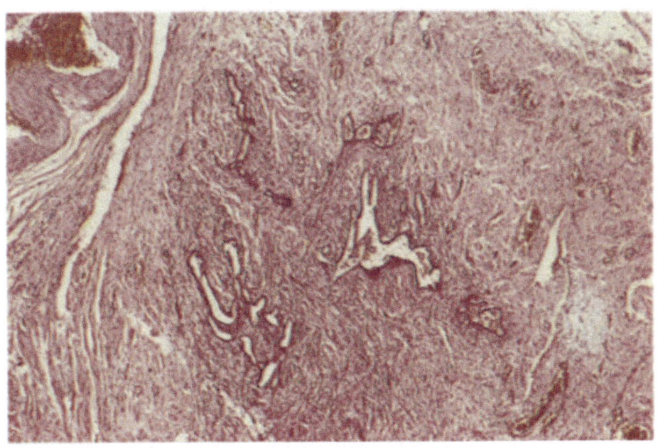

Figure 22.12 Ovary: rete ovarii. Within the ovarian hilum, the rete ovarii forms an irregular cluster of tubules lined by flattened cuboidal cells and surrounded by stroma of ovarian cortical type. H & E x 40

paralutein cells, become particularly large. Hyalinized colloid bodies or droplets appear among the granulosa cells (Figure 22.9), and ultimately calcified foci appear in the same areas[2]. The luteinized cells slowly become hyalinized and the corpus involutes after 2–3 months.

Follicular Atresia

Not all ova pass through the full sequence of the maturational process; the vast majority degenerate at a very early stage of development leaving no visible trace but others become atretic after reaching a considerable degree of development, the exact appearance then depending upon the degree of maturation at the time of its demise (Figure 22.10). As growth ceases, the granulosa cell nuclei become pyknotic, the cumulus sloughs off and floats into the antrum, granulation tissue replaces the lumen and a fibrous scar results, the corpus fibrosa; this is similar to, but smaller and smoother in outline than, the corpus albicans. Theca interna cells are often large and well-developed in these atretic follicles[2].

The Ovary after the Menopause

During the reproductive years, the germ cells are progressively depleted, mainly through the process of atresia, but some by maturation. By the time of the menopause all follicular activity has ceased, the ovarian surface has become wrinkled and the cortex narrow although in some women there is a minor degree of diffuse or nodular cortical thickening. The distinction between this appearance and that of hyperplasia is, to some extent, purely arbitrary.

The Ovarian Hilum

Hilar cells are morphologically similar to the Leydig cells of the testis. They are large cells with round nuclei, and granular eosinophilic cytoplasm in which occasional Reinke crystals occur (Figure 22.11). They lie in one of several clusters around the autonomic nerves, the tubules of the rete ovarii or adjacent to stromal nodules at the ovarian hilum. They may also be seen in the mesovarium.

The tubules of the rete ovarii are small, irregular and lined by a single layer of cubo-columnar cells. The cell margins are clearly defined, the nuclei round to oval and the cytoplasm scanty but sometimes more copious and clear to produce a transitional-like epithelium (Figure 22.12); mitoses are not usually seen. The surrounding tissue may closely resemble ovarian cortex but is separate from the main cortex.

References

1. Blaustein, A. (1982). Anatomy and histology of the human ovary. In Blaustein, A. (ed.). *Pathology of the Female Genital Tract.* 2nd edn. (New York, Heidelberg, Berlin: Springer-Verlag)
2. Scully, R. E. (1979). Tumors of the ovary and maldeveloped gonads. *Atlas of Tumor Pathology. 2nd Series. Fascicle 16.* (Washington, D.C.: Armed Forces Institute of Pathology)

Ovary: Cysts and Tumour-Like Conditions

23

Apart from endometriosis, the non-neoplastic cysts of the ovary develop almost exclusively from either the follicle or the ovarian surface epithelium.

Cysts of Follicular Origin

Follicular Cysts

Follicular cysts occur in the fetus, the neonate and in the prepubertal child but are most common during the reproductive years. Although the follicle includes a cyst or antrum during its normal development, the term follicular cyst is customarily reserved for those cysts exceeding 1 cm in diameter. Such cysts, which are commonly multiple, form in the ovarian cortex and are usually 2–3 cm in diameter but may, rarely, measure up to 10 cm in diameter. They often impart a bosselated appearance to the ovary and may bulge from the surface; they are thin-walled and contain clear, colourless, or faintly yellow, serous fluid. They are lined by multilayered granulosa cells which are small round cells with well-defined, darkly staining, granular nuclei, a high nucleo–cytoplasmic ratio, scanty basophilic cytoplasm and ill-defined cell margins (Figure 23.1). The surrounding thecal stromal cells are spindle-shaped and also have ill-defined cell margins. In practice, follicular cysts are more commonly encountered when they already show evidence of atresia and their granulosa cell lining has become compressed, or has been covered by a layer of granulation or fibrous tissue, (Figure 23.2). During the period of regression, the cyst lumen is filled by a fibrous plug and the granulosa and thecal cells buried in the wall gradually become less distinct, ultimately leaving the small fibrous scar with a smooth or only minimally irregular contour known as a corpus fibrosa.

Luteinized Follicular Cyst

In many cases the follicular cyst shows evidence of luteinization both in the granulosa and thecal cell layers; the granulosa cells thus become a little enlarged, their cytoplasm clear or granular and eosinophilic and the cells of the theca interna are recognized as a continuous layer of large cells with eosinophilic cytoplasm and round, regular central nuclei lying outside the granulosa cell layer (Figure 23.3).

Corpus Luteum Cyst

Haemorrhage normally occurs into the corpus luteum at the time of ovulation, and the cavity later becomes obliterated by fibrous tissue. In some cases this obliteration is slow, regression of the corpus is delayed and the resulting cyst has a wall in which the typical structure of the corpus luteum can be identified (Figure 23.4). Such cysts often continue to secrete progesterone and are associated with abnormalities of the menstrual cycle, including delayed shedding[1].

Corpus Albicans Cyst

If resolution of the corpus luteum cyst is further delayed, and the cavity persists, the luteinized cells within the wall may gradually become hyalinized and a corpus albicans cyst results (Figure 23.5). These cysts have the scalloped margin so typical of the corpus luteum.

Corpus Luteum Cyst of Pregnancy

The corpus luteum of pregnancy, which is frequently cystic, is characterized by the presence of colloid droplets among the luteinized granulosa cells (Figure 23.6) and, later, calcified foci with a similar distribution are seen. The corpus persists for 2–3 months or so before the lutein cells become progressively hyalinized and finally a corpus albicans results.

Large or Giant Luteinized Follicular Cyst of Pregnancy and Puerperium

Young women with this rare condition present with a palpable abdominal mass in pregnancy or the puerperium, or a unilateral ovarian cyst is discovered unexpectedly at Caesarean section[2]. The cysts range in size from 8 to 26 cm, have thin walls and contain clear serous or sero-sanguineous fluid or, occasionally, mucoid material. They are lined by single or multiple layers of luteinized granulosa cells, the cytoplasm of which varies in appearance, some being densely eosinophilic whilst others show cytoplasmic vacuolation. The nuclei are mainly small, round and regular but focal bizarre hyperchromatic nuclei, sometimes exhibiting pleomorphism, are a common finding (Figure 23.7): mitoses are not, however, seen. The luteinized layer is penetrated by capillaries, and where there is shedding of the luteinized cells, the cyst is lined by fibrin or fibrous tissue. The cyst wall is fibrous and contains clusters of luteinized cells similar to those lining the cyst. These cysts differ from the ordinary luteinized follicular cysts in that they show no differentiation into granulosa and thecal cell layers.

Theca-lutein Cyst (*Hyperreactio Luteinalis*)

Lutein cysts occur in normal pregnancy but are more common in multiple pregnancy, hydatidiform mole and choriocarcinoma. The use of ovulation-stimulating hormones has occasionally induced this

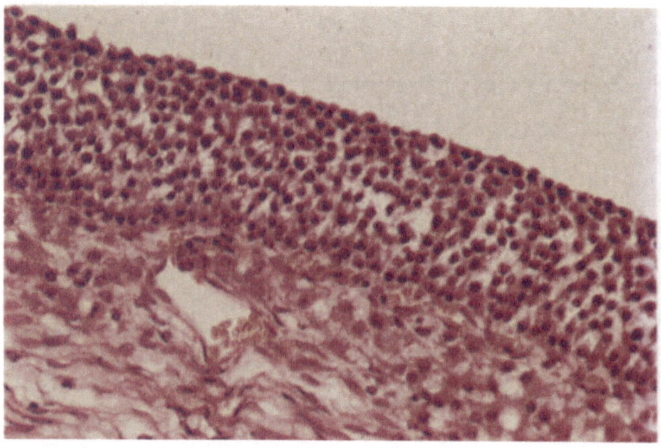

Figure 23.1 Ovary: follicular cyst. The cyst is lined by a broad band of uniform granulosa cells with regular, darkly-staining nuclei, and eosinophilic cytoplasm. The larger, round, pale cells of the theca interna lie deep to the granulosa cell layer. H & E × 250

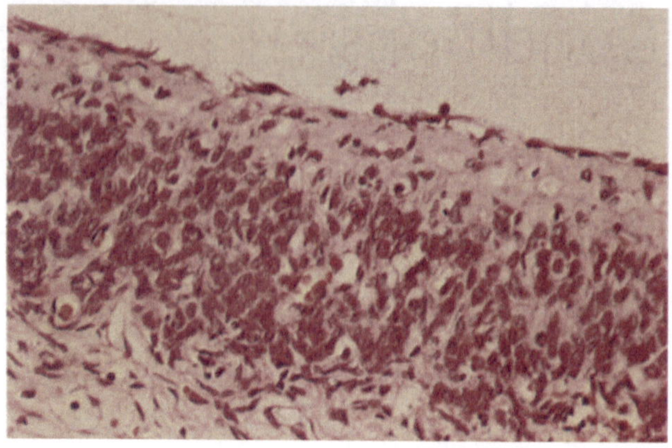

Figure 23.2 Ovary: atretic follicular cyst. The cyst is lined by a flattened layer of cells of indeterminate type but the identifying feature is the band of small, dark granulosa cells with the high nucleo–cytoplasmic ratios which lie deep within the wall. H & E × 25

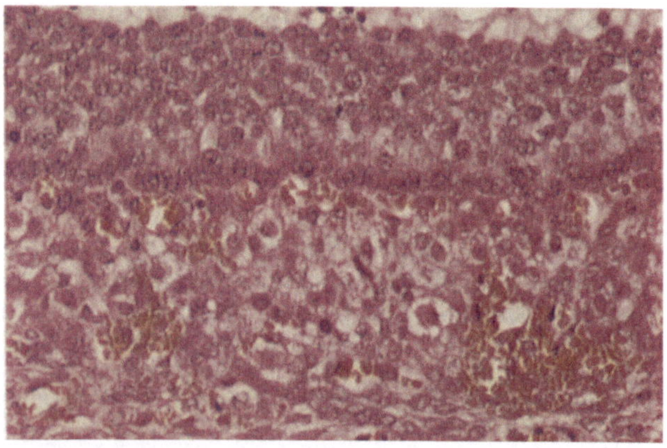

Figure 23.3 Ovary: luteinized follicular cyst. The cyst is lined by granulosa cells which have eosinophilic cytoplasm and regular nuclei; mitoses are present. Immediately deep to the granulosa cells the more conspicuously luteinized cells of the theca interna form a band. Their nuclei are large, round and central and their cytoplasm eosinophilic and focally vacuolated. The cells of the theca externa no longer form a distinct layer. H & E × 250

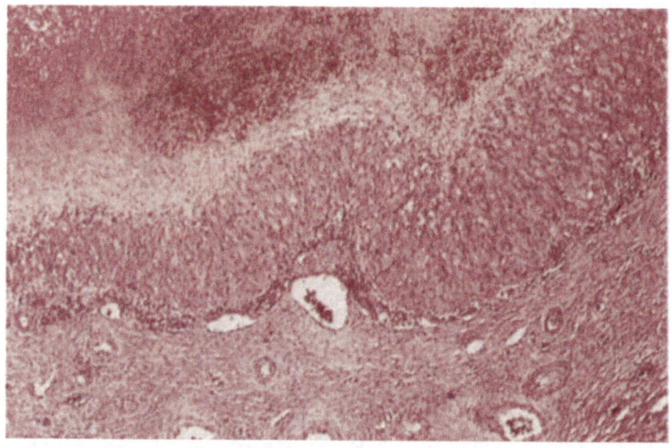

Figure 23.4 Ovary: cystic corpus luteum. The cyst lumen, which contains fibrin and blood, lies to the top of the field. It is lined by a thin layer of fibrous tissue covering an inner band of heavily luteinized granulosa cells with copious eosinophilic cytoplasm and an outer, discontinuous layer of smaller darker luteinized thecal cells. H & E × 40

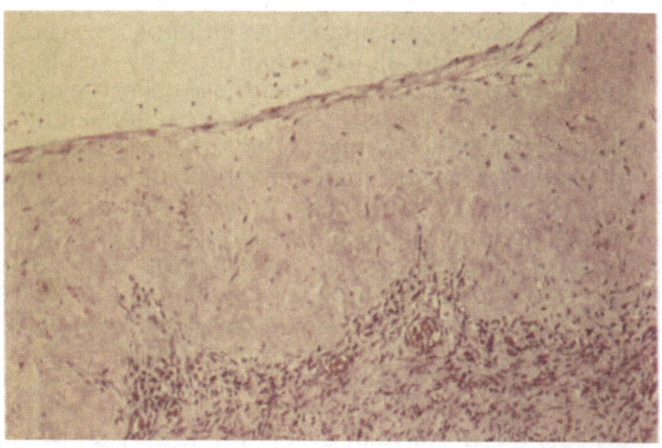

Figure 23.5 Ovary: corpus albicans cyst. The cyst wall is formed by the hyalinized festoons of the corpus albicans and is lined (above) by a thin layer of flattened fibrous tissue. It is not unusual to see calcified foci in the walls of such cysts. H & E × 100

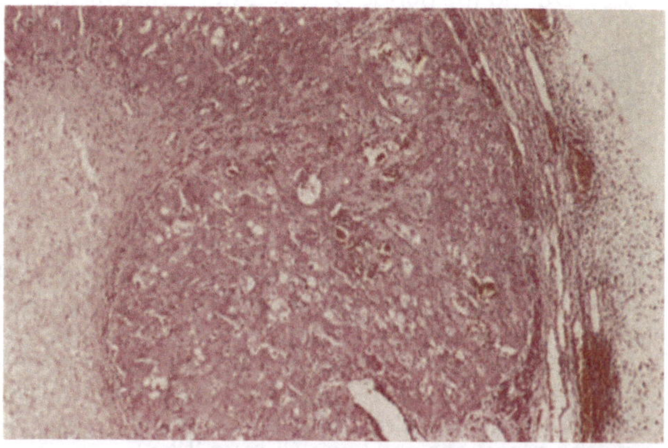

Figure 23.6 Ovary: cystic corpus luteum of pregnancy. This cyst was removed from a patient who had an ectopic pregnancy. The lumen lies to the left and the wall is formed by successive layers of granulation tissue, heavily luteinized granulosa cells and a discontinuous layer of luteinized thecal cells. H & E × 40

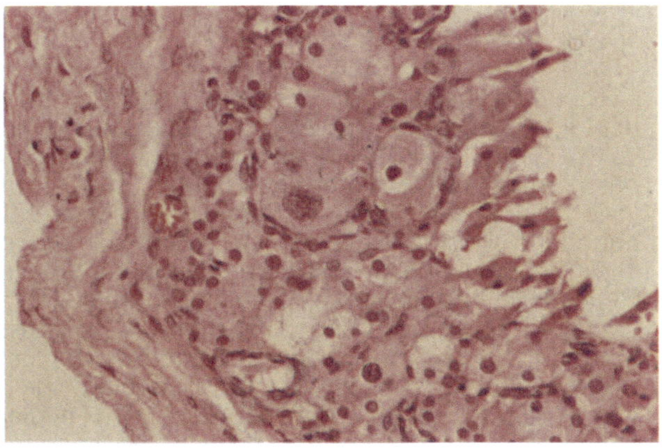

Figure 23.7 Ovary: giant follicular cyst of pregnancy. This cyst was 19 cm in diameter. It is lined (to the right) by several layers of heavily luteinized pleomorphic granulosa cells. The cytoplasm in some cells is densely eosinophilic whilst in others (particularly to the lower left) there is cytoplasmic vacuolation. The degree of nuclear pleomorphism is quite striking. H & E × 250

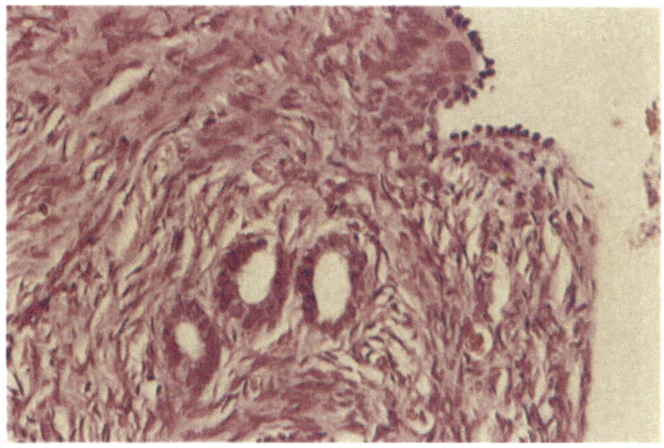

Figure 23.8 Ovary: germinal inclusion cysts. Immediately deep to the surface epithelium lie three germinal inclusion cysts. Their lining epithelium is cubo–columnar in contrast to the flattened cuboidal surface epithelium (to the right) from which they arise. H & E × 250

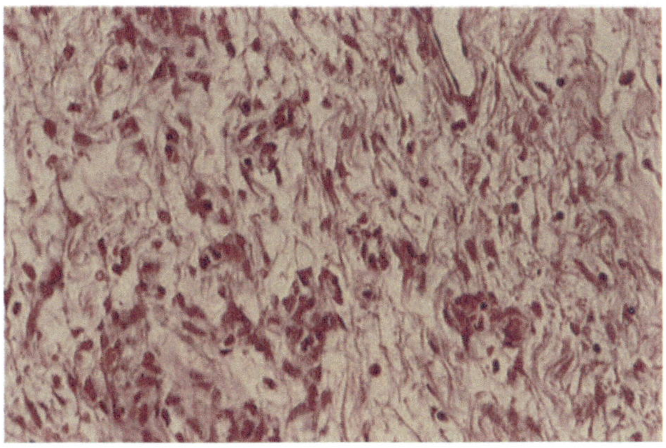

Figure 23.9 Ovary: oedema. The field shows extremely oedematous stroma in which there are clusters of larger cells with eosinophilic cytoplasm and rather ill-defined cell boundaries. These latter cells are luteinized stromal cells. The sprinkling of small cells with darkly staining nuclei are mast cells and macrophages. H & E × 250

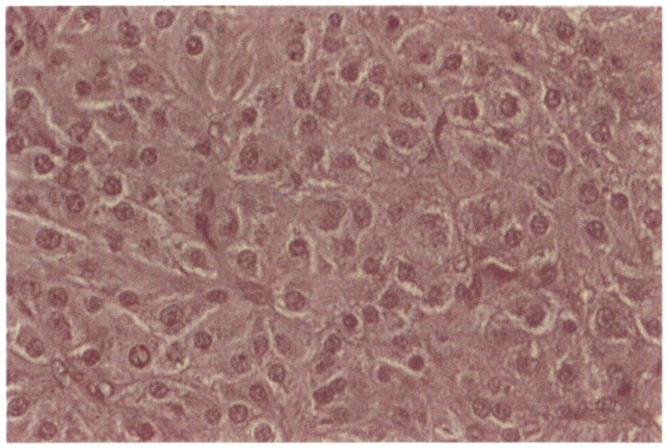

Figure 23.10 Ovary: luteoma of pregnancy. The lesion is composed of lobules formed by large, uniform cells with round, central nuclei and copious eosinophilic cytoplasm. Fine fibrous bands can be seen between the lobules. H & E × 250

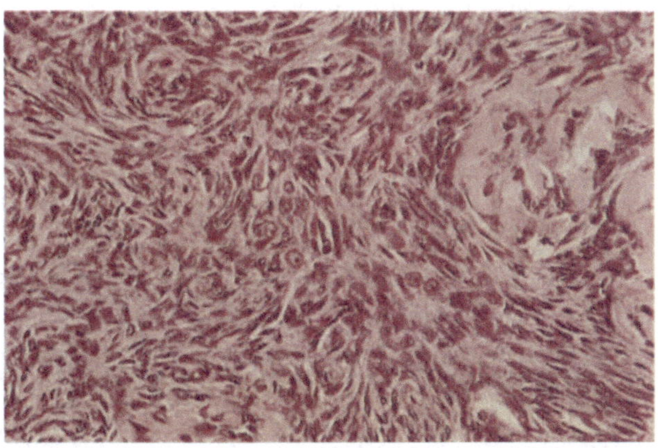

Figure 23.11 Ovary: stromal hyperplasia. This field is typical of the appearance seen in several stromal nodules present in the ovary of a 56-year-old patient who presented with post-menopausal bleeding. The stromal cells have more copious eosinophilic cytoplasm than normal and some are particularly enlarged and rounded. H & E × 250

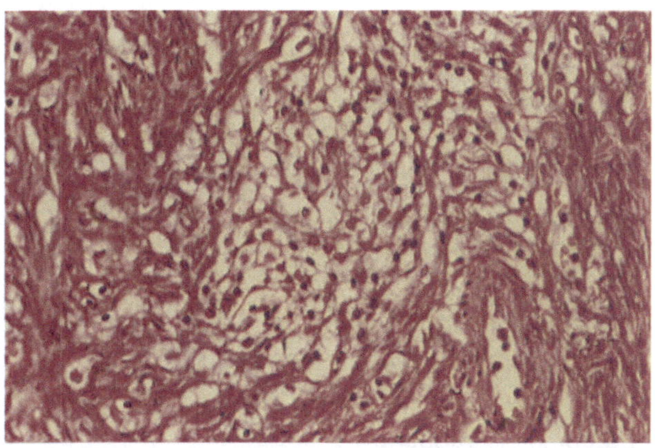

Figure 23.12 Ovary: hyperthecosis. This cluster of larger luteinized cells with clear cytoplasm, distinct cell boundaries and small rather densely staining central nuclei is from the ovarian medulla of a patient with stromal hyperplasia. Many such foci were present. H & E × 250

change, particularly in patients with polycystic ovaries[3] (Stein–Leventhal syndrome).

The lesions usually present late in pregnancy or in the puerperium as bilateral ovarian enlargements, and occasionally there is maternal virilization. The ovaries contain multiple cysts which often contain blood and their walls contain yellowish nodules. Microscopically, there is luteinization of the theca interna and in some instances the granulosa cell layer, although more commonly the granulosa cells are atrophic. Nuclear pleomorphism if present is usually slight.

Germinal Inclusion Cysts

Germinal inclusion cysts occur at all ages but are most common towards the end of the reproductive era. They arise when the surface epithelium of the ovary becomes invaginated and subsequently sequestrated within the ovarian cortex to form a cyst. Such cysts are quite arbitrarily defined as non-neoplastic when their diameter is less than 3 cm whilst cysts of a similar origin greater than 3 cm in diameter are regarded as neoplastic. The cysts lie superficially or deep in the cortex and may be single but more commonly are multiple and of microscopic size. They are lined by flattened or cubo-columnar cells and the epithelium may undergo metaplasia to a serous, mucus-secreting, endometrial or clear cell pattern (Figure 23.8); they usually contain clear serous fluid.

Tumour-like Lesions of the Ovary

Massive Ovarian Oedema

Massive oedema of the ovary is uncommon. It presents in young women or children as an abdominal mass and is usually unilateral[4]. Although menstrual irregularities are frequent, evidence of gross hormonal abnormalities, such as virilization, is less usual.

The finding of incomplete mesovarian torsion in these cases with venous and lymphatic obstruction suggests that ischaemia due to chronic or recurrent torsion may be the main aetiological factor.

The cut surface is white, glistening and moist with cystic spaces containing proteinous fluid. Histologically, eosinophilic oedema fluid is present in the medulla and inner cortex (Figure 23.9), whilst the outer layers of the cortex are spared. Dilated blood vessels are present and focal haemorrhage may occur; collagen fibres are widely separated. Sometimes in the areas where atretic primary and secondary follicles can be identified, the stroma is less oedematous and more cellular. Luteinized cells are seen in clusters throughout the oedematous areas and are particularly marked in those patients with evidence of excess testosterone and oestrogen production; macrophages and mast cells are also often present.

Luteoma of Pregnancy

These tumour-like, hyperplastic lesions are solid, single or multiple, often bilateral, ovarian masses discovered incidentally at the time of Caesarean section or postpartum tubal ligation or sometimes as a mass in the puerperium. They are associated with mild maternal virilization in 30% of cases and female infants are virilized in 30% of such cases[2].

They are believed to develop from the theca minterna[5], and the masses are circumscribed tan, yellow-brown or grey-brown nodules with focal haemorrhages. Histologically (Figure 23.10), the lesion comprises lobules of large round cells with abundant eosinophilic granular, or less commonly, vacuolated cytoplasm and large pleomorphic nuclei. Reticulin stains reveal an alveolar structure. Occasionally the cells are arranged in acinar-like structures around colloid material, and colloid in the cytoplasm is similar to that seen in the corpus luteum of pregnancy. Focal balloon degeneration with nuclear pyknosis and cytoplasmic hyaline degeneration is not uncommon; mitoses are frequent but atypical forms do not occur. These lesions resolve spontaneously and become clinically undetectable within a few weeks or months of the end of the pregnancy.

Stromal Hyperplasia and Hyperthecosis

The distinction between stromal hyperplasia and the minimal stromal proliferation or thickening seen in the normal postmenopausal ovary is to some extent arbitrary and the conditions merge imperceptibly[3], the use of the term hyperplasia often being restricted to stromal foci exceeding 2 mm in diameter[3].

Stromal hyperplasia results in bilateral ovarian enlargement of up to 7 cm in diameter: the ovaries are rounded and the parenchyma is often almost completely replaced by grey-pink or yellow-grey firm tissue. The hyperplastic stroma, which may be diffuse or nodular and is composed of cells similar to, but plumper than, normal stromal cells, is centred mainly in the medulla and fans out towards the cortex where there may be nodules. Within the hyperplastic stroma of the medulla and, to a lesser extent, in the cortex there are frequently clusters of pale luteinized stromal cells (Figure 23.12), this change being termed hyperthecosis. Although foci of luteinized stromal cells occur in the normal ovary it is usually most florid in the hyperplastic ovary. Stromal hyperplasia and hyperthecosis may be associated with features of virilization and the occasional occurrence of oestrogenic phenomena is due to the peripheral conversion of androgens to oestrogens[6].

References

1. Blaustein, A. (1982). Non-neoplastic cysts of the ovary. In Blaustein, A. (ed.) *Pathology of the Female Genital Tract*. 2nd edn. (New York, Heidelberg and Berlin: Springer-Verlag)
2. Clement, P. B. and Scully, R. E. (1980). Large solitary luteinized follicle cyst of pregnancy and puerperium. A clinicopathological analysis of eight cases. *Am. J. Surg. Pathol.*, **4**, 431–438
3. Scully, R. E. (1979). Tumors of the ovary and maldeveloped gonads. *Atlas of Tumor Pathology, 2nd Series, Fascicle 16*. (Washington, D.C.: Armed Forces Institute of Pathology)
4. Spinas, G. A., Heitz, Ph. U., Oberholzer, M., Torhorst, J., Stahl, M. and Girard, J. (1981). Massive ovarian oedema with production of testosterone. *Virch. Arch.* (*Pathol. Anat.*), **390**, 365–371
5. Honoré, L. H., and O'Hara, K. E. (1978). Incidental pregnancy luteoma associated with ectopic tubo-ovarian pregnancy: evidence in favor of origin from theca interna of an atretic follicle. *Eur. J. Obstet., Gynecol. Reprod. Biol.*, **8**, 15–19
6. Aiman, J., Edman, C. D., Worley, R. J., Vellios, F. and Macdonald, P. C. (1978). Androgen and estrogen formation in women with ovarian hyperthecosis. *Obstet. Gynecol.*, **51**, 1–9

Ovary: Miscellaneous Disorders 24

Inflammation

Peri-oophoritis

Inflammatory processes in the pelvic organs often involve the ovaries because of their close proximity. Inflammation reaching the ovary in this fashion may be acute or chronic, is limited to the ovarian surface and immediately contiguous stroma and is termed peri-oophoritis. The most common source of infection is the Fallopian tube but peritonitis secondary to acute appendicitis or diverticular disease of the colon may also involve the ovary.

In the acute phase the ovary is covered by a fibrinous exudate containing neutrophil polymorphs and the adjacent stroma is oedematous; a few acute inflammatory cells may be seen in the cortex. Adhesions tend to form rapidly between the involved structures and if these fail to resolve, as is usually the case, vascular fibrous adhesions or a dense layer of fibrous tissue remain on the ovarian surface (Figure 24.1). The surface epithelium which becomes sequestrated beneath the fibrous tissue may show papillary hyperplasia, reactive cytological changes or metaplasia and can form cysts.

Acute Oophoritis

Acute infection of the ovary occurs most commonly by direct extension from adjacent organs, but may also be due to spread via the blood stream and lymphatics in patients who have had recent surgical procedures elsewhere in the genital tract, and in women with mumps. The ovary is red, oedematous, swollen and covered in fibrin. Histologically, a neutrophil polymorph infiltrate is usually limited to the surface and the superficial part of the cortex (Figure 24.2).

Intraovarian Abscess

Infection can enter the ovary by way of a recently ruptured follicle[1] and may therefore be deep-seated; it is generally caused by a variety of anaerobic organisms. The ovary may appear superficially normal, but on section a unilocular, thick-walled cavity is seen which contains pus, and histologically a neutrophil and fibrinous exudate fills a cavity lined by foamy macrophages, non-specific granulation tissue and fibrous tissue (Figure 24.3). The remnants of a follicle or corpus luteum may form part of the wall. In other cases a tubo-ovarian abscess forms, and a mass develops which so distorts the structures that the exact site of the abscess may only be identified after histological examination.

Infection by *Actinomyces* which may occur via the lower genital tract in IUCD wearers or spread directly from the bowel, although rare, produces a typical yellow-white honeycomb abscess in which the pus contains the classical sulphur granules. Histologically, the locules are filled with neutrophil polymorphs in which there are colonies of the organisms (Figure 24.4), these appear basophilic in haematoxylin and eosin stained sections and Gram stains show blue, filamentous radiating colonies with Gram negative peripheral clubs. The abscess walls are formed by macrophages, often with strikingly clear cytoplasm, granulation tissue and fibrous tissue.

Crohn's Disease

Crohn's disease rarely affects the ovary but when it does so this is usually the consequence of direct spread from adjacent diseased bowel. If there are extensive peritoneal adhesions, or intestinal fistulae, a peri-oophoritis may be apparent with dense fibrous adhesions forming between the bowel and ovary. Histologically, the adhesions may be entirely non-specific but non-caseating, tuberculoid granulomata can occur both in the fibrous tissue and in the ovary (Figure 24.5). The Fallopian tube is usually affected simultaneously.

The Ovary in Infertility

The Polycystic Ovary

The polycystic ovary is the morphological counterpart of the clinical Stein–Leventhal syndrome which consists of oligomenorrhoea, infertility and hirsutism. A series of histological features define the condition but a diagnosis can be made in the absence of the complete picture: the clinical picture also varies considerably, infertility being the most constant component.

Typically there is bilateral ovarian enlargement, although this may be minimal or absent; this is due to an increased number of developing and atretic cystic follicles (Figure 24.6) and to thickening of the cortical and medullary stroma which may show focal luteinization, hyperthecosis; the tunica, or capsule, is collagenized and thickened in most cases. It is not uncommon to see a band of primordial and primary follicles below the thickened capsule (Figure 24.7) although their total number is not increased[2]. In the complete syndrome there is a temporary or permanent absence of ovulation, but in the majority of cases corpora albicantia, indicating previous ovulation, are present and corpora lutea may be seen, reflecting more recent ovulation, in 20% of cases. Theca lutein hyperplasia may occasionally be noted, both developing and atretic follicles being luteinized (Figure

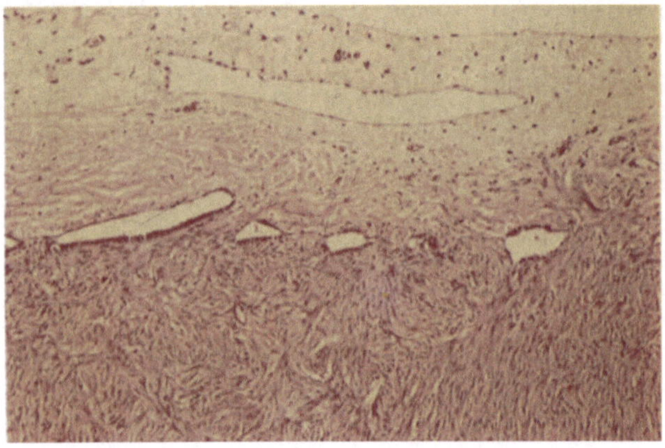

Figure 24.1 Ovary: chronic peri-oophoritis. The ovarian surface is covered by fine fibrovascular adhesions. The surface epithelium of the ovary is sequestrated beneath the adhesions and is forming a series of small cysts, lined by flattened cubo–columnar cells, across the middle of the field. Reactive hyperplasia, metaplasia and cytological atypia in these cysts can be distinguished from neoplasia by the absence of malignant nuclear features and atypical mitoses. H & E × 100

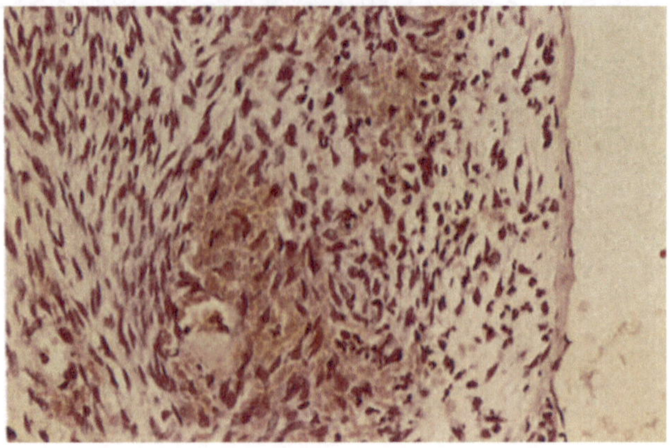

Figure 24.2 Ovary: acute oophoritis. The ovarian surface lies to the right. The surface epithelium has been shed and the superficial part of the stroma is congested and infiltrated by polymorphonuclear leukocytes. The deeper stroma (to the right) is of fairly normal appearance. H & E × 250

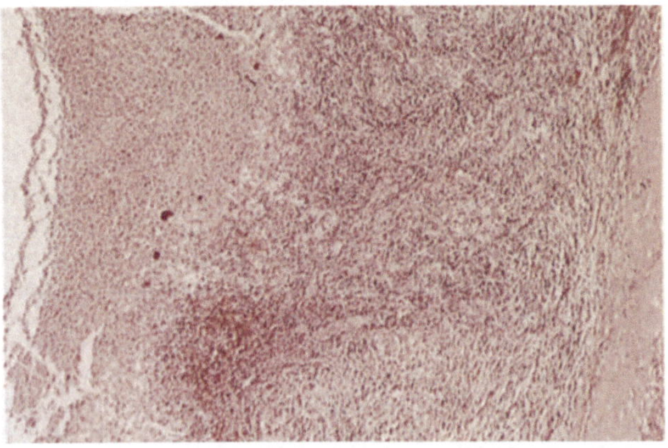

Figure 24.3 Ovary: intraovarian abscess. The specimen came from a young woman who had developed an intraovarian abscess following bilateral acute salpingitis. The abscess cavity, to the left, contains a polymorphonuclear leukocyte exudate and the wall is formed by successive layers of immature and mature granulation tissue and fibrous tissue. H & E × 40

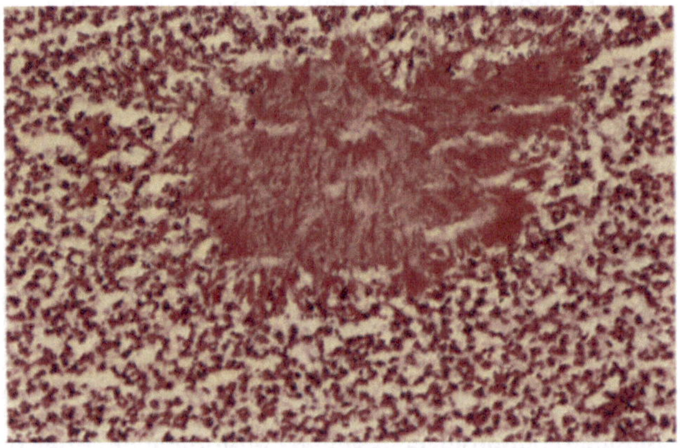

Figure 24.4 Ovary: actinomycotic abscess. This section was taken from the centre of an abscess locule. It shows a typical colony of actinomyces formed by radiating filaments, in the midst of an inflammatory exudate consisting mainly of polymorphonuclear leukocytes and containing a few macrophages. H & E × 250

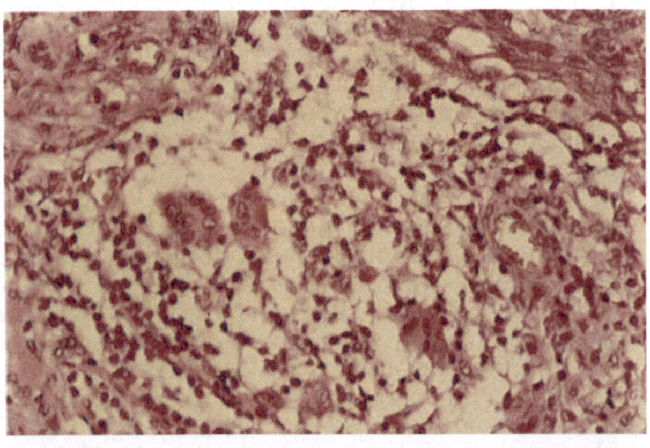

Figure 24.5 Ovary: Crohn's disease. The centre of the field shows a typical non-caseating, tuberculoid granuloma formed by epithelial macrophages, four macrophage giant cells and a cuff of lymphocytes. Many similar granulomata were seen in the rest of the ovary and the adjacent fallopian tube. The patient had suffered from intestinal Crohn's disease for many years. H & E × 250

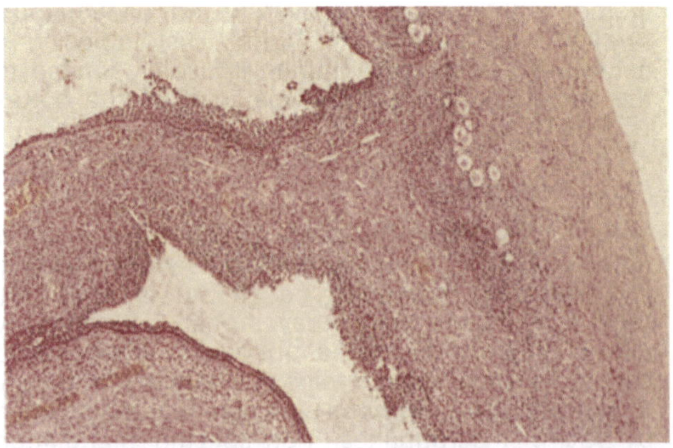

Figure 24.6 Ovary: polycystic ovary. This is a general, and fairly typical example of a polycystic ovary from a woman of 21 years with the clinical features of Stein–Leventhal syndrome. The ovarian capsule (to the right) is collagenized and thickened; primordial follicles are clustered in the cortex and two luteinized follicular cysts are present. H & E × 40

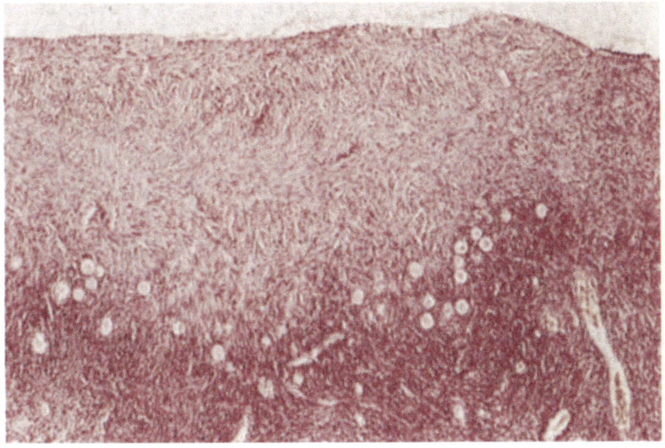

Figure 24.7 Ovary: polycystic ovary. Beneath a heavily collagenized ovarian capsule there are numerous primordial and primary follicles. The biopsy was from a young woman who was being investigated for infertility. H & E x 40

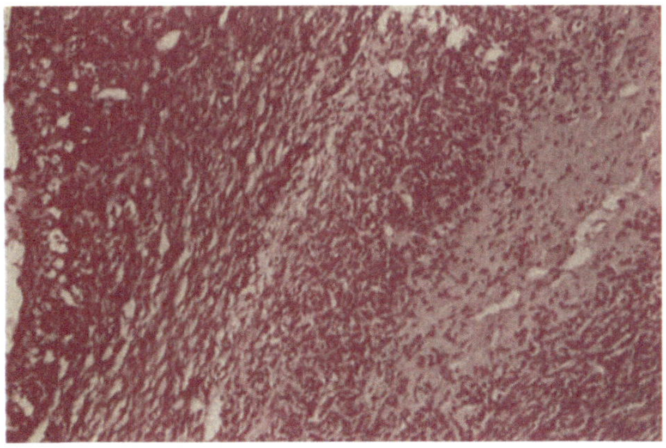

Figure 24.8 Ovary: polycystic ovary. To the right of the field is a corpus fibrosa surrounded by luteinized stromal cells and to the left is an atretic follicular cyst. In the wall of the latter can be seen luteinized granulosa cells, some of which are vacuolated, theca interna and luteinized theca externa cells which lie parallel to the cyst lumen. H & E x 100

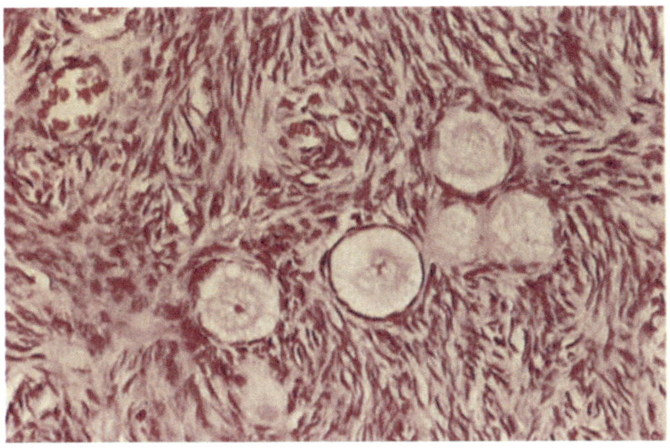

Figure 24.9 Ovary: gonadotrophin-resistant ovary. The ovarian cortex in this case showed numerous primordial follicles such as those seen here. Many show evidence of degeneration and atresia, particularly the three to the right of the field, whilst others appear normal. There is no evidence of previous or current follicular maturation. H & E x 250

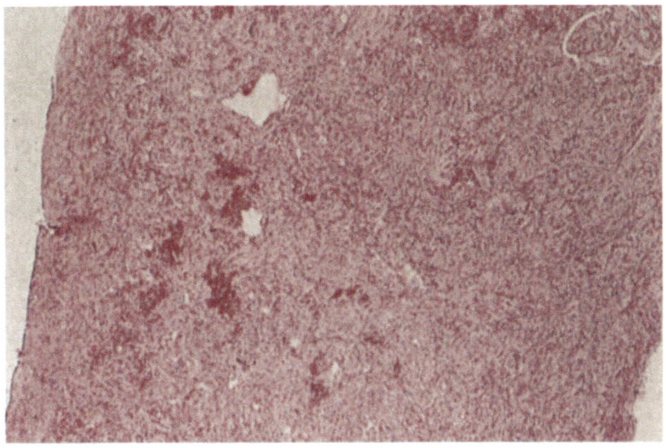

Figure 24.10 Ovary: streak gonad. The full width of the gonad is seen in this field from a laparoscopic biopsy. It is composed of stroma showing a hint of differentiation into a compact cortex and a more loosely organized medulla where there are small, thin-walled vascular channels. There are no follicles, corpora albicantia or corpora fibrosa which would suggest previous follicular activity. H & E x 40

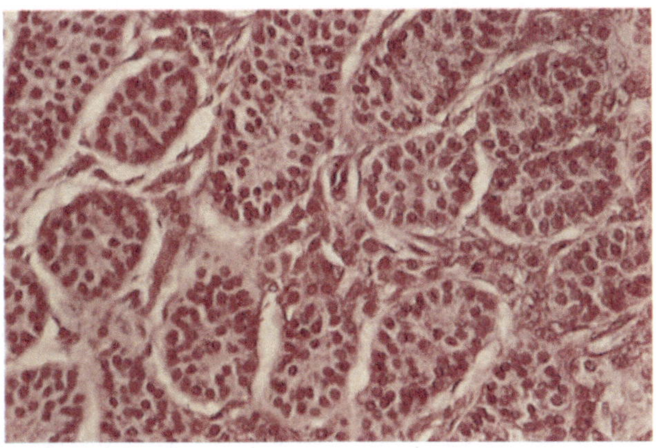

Figure 24.11 Testis: androgen insensitivity. The field shows a group of seminiferous tubules lined only by Sertoli cells. Several clusters of Leydig cells lie between the tubules. H & E x 250

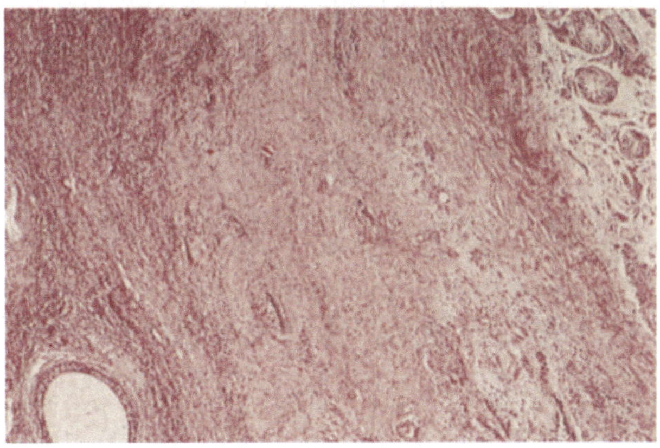

Figure 24.12 Gonad: ovotestis. In this field ovarian stroma to the lower left contains a cystic follicle and to the upper right there are seminiferous tubules lined only by Sertoli cells. Leydig cells are seen between the seminiferous tubules. The ovarian and testicular components of the gonad are separated by fibrous tissue. H & E x 40

24.8), but its reported prominence is probably more commonly a reflection of the increased number of follicles as the degree of luteinization of individual follicles appears to be no greater than normal[2].

Polycystic ovaries become larger the longer the condition persists due mainly to an increase in the quantity of cellular stroma[2].

Gonadotrophin Resistant Ovary

The histological features of the ovary in this syndrome are the presence of numerous primordial follicles showing no evidence of maturation or development (Figure 24.9) and a complete absence of corpora albicantia[3]. It is believed that the condition results from an absence of gonadotrophin receptors although this has not yet been proved.

Premature Menopause

The menopause is regarded as premature when it occurs before the age of 35 years. The appearance of the ovary in this condition is unremarkable and similar to that seen after a menopause occurring at the normal age. The ovary is small, the cortex narrow and corpora albicantia and fibrosa are present. In some patients the presence of few such structures may be a reflection of the primary paucity of germ cells which is believed to be the underlying abnormality in these patients[4].

Abnormal Gonadal Differentiation

Streak Gonad

In patients with gonadal dysgenesis, the most common form of which is Turner's syndrome (genotype 45 XO), the ovaries in the adult are represented only by a strip or nodule of grey-white fibrous tissue. Histologically, the gonad consists of whorls and sheets of fibrous tissue which may be randomly arranged but which in some cases show differentiation into an abortive cortex and medulla (Figure 24.10); cysts resembling germinal inclusion cysts lined by cuboidal epithelium may be present. There are no germ cells in the adult but in the fetus, and until the time of puberty, germ cells may be seen[5].

In patients with a 45 XO/46 XX genotype (Turner's mosaic) follicular development may occur, this possibly explaining the occurrence of pregnancy in occasional cases of apparent Turner's syndrome[6].

Androgen Insensitivity Syndrome (Testicular Feminization)

Patients with a 46 XY genotype, testes and a failure of end organ androgen receptors present as phenotypic females with breast development but no axillary or pubic hair. The structures derived from the Müllerian system, i.e. the cervix, uterus and Fallopian tubes are absent as there is no abnormality of Müllerian inhibitory factor production.

The gonads may lie in the abdominal cavity, in the inguinal region or in an inguinal hernial pouch; they are small and tend to have a somewhat bosselated appearance. On section, yellow-brown testicular tissue is contained within a tunica albuginea and grey-white, well-demarcated nodules may lie within the parenchyma. Histologically, the seminiferous tubules are small, narrow and lined only by Sertoli cells; spermatogenesis is absent. Leydig cells are numerous and normally disposed, the whole resembling the fetal testis (Figure 24.11). The nodules noted macroscopically are foci of tubular hyperplasia or tubular adenomata which form non-encapsulated but sharply demarcated clusters of enlarged seminiferous tubules lined by tall columnar Sertoli cells with clear cytoplasm. Leydig cells are absent from the nodules.

Ovotestis

In a true hermaphrodite both ovarian and testicular tissue is present; there may be a testis on one side and an ovary on the other, or a single gonad may contain a combination of ovarian and testicular tissue forming an ovotestis.

The ovarian tissue contains follicles in different stages of development and regression whilst the testicular tubules are lined only by Sertoli cells and primary spermatocytes (Figure 24.12), there being no spermatogenesis.

References

1. Blaustein, A. (1982). Inflammatory diseases of the ovary. In Blaustein, A., (ed.). *Pathology of the Female Genital Tract.* 2nd edn. (New York, Heidelberg and Berlin: Springer-Verlag)
2. Hughesdon, P. E. (1982). Morphology and morphogenesis of the Stein–Leventhal ovary and of so-called 'Hyperthecosis'. *Obstet. Gynecol. Surv.*, **37**, 59–77
3. Dalemans, P., Buytaert, P. and Meulyzer, P. (1979). The gonadotropin-resistant ovary syndrome in association with secondary amenorrhea. *Eur. J. Obstet. Gynecol. Reprod. Biol.*, **9**, 327–334
4. Board, J. A., Redwine, F. O., Moncure, C. W., Frable, W. J. and Taylor, J. R. (1979). Identification of differing etiologies of clinically diagnosed premature menopause. *Am. J. Obstet. Gynecol.*, **134**, 936–941
5. Singh, R. P. and Carr, D. H. (1966). The anatomy and histology of XO human embryos and fetuses. *Anat. Rec.*, **153**, 369–383
6. Nielsen, J., Sillesen, I. and Hansen, K. B. (1979). Fertility in women with Turner's syndrome: case report and review of literature. *Br. J. Obstet. Gynaecol.*, **86**, 833–835

Ovary: Benign Epithelial Neoplasms **25**

The epithelial group of ovarian tumours accounts for 60% of all primary neoplasms of the ovary. All are thought usually to originate from cells in the surface epithelium of the ovary, either arising directly from that epithelium or from epithelial fragments sequestrated into the ovarian cortex to form inclusion cysts[1]. The ovarian surface epithelium is the adult equivalent, and direct descendant, of the coelomic epithelium which, during embryonic life, overlies the nephro-genital ridge, and from which are derived the Müllerian ducts and the structures to which these give rise. It is believed that undifferentiated cells in the surface epithelium of the postnatal ovary retain a latent capacity to differentiate along the same pathways as do their embryonic precursors, and hence a neoplasm derived from these cells can differentiate along various Müllerian pathways, those differentiating along tubal epithelial lines forming the serous group of neoplasms, those following an endocervical route being the mucinous tumours and those differentiating along an endometrial pathway forming the endometrioid group of neoplasms. The Brenner tumour usually originates from the surface epithelium but is, however, non-Müllerian in nature for the epithelial component of these neoplasms is identical with uroepithelium[2]: this indicates that cells in the surface epithelium also have a residual capacity for Wolffian differentiation, a not surprising potentiality in view of the close embryological relationships between Wolffian and Müllerian systems. The mesonephroid group of tumours, so called because of a historical misinterpretation of their origin, is still of slightly controversial nature; many, probably most, are of Müllerian type[3] and represent a variant form of endometrial differentiation, but it remains possible that some are mesotheliomata[4]: it should be remembered in this respect that all these neoplasms, derived as they are from serosa, are in essence mesotheliomata though their true nature is usually concealed by various degrees of Müllerian or Wolffian differentiation. Certainly a true mesothelioma can, very rarely, develop from the ovarian surface epithelium[5].

Although this unitary concept of the histogenesis of epithelial neoplasms is generally correct a proportion of epithelial neoplasms arise in a different manner. Thus, some mucinous tumours are formed, not of endocervical-type epithelium, but of gastro-intestinal-type epithelium, such neoplasms probably being of teratomatous origin[6]. Further, a minority of endometrioid neoplasms arise, not from the surface epithelium, but from pre-existent foci of ovarian endometriosis, whilst some Brenner tumours originate in the hilum, probably from structures of mesonephric origin such as the epoophoron or epigenital tubules. Despite these exceptions the vast majority of epithelial neoplasms are derived from the surface epithelium and all can exist in benign, borderline or malignant forms.

Benign Serous Tumours

These are common and show three basic patterns which may occur separately or in combination, these being the cystic, papillary and adenofibromatous forms. The cystic variety, the serous cystadenoma, usually occurs as a unilocular cyst containing thin straw-coloured fluid: they range in size from 3 to 30 cm in diameter (lesions less than 3 cm across being regarded as inclusion cysts). The papillary type of benign serous tumour can occur in combination with a cyst thus forming the papillary serous cystadenoma: the papillae may be on the outer or inner surface of the cyst and may be few, small and semi-sessile or numerous, large and pedunculated. The papillary form also occurs without any cyst formation, as finger-like or warty projections from the ovarian surface, this being the serous surface papilloma. The third form, the serous adenofibroma, occurs as a lobulated, knobbly, hard mass which may develop in isolation or as a nodule in the wall of a cyst: on section, tiny microcysts may be seen in the largely solid mass.

Histologically, the cysts are often lined by, and the papillae covered with, a single layer of flattened or cuboidal cells (Figure 25.1) but in places the epithelium is more columnar and can, under favourable conditions, be recognized as being similar to that of the Fallopian tube (Figure 25.2) The stroma of the papillae is usually abundant and may be dense and collagenous or oedematous; psammoma bodies, which are small calcified microspherites, are often seen in the papillary tumours but their presence is neither specific to the serous group of neoplasms nor an indication of malignancy.

The serous adenofibroma is essentially a fibrous neoplasm in which are embedded small cystic, gland-like spaces which are lined either by a flattened or cuboidal epithelium or by an epithelium showing tubal characteristics.

Benign Mucinous Tumours

These frequently encountered neoplasms usually take the form of a mucinous cystadenoma which is characteristically a large multilocular cystic neoplasm containing mucoid fluid. Sometimes the neoplasm consists of one major cyst with a number of smaller satellite locules, whilst closely packed small locules

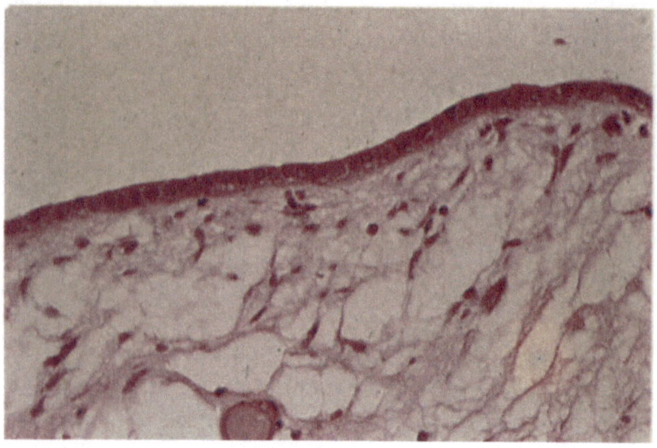

Figure 25.1 Ovary: benign serous tumour. This serous cyst is lined by flattened cuboidal cells. The underlying tissue is oedematous fibrous stroma. In many cases the epithelium may be even more flattened and careful sectioning of the tissue is necessary to preserve the rather delicate monolayer. H & E × 250

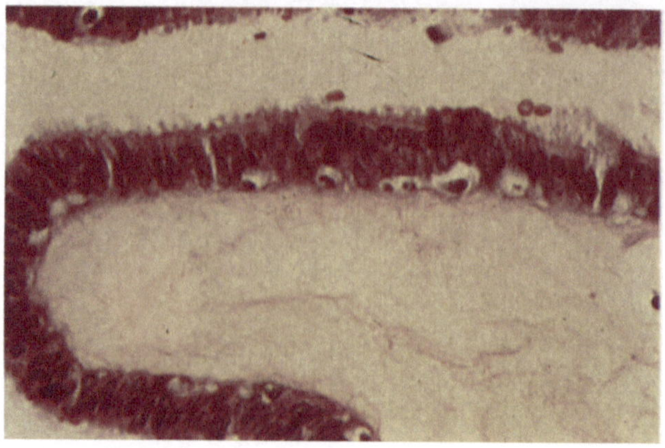

Figure 25.2 Ovary: benign serous tumour. The epithelium covering the serous papillae in a cystadenoma is a single layer of cubo–columnar cells similar to those seen in the Fallopian tube. Ciliated cells with round nuclei, secretory cells with elongated or oval nuclei lying near the epithelial surface and intercalary ('peg') cells can be seen. The underlying stroma is almost acellular and oedematous in this example. H & E × 400

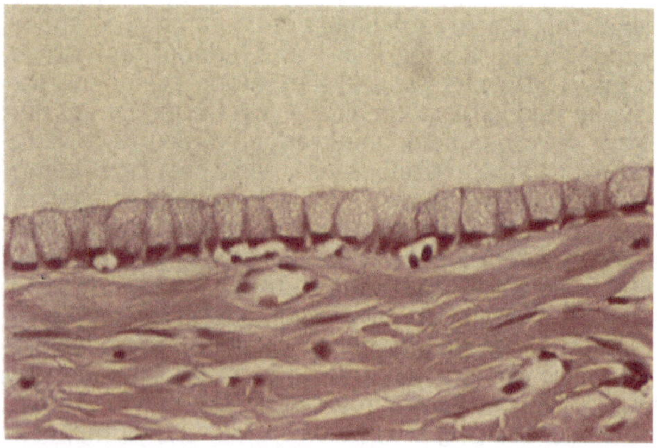

Figure 25.3 Ovary: mucinous cyst. The lining of this locule is formed by a single layer of tall, mucus-secreting cells with granular weakly basophilic cytoplasm and compressed basal nuclei. The wall is fibrous. H & E × 400

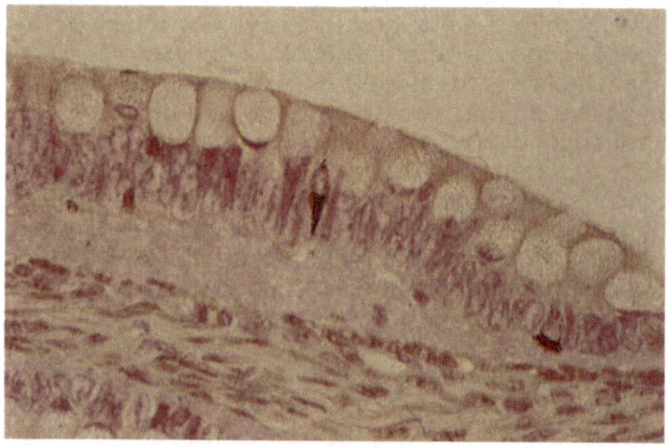

Figure 25.4 Ovary: mucinous cyst of enteric type. The cyst locules are lined by mucus-secreting epithelium similar to that seen in Figure 25.3. In addition goblet cells and argyrophil cells with black and brown staining intracytoplasmic granules are also present indicating the enteric nature of the cyst. Grimelius × 400

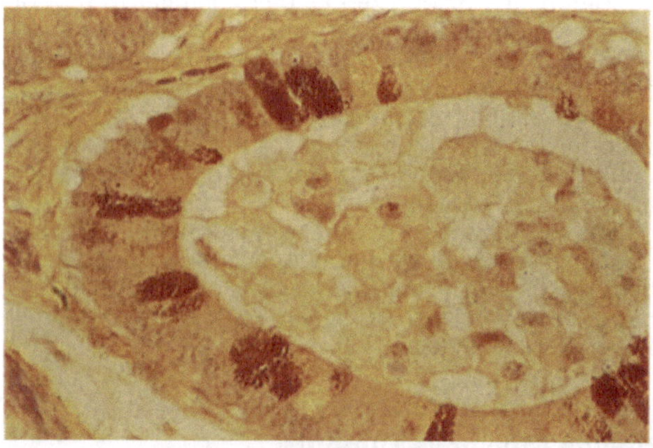

Figure 25.5 Ovary: mucinous cyst of enteric type. A locule from the same tumour as that shown in Figure 25.4. Paneth cells with their basal nuclei and intensely eosinophilic intracytoplasmic granules can be seen amongst the mucus-secreting cells. Phloxine Tartrazine × 400

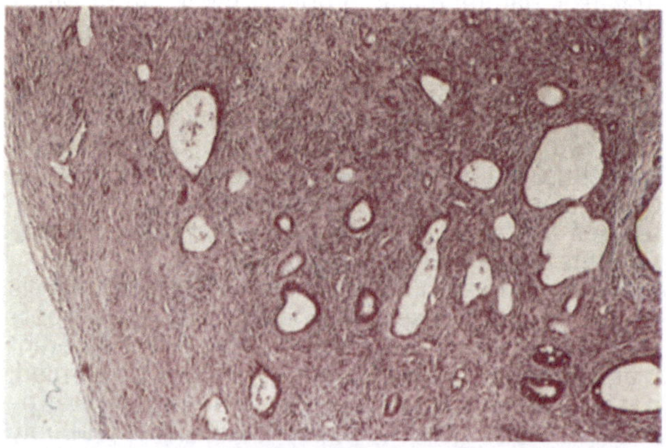

Figure 25.6 Ovary: endometrioid adenofibroma. This is a predominantly solid, fibrous neoplasm in which there are small cystic glandular spaces lined by epithelium of endometrial type. It is not unusual to see foci of intraglandular squamous metaplasia similar to those shown in Figure 13.3. H & E × 40

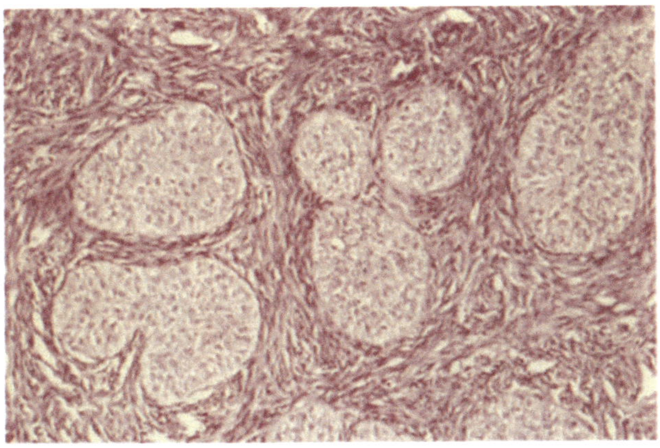

Figure 25.7 Ovary: Brenner tumour. The neoplasm consists of well-defined islands of pale-staining epithelial cells set in a dense fibrous stroma. H & E × 100

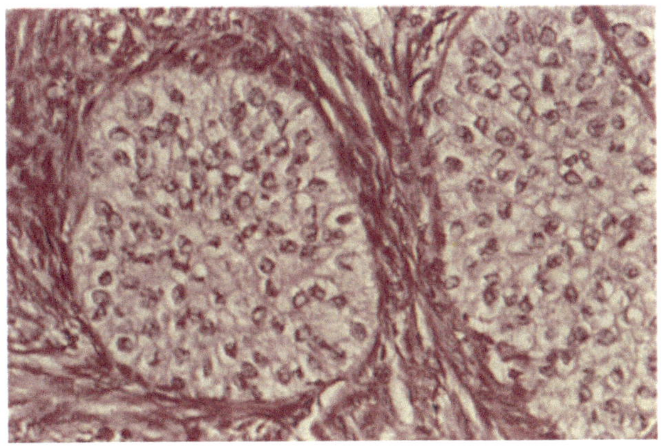

Figure 25.8 Ovary: Brenner tumour. The epithelium consists of polygonal and rounded cells with clearly defined cell boundaries, plentiful eosinophilic cytoplasm and round or ovoid nuclei. Many of the nuclei are grooved longitudinally. H & E × 250

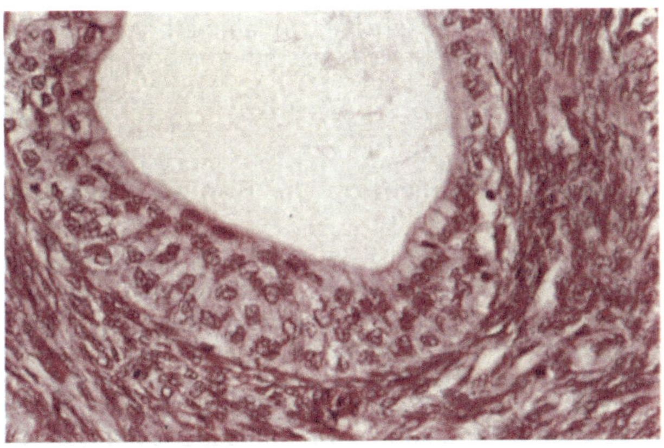

Figure 25.9 Ovary: Brenner tumour. In this nest of epithelial cells a cyst has formed. It is lined by a single layer of flattened endothelial-like cells, cuboidal cells and mucus-secreting columnar cells which are most clearly seen in the lower right. Between the cyst lining and the margins of the nest there is a band of cells similar to those seen in the common form of Brenner tumour (Figures 25.7 and 25.8). H & E × 250

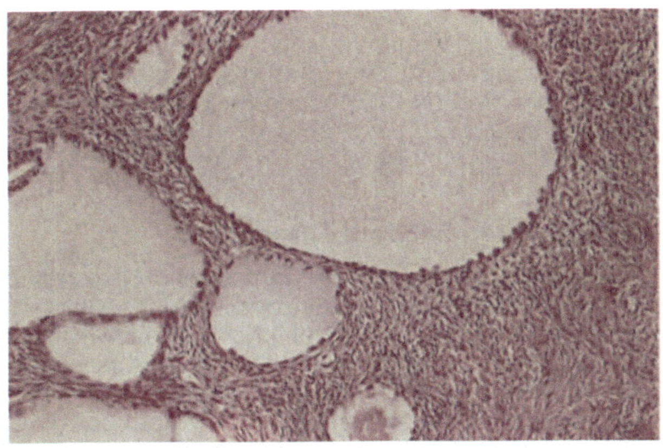

Figure 25.10 Ovary: mesonephroid adenofibroma. The solid fibrous stroma contains numerous cystic spaces which vary in size and are lined by a single layer of cuboidal cells with prominent hobnail nuclei. There is no cellular atypia and mitoses are absent. H & E × 100

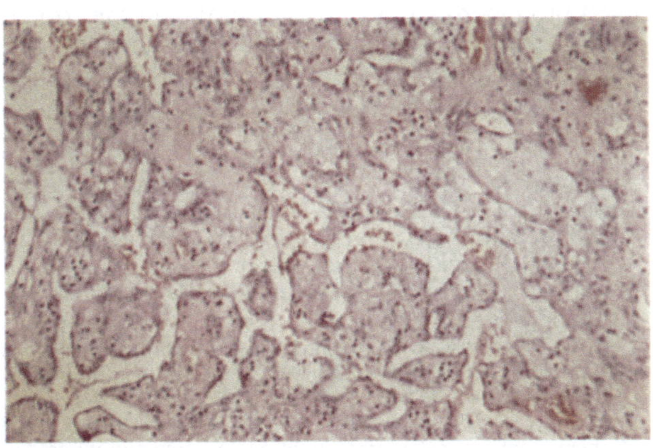

Figure 25.11 Ovary: mesothelioma. The tumour is composed of papillae with oedematous fibrous cores covered by a single layer of flattened and low cuboidal cells with eosinophilic cytoplasm and regular ovoid nuclei. Strands of similar cells lie in the fibrous stroma of the more solid areas and also line fissures. There is no cellular atypia and abnormal mitoses are absent. Throughout, there is a scattering of chronic inflammatory cells. H & E × 100

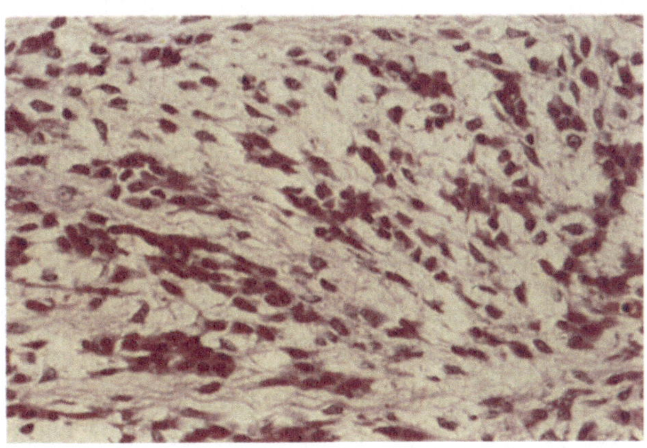

Figure 25.12 Ovary: stromal luteinization. This rather oedematous area of stroma contains clusters of conspicuous cells with dense eosinophilic cytoplasm and oval or round nuclei. They are typical of the luteinized cells which can be found in the stroma of many ovaries in which there is an expansile lesion. H & E × 250

may impart a semi-solid appearance to parts of the tumour. Histologically, the walls of the locules are formed by fibrous tissue and the cyst is lined by an epithelium of strikingly uniform appearance, consisting of a single layer of tall columnar cells with regularly arranged, darkly staining, basal nuclei and abundant, glassy, weakly basophilic cytoplasm (Figure 25.3) which stains positively for mucin. In the less common enteric type of mucinous cystadenoma the columnar cells are interspersed with goblet cells of intestinal type: argyrophil cells are usually present (Figure 25.4) and Paneth cells are occasionally found (Figure 25.5). Those mucinous cystadenomata which are associated with a mature cystic teratoma (a not uncommon combination) are invariably of enteric type whilst carcinoid tumours and, very rarely, Paneth cell neoplasms may arise from enteric type mucinous cystadenomata: there have been occasional instances of a Zollinger–Ellison syndrome complicating, and apparently being due to, a mucinous cyst of enteric type in which numerous gastrin-containing cells were present.

A rare type of benign mucinous tumour is the mucinous adenofibroma; this resembles grossly its serous counterpart, but the gland-like structures within the fibrous tumour are lined by a mucinous type epithelium.

Benign Endometrioid Tumours

These are extremely rare though occasional examples of an endometrioid adenoma, which tends to resemble an endometrial polyp, and of endometrioid adenofibroma, which resembles the serous adenofibroma but in which the gland-like spaces are lined by endometrial-type epithelium (Figure 25.6), do occur. The rarity of benign endometrioid neoplasms may be more apparent than real for it has been suggested, not without some validity, that many examples of presumed ovarian endometriosis are in reality benign endometrioid neoplasms.

Brenner Tumours

Nearly all Brenner tumours are benign and many are of only microscopic size with the vast majority measuring less than 2 cm in diameter and only occasional examples attaining a diameter of 10 cm. The neoplasm is usually well circumscribed with a smooth or bosselated surface and a hard, slightly whorled, whitish-grey cut surface. Sometimes Brenner tumours occur in the wall of a mucinous cystadenoma or, less commonly, of a mature cystic teratoma or serous cystadenoma and are then seen as localized, firm, white, intramural nodules. Histologically, the tumour consists of well demarcated nests and branching columns of epithelial cells set in a fibrous stroma (Figure 25.7). The sharply delineated epithelial component is formed of round or polygonal cells with clearly defined margins, abundant clear, or weakly eosinophilic cytoplasm and round or ovoid vesicular nuclei which often, but not invariably, show a well marked longitudinal groove (Figure 25.8). Frequently, the central part of the epithelial nests becomes cystic (Figure 25.9). The fibrous stroma varies in cellularity and often shows focal, but widespread, hyalinization and calcification: not infrequently, a definite collar of hyalinized tissue surrounds individual epithelial cell nests. Occasionally the stroma is markedly cellular and may be of a pleomorphic 'pseudosarcomatous' appearance.

Mesonephroid Tumours

Benign mesonephroid tumours are represented only by the rare mesonephroid adenofibroma which microscopically resembles other adenofibromata but in which the gland-like spaces are lined by cells with clear cytoplasm or 'hob-nail' nuclei (Figure 25.10).

Mesothelioma

A true mesothelioma arising from the ovarian surface epithelium is an extreme rarity and takes the form of a papillary or tubulo-papillary lesion with less prominent more solid areas (Figure 25.11) Sheets of mesothelial cells may also be seen. A stromal infiltrate with non-specific chronic inflammatory cells is a characteristic feature and psammoma bodies may be present.

Stromal Luteinization in Benign Epithelial Neoplasms

Focal luteinization of the non-neoplastic stroma (Figure 25.12) can occur in almost every type of ovarian neoplasm, whether these be epithelial or non-epithelial, benign or malignant, primary or metastatic. Nevertheless, this phenomenon is encountered most commonly in the benign epithelial neoplasms of the ovary, and is believed to be responsible for the oestrogenic, or less commonly androgenic, manifestations sometimes displayed by these tumours. Stromal luteinization is thought to occur because the ovarian stroma appears to respond to any enlarging intraovarian lesion as it would to a developing follicle[7]: this concept has been criticized as an over-simplification[3] but multifocal lesions with a high surface area to volume ratio, e.g. Brenner tumours and some metastatic tumours, often appear to provoke the most prominent stromal luteinization and this would accord with a mechanistic interpretation of this response.

References

1. Fox, H. and Langley, F. A. (1976). *Tumours of the Ovary.* (London: Heinemann Medical Books)
2. Roth, L. M. (1971). Fine structure of the Brenner tumor. *Cancer*, **27**, 1482–1488
3. Scully, R. E. (1979). Tumors of the Ovary and Maldeveloped Gonads. *Atlas of Tumor Pathology, 2nd Series, Fascicle 16.* (Washington DC: Armed Forces Institute of Pathology)
4. Okagi, J. and Richart, R. M. (1970). Mesonephroma ovarii (hypernephroid carcinoma): light microscopic and ultrastructural study of a case. *Cancer*, **26**, 453–461
5. Addis, B. J. and Fox, H. (1982). Papillary mesothelioma of the ovary. *Histopathology*, **6** (in press)
6. Fox, H., Kazzaz, B. and Langley, F. A. (1964). Argyrophil and argentaffin cells in the female genital tract and in ovarian mucinous cysts. *J. Pathol. Bacteriol.*, **88**, 479–488
7. Hughesdon, P. E. (1958). Thecal and allied reactions in epithelial ovarian tumours. *J. Obstet. Gynaecol. Br. Emp.*, **65**, 702–709

Ovary: Epithelial Neoplasms of Borderline Malignancy

26

These neoplasms have also been called 'proliferating tumours' or 'carcinomas of low malignant potential', but the term 'tumour of borderline malignancy' most aptly indicates their rather equivocal biological status. Categorization of an ovarian tumour as being of borderline malignancy should not, however, be taken as implying diagnostic indecision on the part of the pathologist: it is a specific and positive diagnosis which is based solely on the histological findings and which takes no account as to whether or not there is extra-ovarian spread.

Ovarian tumours of borderline malignancy are defined as ones in which the epithelium shows some, or all, of the features of malignancy, e.g. multilayering, irregular budding, pleomorphism, nuclear hyperchromatism, but in which there is no stromal invasion. The emphasis on lack of stromal invasion as a defining characteristic indicates that these tumours have to be extensively sampled, and that there must be a readiness to resort to serial sectioning. Nevertheless, it can be very difficult to be sure that stromal invasion is not occurring: this is so in all types of ovarian tumour of borderline malignancy but applies with most force to those in which there are epithelial outpouchings or the formation of secondary cysts or glands. Features suggestive of invasion, rather than inclusion, are an irregular contour or outline of the glandular structures, a focal chronic inflammatory cell infiltration around the invading cells, the presence of immature-type stroma at the site of invasion and a local desmoplastic reaction to the infiltrating neoplasm[1]: certainly there can be little doubt that invasion is occurring if single cells, nests of cells or cellular cords are seen infiltrating the stroma.

The definition of prognostic criteria for ovarian tumours of borderline malignancy offers an as yet unsolved challenge to the pathologist, for while the majority of these neoplasms behave in an apparently benign fashion others, between 5 and 15%, pursue a malignant course, albeit a rather leisurely and indolent one. Attempts at grading these tumours in terms of the degree of epithelial abnormality have proved to be of prognostic value in some hands[1] but not in others[2,3].

Serous Tumours of Borderline Malignancy

These are relatively common for about 8% of all serous neoplasms fall into this category: most present as a papillary cystic tumour though a few resemble a papillary surface tumour. Histologically, fine branching papillae with well formed fibrous cores are covered by an irregular cellular mantle (Figure 26.1): the epithelium (Figure 26.2) shows a variable degree of multilayering, and has a marked tendency to form cellular buds which may break off to float freely within the cyst or can fuse to produce a honeycomb pattern: nuclear crowding, atypia and hyperchromatism are of variable degree but nucleoli are not prominent and whilst mitotic figures are not infrequent they are rarely of abnormal form. There is usually a sharp junction between epithelium and stroma and the possibility of stromal invasion can often be excluded with relative ease: epithelial invaginations into the stroma do, however, occur in some tumours and pose a diagnostic difficulty which is commonly, though not invariably, resolved by serial sectioning. In general, all serous tumours of borderline malignancy have a very similar and easily recognized appearance: they also tend, except in those showing only minimal epithelial abnormalities, to have a relatively uniform pattern throughout, it being unusual to find areas of benign epithelium alternating, or admixed, with epithelium showing malignant features.

Serous tumours are often bilateral, and it is not uncommon for there to be multiple apparent seedling deposits in the pelvic peritoneum at the time of initial diagnosis. Histologically, many of these are deep to, rather than on the surface of, the peritoneum and most will show either a benign or a borderline appearance, it being relatively rare for there to be an overtly carcinomatous picture (Figure 26.3). Some of these peritoneal lesions do progress, though rather slowly, but many either remain stationary or regress, and it appears likely that most are not true implants but represent multiple foci of neoplastic transformation, not necessarily or even usually of a malignant nature, within peritoneal mesothelium: indeed they can often be regarded as a form of endosalpingiosis.

Mucinous Tumours of Borderline Malignancy

These neoplasms, which constitute about 20% of all ovarian mucinous tumours, usually present as large multilocular cysts with either focal mural thickening, mural nodules or endophytic nodulo–papillary projections. They differ from their serous counterparts in showing a much less uniform appearance, areas of fully benign epithelium mingling with others in which there is a variable degree of epithelial abnormality: furthermore, the atypical epithelium is often very focal and sharply circumscribed (Figure 26.4), and hence the necessity for thorough sampling of all tumours of mucinous type.

In the areas of borderline malignancy the epithelium may show a complex glandular pattern (Figure 26.5), but is often characterized by short papillary infoldings which impart to the epithelium a somewhat

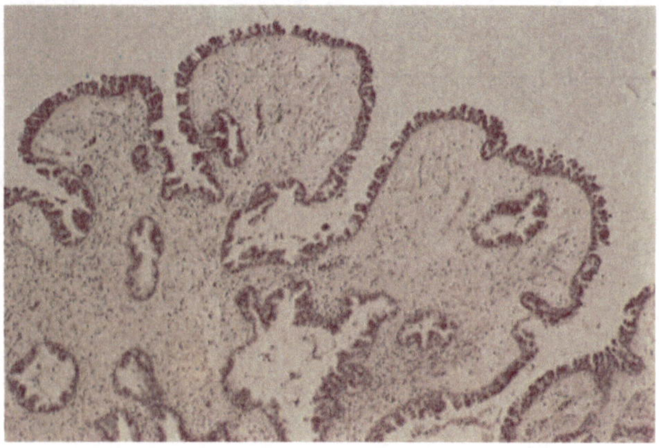

Figure 26.1 Ovary: serous tumour of borderline malignancy. The fibrous stroma is covered by epithelium showing variable multilayering, tufting and papillae formation. There is no evidence of stromal invasion. H & E × 40

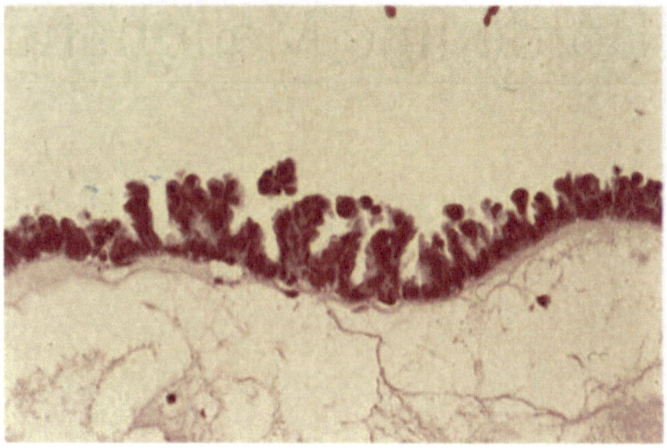

Figure 26.2 Ovary: serous tumour of borderline malignancy. The epithelium lining this locule is multilayered and shows budding. The cells are crowded and their nuclei hyperchromatic. Note that the atypical features are limited to the epithelial component, the fibrous stroma being entirely bland and rather oedematous. H & E × 250

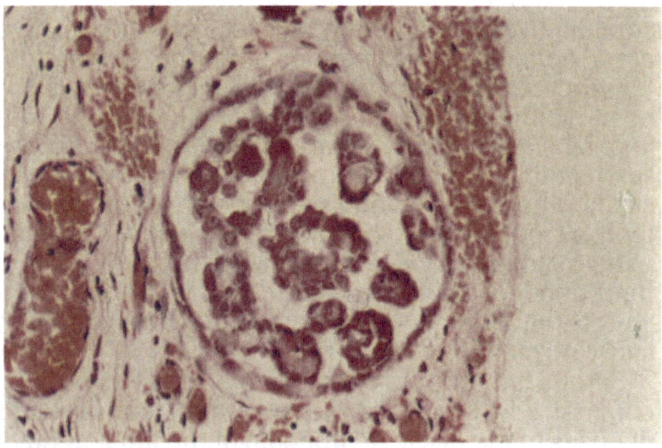

Figure 26.3 Omentum: peritoneal implants. A fragment of serous, papillary cystadenoma lies within the omentum. The epithelium lining the cyst and covering the papillae is cuboidal and shows neither cellular nor nuclear atypia. Note the psammoma bodies and total absence of mitotic activity. H & E × 250

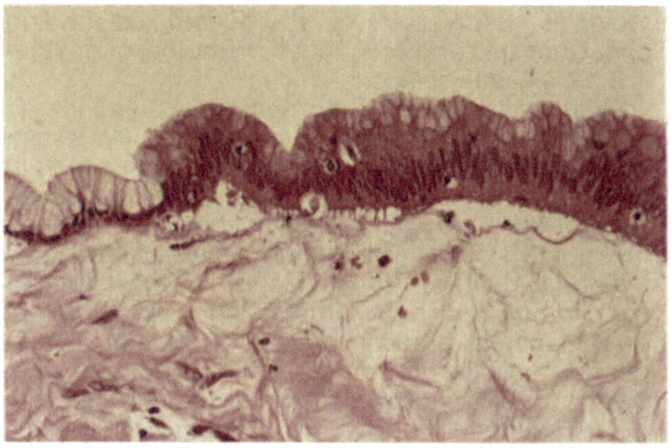

Figure 26.4 Ovary: mucinous tumour of borderline malignancy. To the left, the epithelium lining the cyst locule is tall and columnar, has basal nuclei and clear or faintly granular cytoplasm. To the right there is an abrupt transition to a multilayered columnar epithelium with larger, elongated nuclei and minimal mucus secretion. There is no evidence of stromal invasion. H & E × 250

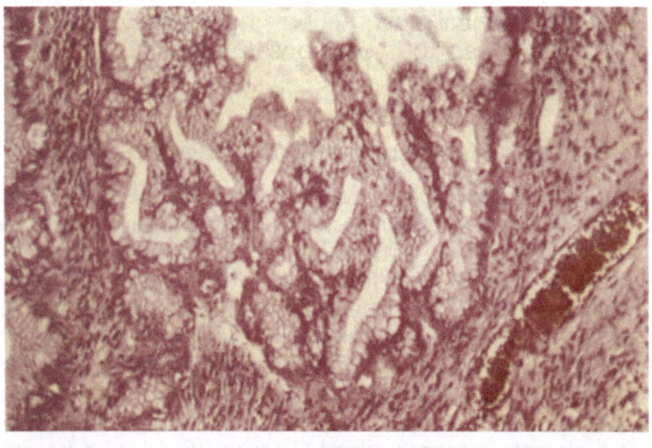

Figure 26.5 Ovary: mucinous tumour of borderline malignancy. The epithelium in this example is forming a complex glandular pattern. Although the individual cells show minimal atypia, there is a minor degree of multilayering. Undoubtedly in some instances this appearance is the result of tangential cutting across complex papillae and infoldings of the epithelium; nonetheless it is a typical appearance and a common problem in these neoplasms. H & E × 100

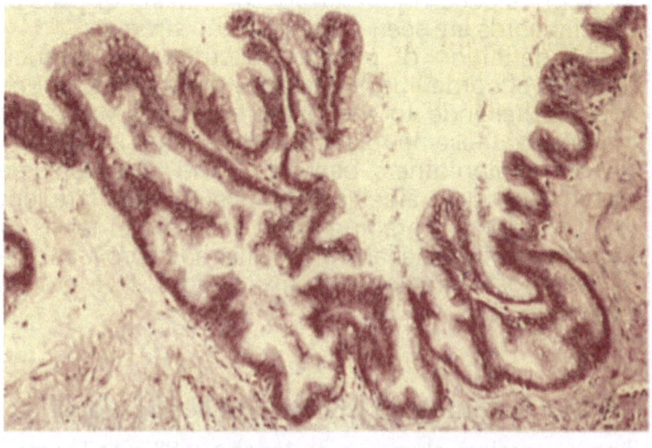

Figure 26.6 Ovary: mucinous tumour of borderline malignancy. The focally multilayered epithelium is here forming short papillary infoldings producing a somewhat serrated margin to the cyst locule. H & E × 100

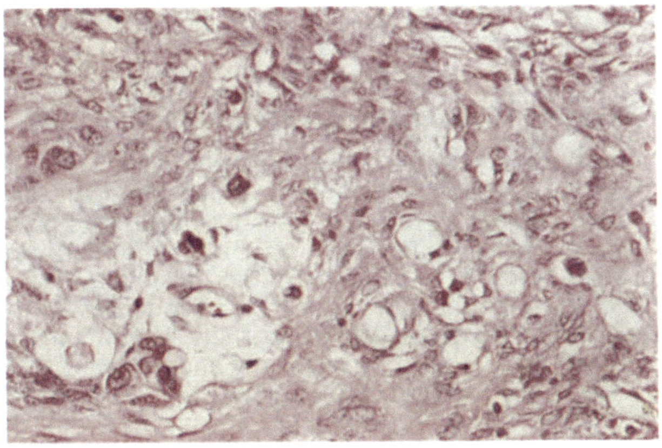

Figure 26.7 Ovary: pseudomyxoma peritonei. The acini in this borderline mucinous tumour have ruptured and mucus has leaked into and accumulated in the stroma. Within the pools of mucus are fragments of epithelium and single mucinous cells. The condition can be differentiated from infiltrating carcinoma by the absence of atypical mitoses and nuclear chromatin irregularities. H & E × 250

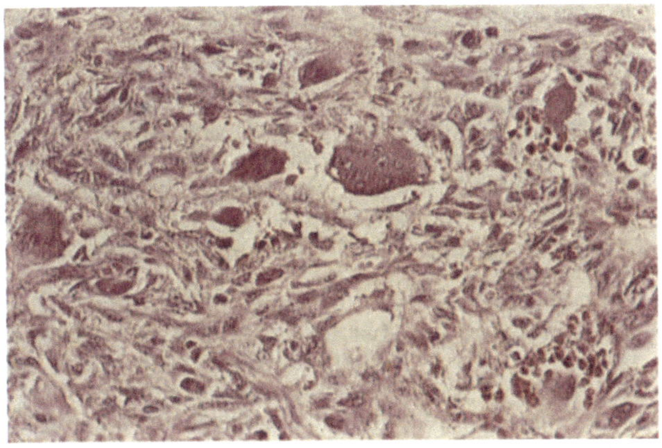

Figure 26.8 Ovary: pseudosarcoma. This is a section taken from a thickened area in the wall of a mucinous tumour of borderline malignancy. It is formed by a mesh of spindle cells between which there are histiocytes of varying appearance; some are small and have foamy cytoplasm whilst others are multinucleate. The largest of these cells (of which there are several) resemble osteoclasts, having rather serrated margins and scattered nuclei. There are focal collections of chronic inflammatory cells. H & E × 250

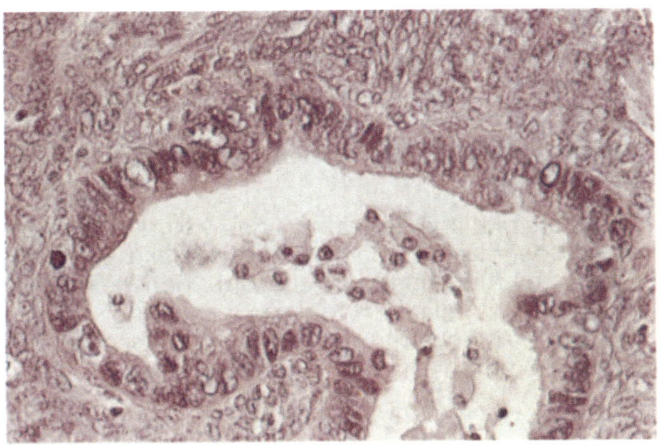

Figure 26.9 Ovary: endometrioid tumour of borderline malignancy. The cells forming the epithelial lining of this acinus are pleomorphic, multilayered, irregular in outline and show loss of polarity. There are mitoses but there is no evidence of stromal invasion. H & E × 250

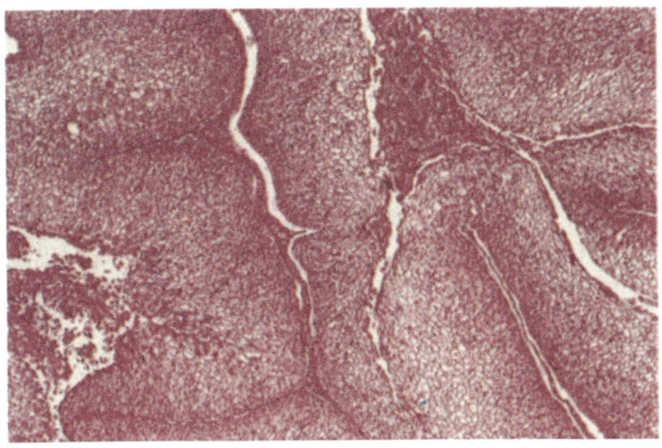

Figure 26.10 Ovary: Brenner tumour of borderline malignancy (proliferating Brenner tumour). Part of the wall of a cyst locule showing the characteristic folds of transitional-type epithelium with fine fibrovascular cores. H & E × 40

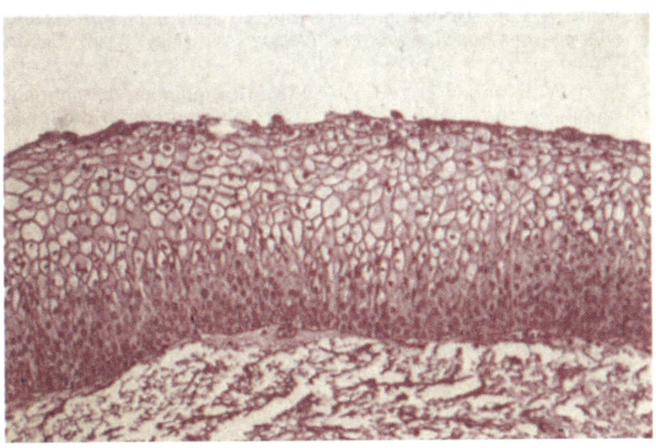

Figure 26.11 Ovary: Brenner tumour of borderline malignancy (proliferating Brenner tumour). A detail of the epithelium from the tumour shown in Figure 26.10. The cells are a little pleomorphic and there is loss of nuclear polarity but no hyperchromatism or atypical mitoses. H & E × 100

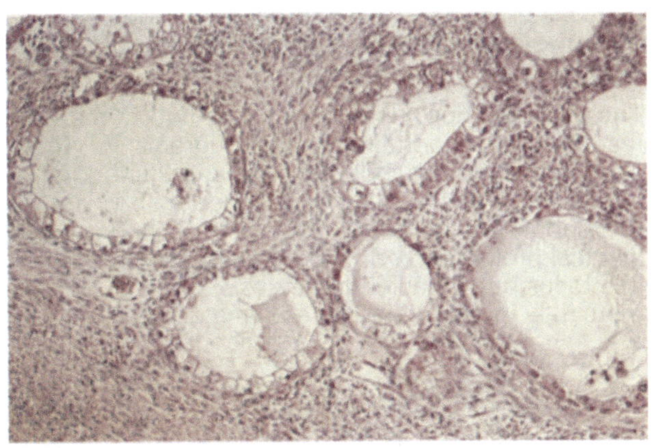

Figure 26.12 Ovary: mesonephroid tumour of borderline malignancy. The tumour acini are set in a fibrous stroma and are lined by cells with clear cytoplasm and well-defined cell boundaries. In the acinus above and to the right of centre the cells are rather pleomorphic, show nuclear enlargement and some loss of cellular polarity. Compare the appearances with the mesonephroid adenofibroma in Figure 25.10. H & E × 100

serrated appearance (Figure 26.6). There are varying degrees of multilayering, loss of polarity and cellular atypia whilst mitotic figures are seen with some frequency: with increasing degrees of atypia the cytoplasm of the epithelial cells becomes progressively more basophilic and the amount of intracellular mucus declines.

It is in the mucinous tumours of borderline malignancy that the greatest difficulty is encountered in excluding the possibility of stromal invasion, and this has led some to maintain that mucinous neoplasms should be regarded as adenocarcinomata if there are severe epithelial abnormalities, even in the absence of obvious stromal invasion[4]: thus it has been suggested that a diagnosis of mucinous adenocarcinoma can be made if there are striking nuclear abnormalities, marked overgrowth of atypical epithelial cells, formation of papillae without a stromal support or stratification of atypical epithelial cells exceeding three cell layers in thickness. These criteria of malignancy have been widely accepted in the United States but have not gained extensive support elsewhere, largely because it has not been fully shown that their adoption is accompanied by any increased prognostic precision[1].

The histological appearances of a mucinous tumour of borderline malignancy can be complicated by two features which can occur in any type of ovarian mucinous neoplasm, but which tend to be seen with greatest frequency in those of borderline malignancy. The first of these is pseudomyxoma ovarii in which disruption of glandular acini results in leakage of mucus into the stroma where it collects in pools (Figure 26.7), inflammatory cells, isolated tumour cells or clumps of neoplastic cells often being seen floating in the mucoid lakes: in a significant proportion of cases this lesion progresses to a pseudomyxoma peritoneii. The second feature is the formation of reactive pseudosarcomatous nodules, possibly also as a result of seepage of mucus: these occur as sharply demarcated mural nodules which on histological examination are seen to show various permutations of osteoclast-like giant cells (Figure 26.8), pleomorphic spindle cells, large histiocytic cells and chronic inflammatory cells[5].

Endometrioid Tumours of Borderline Malignancy

These uncommon tumours occur in two forms. The first is as an endometrioid adenofibroma in which endometrial-type glands showing irregular budding, stratification and nuclear atypia (Figure 26.9) are set in an abundant fibrous stroma[6]. The second is as an atypical proliferation of endometrial glandular tissue in a focus of ovarian endometriosis; this is discussed more fully in the section on endometriosis.

Brenner Tumours of Borderline Malignancy

These are usually fairly large, partially cystic tumours: the cystic portion is characteristically multilocular and the locules have a papillary, velvety lining. Histologically, areas of typical benign Brenner tumour are usually present but this is not an invariable finding and not one which is a necessary prerequisite for the diagnosis. In the papillary portion of the tumour the epithelium is thrown up into multilayered folds which are supported by thin connective tissue stalks, the appearances in these areas having an unmistakable resemblance to those of a Grade I transitional cell carcinoma of the bladder (Figure 26.10). Focal cellular and nuclear atypia are usually present (Figure 26.11), and there is often a sprinkling of mitotic figures: stromal invasion, which is easy to assess in these neoplasms, is absent.

The diagnosis of a Brenner tumour of borderline malignancy rarely presents any great diagnostic difficulty, but if areas of more typical benign Brenner tumour are absent the possibility of a metastatic deposit from a primary transitional cell carcinoma of the bladder has to be borne in mind.

Mesonephroid Tumours of Borderline Malignancy

These are rare and appear invariably to take the form of an adenofibroma in which gland-like or microcystic structures lined by cells with 'hob-nail' nuclei or abundant clear cytoplasm, showing varying degrees of irregularity or atypia, are embedded in a plenteous fibrous stroma (Figure 26.12).

References

1. Russell, P. (1979). The pathological assessment of ovarian neoplasms. II. The proliferating 'epithelial' tumours. *Pathology*, **11**, 5–26
2. Katzenstein, A. A., Mazur, M. T., Morgan, T. E. and Kae, M. (1978). Proliferative serous tumors of the ovary: histologic features and prognosis. *Am. J. Surg. Pathol.*, **2**, 339–355
3. Fox, H. (1982). Ovarian tumors of borderline malignancy. In Morrow, C. P., Bonnar, J. and O'Brien, T. (eds.). *Diagnosis and Management of Gynecologic Neoplasms.* (New York: Raven Press)
4. Hart, W. R. and Norris, H. J. (1975). Borderline and malignant mucinous tumors of the ovary: histologic criteria and clinical behaviour. *Cancer*, **31**, 1031–1045
5. Prat, J. and Scully, R. E. (1979). Ovarian mucinous tumors with sarcoma-like mural nodules: a report of seven cases. *Cancer*, **44**, 1332–1344
6. Roth, L. M., Czernobilsky, B. and Langley, F. A. (1980). Ovarian endometrioid adenofibromatous and cystadenofibromatous tumors: benign, proliferating and malignant. *Cancer*, **48**, 1838–1845

Ovary: Malignant Epithelial Neoplasms

27

The malignant forms of the epithelial tumours of the ovary present as bulky, partially cystic or solid neoplasms which are often collectively referred to as 'ovarian adenocarcinoma'. An attempt should be made in all cases to make a more precise histological identification of individual malignant epithelial neoplasms, e.g. as 'serous' or 'mucinous', for their consideration as a single entity probably conceals subtle differences in aetiology, epidemiology, mode of spread and therapeutic response. It is recognized, however, that not all malignant epithelial neoplasms can be accurately categorized. Some are so poorly differentiated that no diagnosis more specific than 'undifferentiated carcinoma' can be made whilst others, though better differentiated, do not show features which allow for them to be identified in specific terms, these being classed as 'adenocarcinoma of unspecified type'. Furthermore, a significant proportion of malignant epithelial neoplasms contain more than one type of epithelium: it is, for instance, not uncommon to encounter tumours containing a mixture of serous and mucinous epithelia or ones in which there is an admixture of endometrioid and mucinous epithelia. Such carcinomata are classified in terms of the predominant type of epithelium present and are only diagnosed as 'mixed' if the second epithelial component is a prominent feature of the tumour.

Serous Adenocarcinoma

Adenocarcinomata of this type account for between 40 and 50% of all malignant epithelial ovarian tumours. The striking histological resemblance of the tumour epithelium to that of the Fallopian tube which characterizes the benign serous neoplasms is not found in even the best differentiated serous adenocarcinomata: nevertheless, the presence, in many cases, of ciliated cells, small dark cells with a nucleus almost filling the cell and large clear cells with abundant cytoplasm results in an anarchic resemblance to tubal epithelium and a marked mimicry of a tubal carcinoma. In well differentiated serous adenocarcinomata (Figure 27.1) discrete, slender, branching papillae with a prominent fibrous stalk are covered by an epithelium showing cellular and nuclear atypia with irregular multilayering and the formation of cellular bridges which link adjacent papillae, stromal invasion is present. In less well differentiated neoplasms (Figure 27.2) the papillae are crowded together, irregular, and often lack a mesenchymal stalk: the epithelial cells are more pleomorphic and tend to have vesicular nuclei with prominent nucleoli: stromal invasion is both obvious and extensive. Poorly differentiated serous adenocarcinomata are formed largely of sheets of highly pleomorphic, sometimes anaplastic, cells in which only the presence of occasionally poorly formed papillary or glandular structures offers a clue to the correct diagnosis: mitotic figures are frequent in such neoplasms, nucleoli are large and multinucleated cells are occasionally seen.

Psammoma bodies are present in about one third of serous adenocarcinomata, usually in the well differentiated forms, whilst a little mucus may be present within cyst cavities and in the apical portions of the epithelial cells: rounded extracellular hyaline globules are sometimes encountered.

Mucinous Adenocarcinoma

Although malignant mucinous tumours, which form between 5 and 15% of ovarian adenocarcinomata, may present as bulky masses they sometimes occur as mural nodules in an otherwise benign mucinous cystadenoma or in a tumour which is otherwise of only borderline malignancy. Histologically, these neoplasms show a wide range of differentiation. Some are very well differentiated (Figure 27.3) and are formed of clearly defined glandular acini with little intervening stroma: the acini are lined by tall, columnar, mucus-containing cells with basal nuclei, and often it is only the presence of stromal invasion, moderate cellular atypia, a degree of nuclear pleomorphism, a tendency towards multilayering and the presence of mitotic figures which distinguishes these well differentiated mucinous adenocarcinomata from a benign mucinous cystadenoma. The distinction between a well differentiated mucinous adenocarcinoma and a mucinous tumour of borderline malignancy often rests solely upon a difficult decision as to whether stromal invasion is present or not, and is therefore sometimes a matter of opinion rather than of fact. In less well differentiated mucinous adenocarcinomata (Figure 27.4), glandular acini are poorly formed or markedly irregular, the cells are larger and show a greater degree of pleomorphism, mitotic figures are more numerous and intracellular mucus is less conspicuous: stromal invasion is obvious. Poorly differentiated forms of this neoplasm may consist largely of sheets of pleomorphic cells containing little mucus, and a specific diagnosis is often dependent upon finding focal areas of better differentiated, or more overtly mucinous, epithelium.

Endometrioid Adenocarcinoma

Between 16 and 30% of ovarian adenocarcinomata are of this type. Most are well differentiated tumours

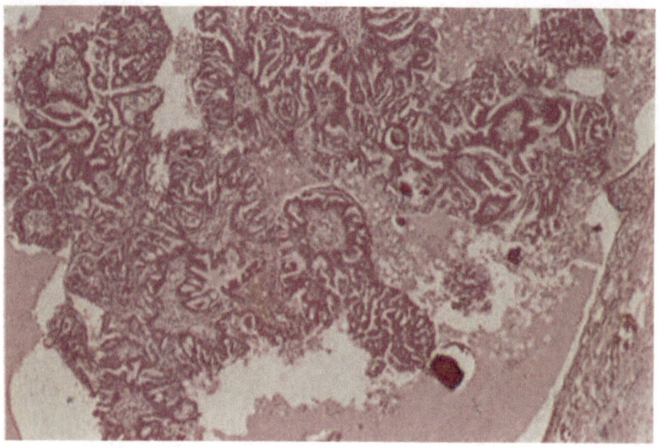

Figure 27.1 Ovary: serous adenocarcinoma. In this papillary area from a well-differentiated tumour the fibrous cores of the papillae and their mantle of epithelium is clearly seen; there are numerous foci of stromal invasion. Several psammoma bodies, which appear as irregular, laminated, eosinophilic bodies and have fragmented on sectioning, are seen to the right of the field. H & E x 40

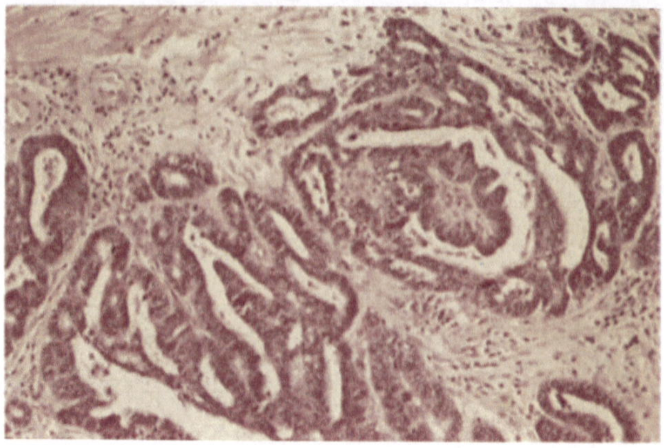

Figure 27.2 Ovary: serous adenocarcinoma. The papillae are smaller, the epithelium less well-differentiated and the acini smaller and more complex than in Figure 27.1. To the left the epithelium is heaped and there are epithelial bridges unsupported by fibrous tissue. Note the small peripheral infiltrating glandular acini. There is a scanty, stromal, chronic inflammatory cell infiltrate. H & E x 100

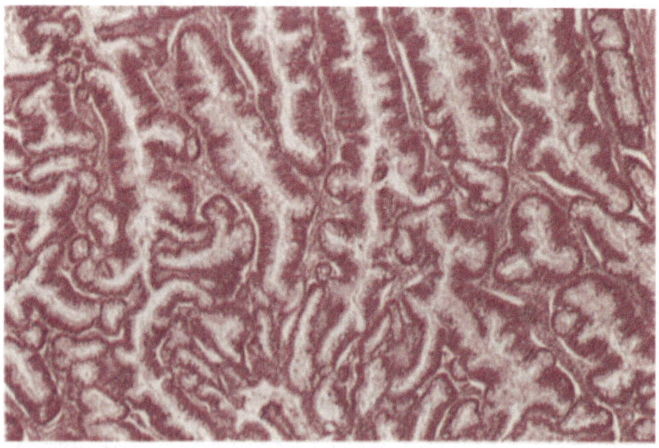

Figure 27.3 Ovary: mucinous adenocarcinoma. This field from a well-differentiated neoplasm shows well-formed glandular structures lined by multilayered, mucus-secreting epithelium. Stroma is scanty and stromal invasion is apparent in many areas. There was also lymphatic spread in the tumour capsule and mesovarium. H & E x 40

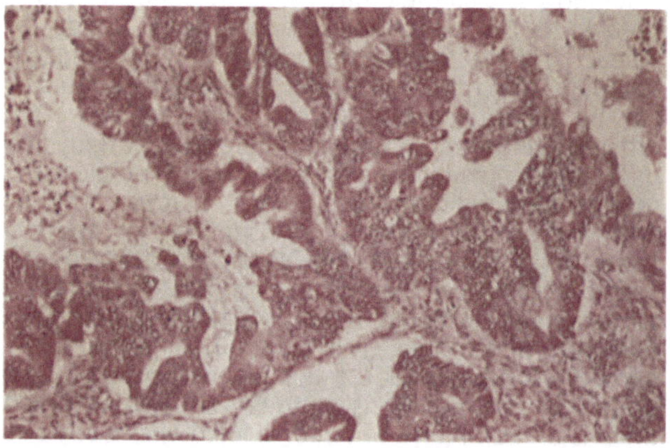

Figure 27.4 Ovary: mucinous adenocarcinoma. This tumour is much less well-differentiated than that seen in Figure 27.3. The epithelium lining the tumour acini is multilayered, shows very little evidence of mucus secretion, is markedly pleomorphic and has lost its nuclear polarity. H & E x 100

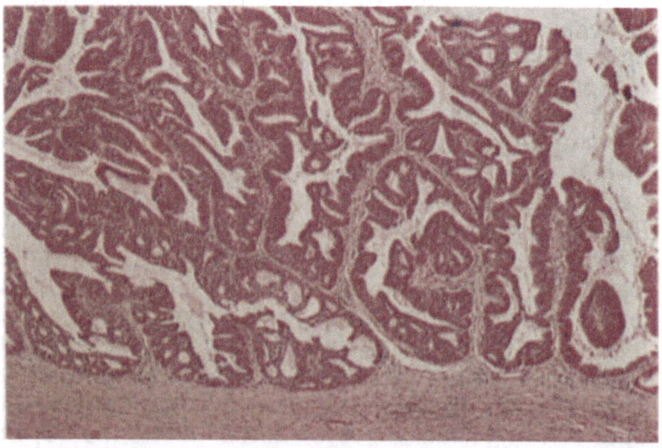

Figure 27.5 Ovary: endometriod adenocarcinoma. This cystic neoplasm is lined by fronds of tumour and solid blunt papillae. The papillae are covered and the acini lined by a cubo–columnar epithelium of endometrial type. The tumour closely resembles that seen in the endometrium (Figure 15.1). H & E x 40

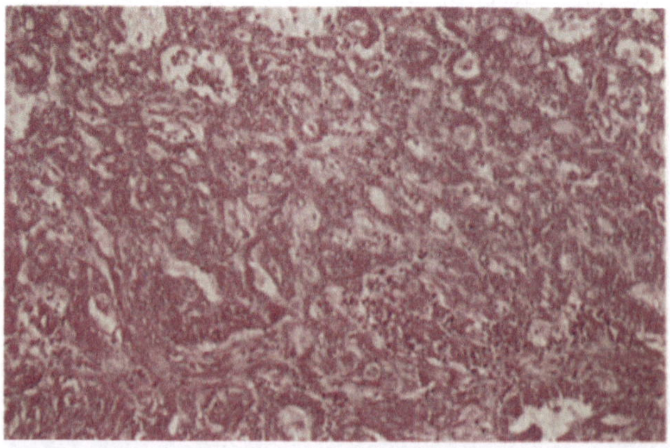

Figure 27.6 Ovary: endometrioid adenocarcinoma. In the less well-differentiated tumour there is a pattern of closely packed, poorly formed acini and small fibrous papillary cores covered by cuboidal cells. H & E x 100

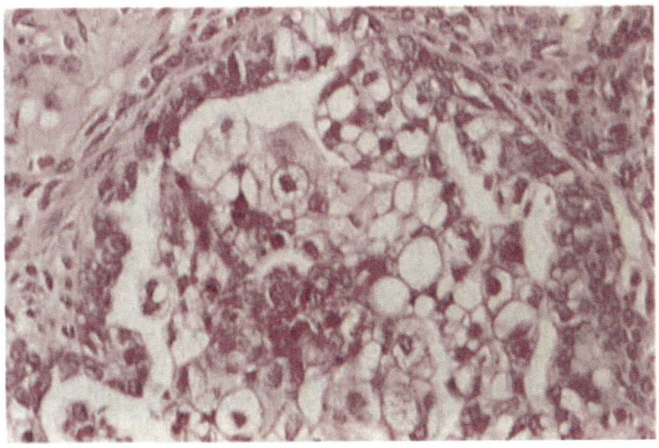

Figure 27.7 Ovary: endometrioid carcinoma. In this otherwise typical endometrioid adenocarcinoma there were foci and sheets of clear cells such as those shown here. The cells are large, their cytoplasm clear or faintly staining and granular and their nuclei large, vesicular and moderately pleomorphic. H & E × 250

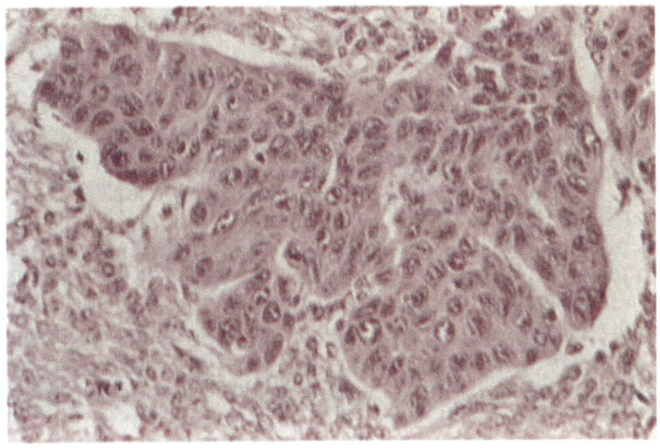

Figure 27.8 Ovary: malignant Brenner tumour. This infiltrating island of highly atypical transitional epithelium is characteristic of one pattern of malignant Brenner tumour. The cells are large, and their nuclei pleomorphic with irregularly distributed chromatin; nucleoli are conspicuous. H & E × 250

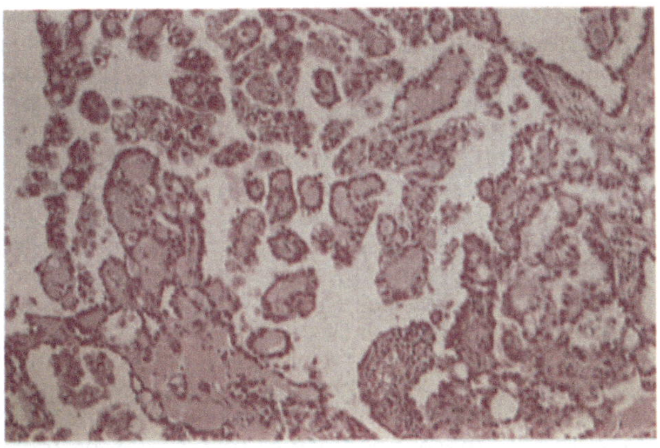

Figure 27.9 Ovary: mesonephroid carcinoma. This field shows the papillary pattern, the papillary cores being fibrous and partly hyalinized. The epithelial cells vary, some having hobnailed nuclei and scanty cytoplasm as in Figure 27.11 whilst others have copious clear cytoplasm and large central hyperchromatic nuclei. H & E × 100

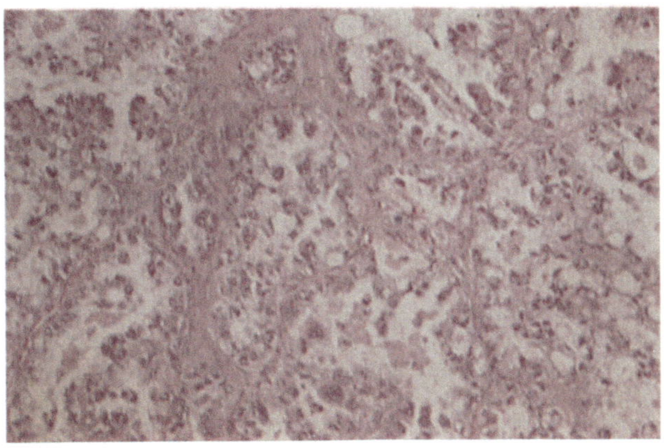

Figure 27.10 Ovary: mesonephroid carcinoma. In this tumour the glandular acini and cysts are lined by epithelial cells with copious clear cytoplasm, ovoid pleomorphic nuclei and well-defined cell boundaries. H & E × 100

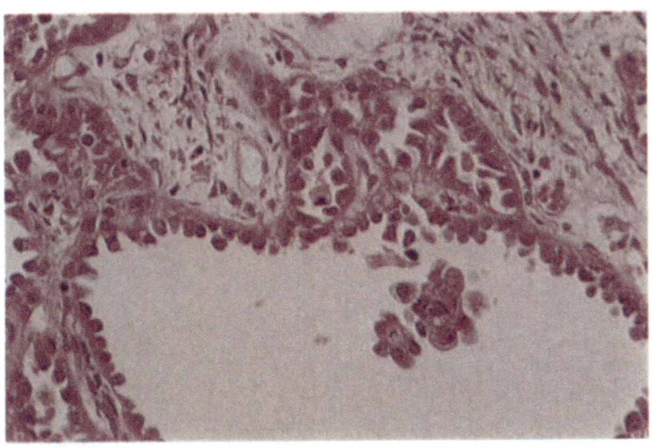

Figure 27.11 Ovary: mesonephroid carcinoma. In this predominantly cystic neoplasm, the cysts are lined by pleomorphic cells with large hyperchromatic, hobnailed nuclei, scanty cytoplasm and ill-defined cell boundaries. It is usual to find a combination of patterns in mesonephroid carcinoma though one may predominate. H & E × 250

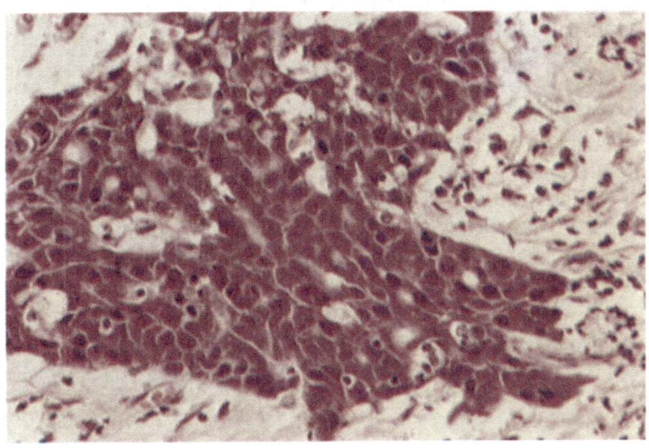

Figure 27.12 Ovary: undifferentiated carcinoma. This is part of the wall of an ovarian cyst lined by sheets of carcinoma. The cells are undifferentiated and have a very high nucleo–cytoplasmic ratio: atypical mitoses are frequent. Tumours such as this are sometimes regarded as serous although there is no justification for this other than a rather superficial resemblance to some serous tumours. H & E × 250

(Figure 27.5) with cuboidal or columnar epithelial cells arranged in a well defined glandular or acinar pattern: the appearances mimic exactly those of a well differentiated adenocarcinoma of the endometrium and, indeed, it is this resemblance to an endometrial neoplasm which is the defining characteristic of the endometrioid adenocarcinoma. Pleomorphism, cellular atypia, mitotic activity and stromal invasion are usually apparent in even the best differentiated endometrioid adenocarcinomata in which, however, the appearances may be modified by a papillary pattern, occurring either focally or predominantly; the papillae tend to be blunt and thus differ from the fine branching structures seen in serous adenocarcinomata. An uncommon, but confusing, pattern is that in which the glandular acini are small, rounded and almost solid, the appearances having some resemblance to a serous cell neoplasm (Figure 27.6). In less well differentiated endometrioid adenocarcinomata the acini are irregular and often poorly formed, whilst in poorly differentiated cases the tumour may consist largely of sheets of cells.

A particular problem with endometrioid adenocarcinoma is that its resemblance to an endometrial neoplasm is usually only readily apparent in well differentiated examples and there is, therefore, a reluctance to diagnose poorly differentiated endometrioid adenocarcinomata. However, there are two clues to the diagnosis of an endometrioid tumour which may be present in less well differentiated cases. The first of these is squamous metaplasia which is common and usually intraglandular: this may be a prominent or an inconspicuous feature. A second feature of many endometrioid tumours is the presence of cells with clear or vacuolated cytoplasm (Figure 27.7): these are typically arranged in sheets and, although often inconspicuous, may be the predominant cell type present: extensive sampling of largely clear celled tumours will, however, usually reveal areas of more conventional endometrioid adenocarcinoma.

Small amounts of extra- or intracellular mucus are present in many endometrioid adenocarcinomata whilst psammoma bodies are by no means rare. It is of importance to bear in mind that an associated adenocarcinoma of the endometrium is present in between 15 and 25% of cases[1,2]: there is considerable evidence to suggest that nearly all such cases are examples of synchronous development of two independent primary tumours.

The term 'malignant endometrioid neoplasm' encompasses any tumour which can occur in the endometrium and hence adeno-squamous carcinomata, carcinosarcomata, mixed Müllerian tumours of both high and low grade malignancy and endometrial stromal sarcomata can all occur in the ovary as variants of a malignant endometrioid neoplasm: all are rare though the mixed Müllerian tumour of high grade malignancy, which is histologically identical to its endometrial counterpart, is probably the least uncommon representative of this group.

Malignant Brenner Tumour

The rare malignant Brenner tumour is characterized by a marked overgrowth of the epithelial component, the epithelial cells showing nuclear hyperchromatism, prominent nucleoli, pleomorphism and mitotic activity, all features conspicuously lacking from the benign Brenner tumour[3]. Two types can be recognized: the first (Figure 27.8) is a clearly malignant infiltrating neoplasm which is similar to a transitional cell carcinoma, the cells growing in irregular sheets and often having a rather squamoid appearance. If a metastatic lesion from a primary carcinoma of the bladder can be confidently excluded the true nature of such a neoplasm can be assumed from the transitional nature of the malignant cells, but can only be proven if areas of more typical benign Brenner tumour are present in close proximity to the malignant neoplasm, preferably with evidence of transition or blending. The other form is that in which the neoplasm is clearly of Brenner type with epithelial islands set in a fibrous stroma but with marked cellular atypia and mitotic activity in the epithelial component and with stromal invasion.

Mesonephroid (Clear Cell) Adenocarcinoma

Most mesonephroid adenocarcinomata have a complex histological appearance (Figure 27.9) and contain tubules, cystic structures, simple or complex papillae and solid sheets of cells in various combinations and proportions. The cells lining the tubules and cysts may have abundant clear cytoplasm (Figure 27.10) or can show a 'hob-nail' appearance (Figure 27.11) with darkly staining, prominent, apparently almost naked, nuclei protruding into the lumen: some sometimes the epithelial lining of the cysts or tubules consists, however, of rather nondescript cubiform or flattened cells with clear or palely eosinophilic cytoplasm. Polygonal cells with well defined limiting membranes and abundant clear cytoplasm are often seen in sheets or solid aggregates whilst any papillae present commonly have a 'glomeruloid' appearance. In many of these neoplasms, foci of rather more straightforward adenocarcinoma, having a somewhat endometrioid appearance, are found. Small masses of hyaline eosinophilic extracellular material are frequently present, psammoma bodies are occasionally encountered and extracellular mucus is often apparent.

Undifferentiated Adenocarcinoma

Between 15 and 30% of ovarian adenocarcinomata are too poorly differentiated to be specifically identified (Figure 27.12). Histologically, it is usual to find sheets, solid masses or irregular nests of malignant cells showing considerable pleomorphism and mitotic activity: the nuclei tend to be large, vesicular and contain prominent nucleoli.

References

1. Czernobilsky, B., Silverman, B. and Mijuta, J. J. (1970). Endometrioid carcinoma of the ovary: a clinicopathologic study of 75 cases. *Cancer*, **26**, 1141–1152
2. Klemi, P. J. and Grönroos, M. (1979). Endometrioid carcinoma of the ovary: a clinicopathologic histochemical and electron microscopic study. *Obstet. Gynecol.*, **53**, 572–579
3. Woodruff, J. D., Dietrich, D., Genadry, R. and Palmley, T. H. (1981). Proliferative and malignant Brenner tumors: review of 47 cases. *Am. J. Obstet. Gynecol.*, **141**, 118–125

Ovary: Germ Cell Neoplasms

Tumours derived from ovarian germ cells may be dysgerminomata, which show no evidence of either embryonic or extraembryonic differentiation; they may show minimal differentiation into primitive embryonic-type cells to form the embryonal carcinoma, may differentiate along embryonic lines to produce the various types of teratoma or can differentiate along extraembryonic pathways, either into trophoblast to produce a choriocarcinoma or into yolk sac structures to give a yolk sac tumour. Many germ cell tumours are, however, mixed, varying combinations and permutations of dysgerminoma, embryonic tissues and extraembryonic elements being found in individual neoplasms.

Dysgerminomata

These neoplasms are formed of cells which acutely resemble, in all respects, primordial germ cells. They are large, round, ovoid or polygonal, with well defined limiting membranes, abundant clear or slightly eosinophilic cytoplasm and large, round or flattened, central vesicular nuclei with one or more prominent nucleoli. These cells are commonly arranged in alveoli separated by delicate fibrous septa (Figure 28.1) but may form strands or cords embedded in a fibrous stroma (Figure 28.2): occasionally they form solid sheets with little evidence of intervening stroma. A stromal lymphocytic infiltration, sometimes with germinal follicle formation, is a characteristic feature as is, less commonly, the presence of sarcoid-like granulomata: scattered multinucleated cells which contain hCG are occasionally seen.

A rare variant of this tumour is the 'anaplastic dysgerminoma' which is characterized by marked cellular pleomorphism, abundant mitotic activity and extensive multinucleation.

The vast majority of dysgerminomata are found in otherwise fully normal adolescent girls and young women: the tumour is malignant but markedly radiosensitive, and features suggestive of a good prognosis are an intact tumour capsule, a marked stromal lymphocytic infiltrate, a low mitotic figure count and minimal atypia of the tumour cells.

Embryonal Carcinomata (Figure 28.3)

These extremely rare neoplasms, more commonly seen as a component of a mixed tumour than in pure form, are formed of sheets of large primitive, pleomorphic, epithelial-like cells with vacuolated cytoplasm and vesicular nuclei containing one or more nucleoli: clefts or gland-like spaces may be present and, occasionally, solid papillae are formed. Multinucleated, hCG-containing, cells and mononuclear cells, containing hyaline droplets which give a positive reaction for α-fetoprotein, are usually also present and mitotic figures are frequent. This highly malignant neoplasm appears to consist, therefore, of cells showing a minimal degree of differentiation into both embryonic and extraembryonic tissues.

Yolk Sac Tumours

The concept that these tumours represent germ cell differentiation into extra embryonic mesoblast and yolk sac mesoderm has been strengthened by the demonstration of their shared ability with the yolk sac to produce α-fetoprotein. The tumours, which occur most commonly during the second decade, have a complex histological appearance with a number of patterns, any one of which may predominate in a given tumour. A loose, vacuolated, labyrinthine network containing microcysts lined by flattened cells is a characteristic feature, as is also the presence of Schiller–Duval bodies which have a mesenchymatous core containing a central blood vessel and an outer investment of cuboidal or columnar cells (Figure 28.4): gland-like structures are often present as are elongated anastamosing channels lined by cuboidal, flattened, columnar or 'hob-nail' cells. Groups or sheets of stellate cells of an indifferent nature may be a conspicuous feature. Small cyst-like structures lined partially by flattened mesothelial cells and partly by columnar cells are frequently seen: these are polyvesicular vitelline structures, and the biphasic lining epithelium is thought to correspond to the transformation of primary yolk sac endoderm into secondary endoderm. Sometimes these structures predominate or are the sole pattern present, the neoplasm then being classed as a polyvesicular vitelline tumour (Figure 28.5).

Yolk sac tumours are extremely malignant but many respond well to modern chemotherapeutic regimes.

Choriocarcinomata

Ovarian choriocarcinomata are occasionally encountered in pure form but are more commonly seen as a component of a mixed tumour: the pure choriocarcinoma is histologically identical with a uterine choriocarcinoma. The derivation of an ovarian choriocarcinoma from germ cells can only be assumed in women during the non-reproductive years of their lives for during the reproductive years the neoplasm could arise from a primary intra-ovarian pregnancy.

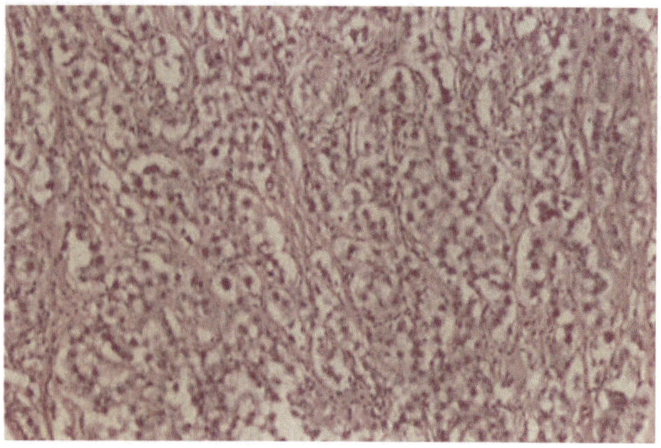

Figure 28.1 Ovary: dysgerminoma. Large cells with prominent round nuclei and clear cytoplasm are growing in an alveolar pattern with fine but distinct fibrous septa between the alveoli. There is a scattering of lymphocytes in the septa and a single ill-formed sarcoid-like granuloma in the upper centre of the field. H & E x 100

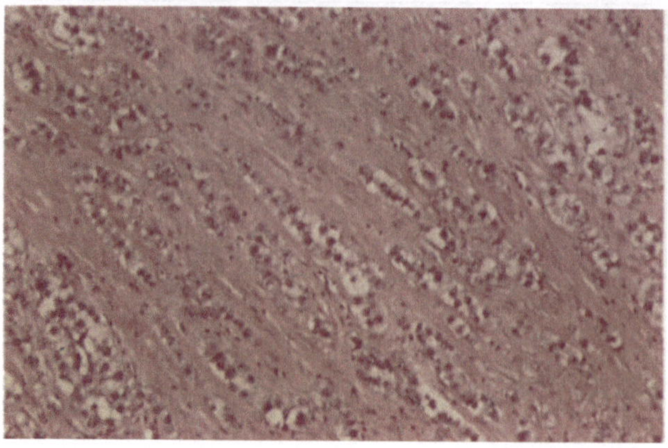

Figure 28.2 Ovary: dysgerminoma. In this example the neoplastic cells are growing in fine strands and cords within dense fibrous tissue. Occasional lymphocytes are present in the stroma. H & E x 100

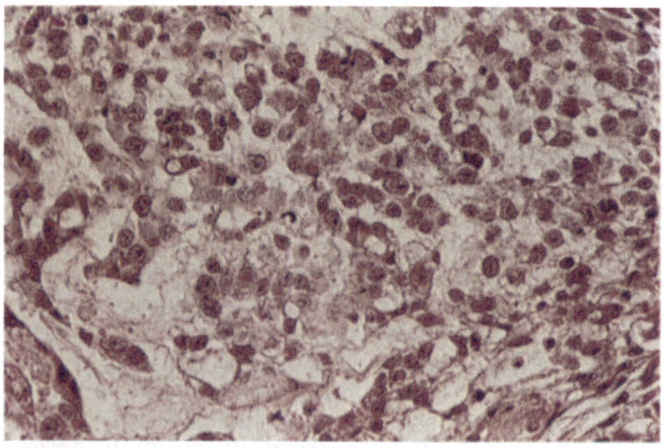

Figure 28.3 Ovary: embryonal carcinoma. An area of tumour with a mainly solid pattern, to the right, and forming clefts, to the left. The cells are large, pleomorphic, have vesicular or hyperchromatic nuclei and pale, eosinophilic granular cytoplasm; they tend to form a syncytium. H & E x 250

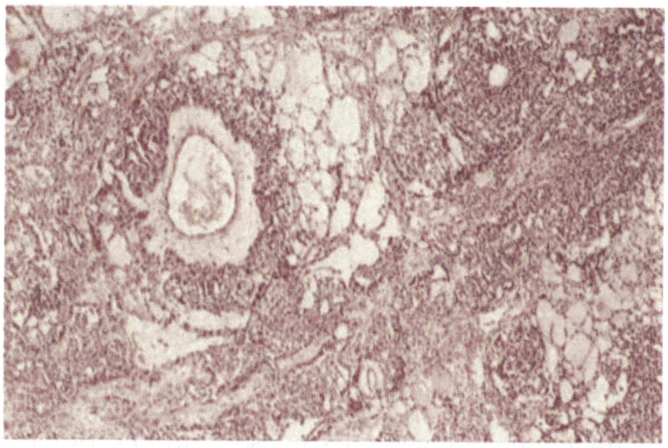

Figure 28.4 Ovary: endodermal sinus tumour. The tumour pattern is that of a loose cellular network forming a finely microcystic mesh. In the upper left of the field there is a Schiller–Duval body. The structure has a central blood vessel around which there is first a layer of loose, relatively acellular mesenchyme and then a dense layer of cubo–columnar cells forming papillae and incorporating small glandular structures. H & E x 40

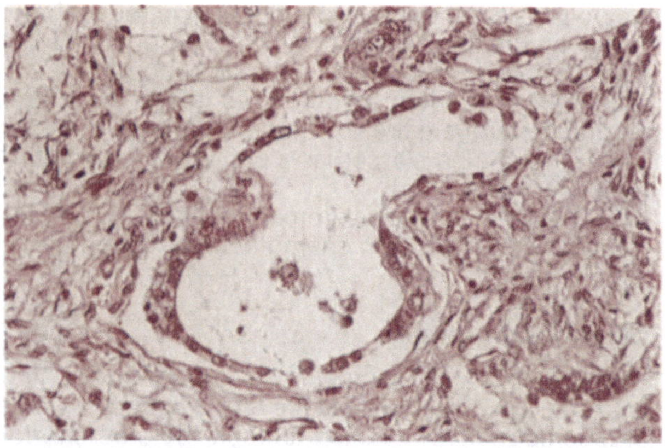

Figure 28.5 Ovary: polyvesicular vitelline tumour. The tumour is composed of cyst-like or vesicular structures, similar to this one, set in a fibrous stroma. The vesicle, which is lined at one end by flattened mesothelial-like cells and at the other by cubo–columnar cells, has a constriction in its midzone which marks the transition from one epithelium to the other. H & E x 250

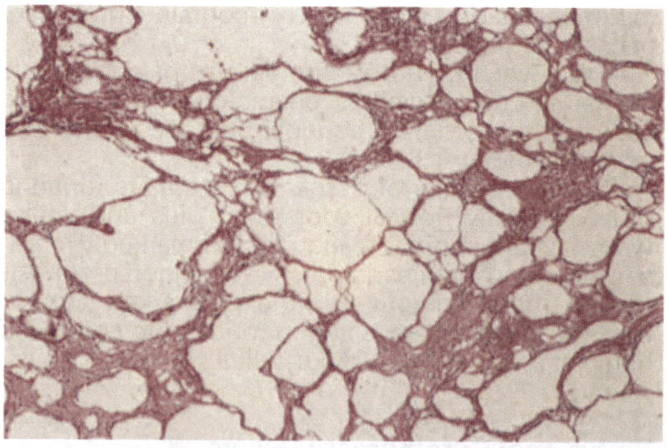

Figure 28.6 Ovary: mature cystic teratoma, sieve-like area. This is the wall of a cystic teratoma which had partially ruptured. It shows spaces around which there is fibrous tissue containing foamy histiocytes and macrophage giant cells. It is usual to find a few lymphocytes as well. H & E x 40

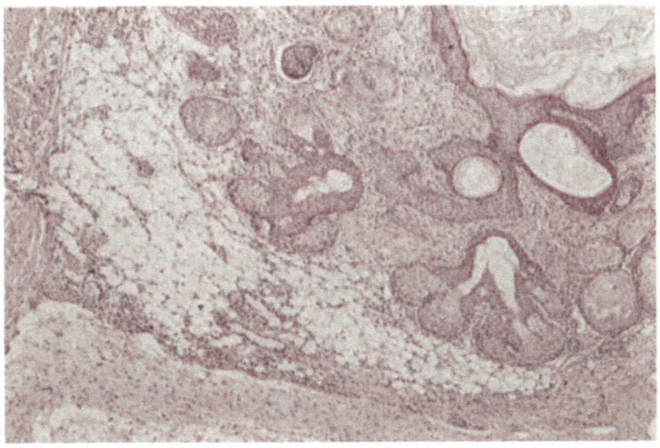

Figure 28.7 Ovary: mature solid teratoma. This field is representative of many such tumours. To the upper right there is a small cyst lined by mature keratinizing squamous epithelium surrounding which there are sebaceous gland units; centrally there is adipose tissue and below and to the left there is mature neural tissue. Cartilage and bone were present elsewhere in the tumour. H & E × 40

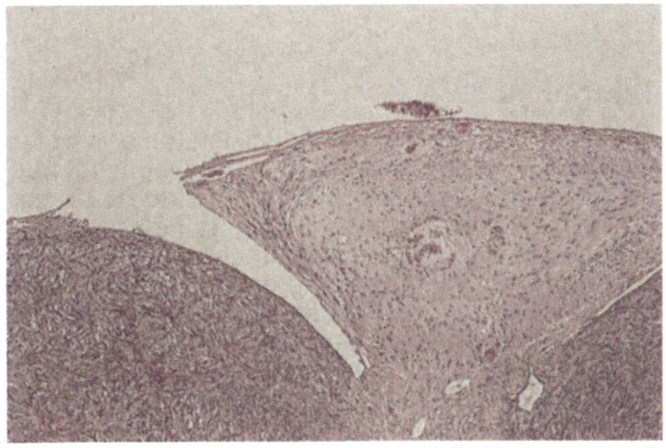

Figure 28.8 Ovary: glial implants. In this example implantation of glial tissue has occurred on the ovarian surface; similar deposits were present in the pelvic peritoneum. The glial tissue is mature and shows no evidence of infiltration into the ovarian stroma (below). H & E × 40

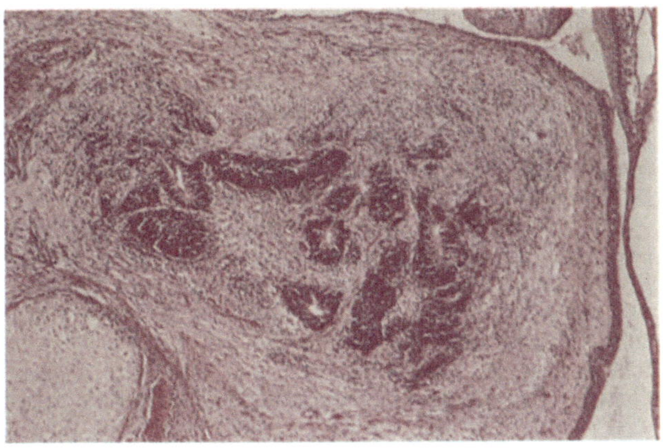

Figure 28.9 Ovary: immature solid teratoma. The centre of the field is occupied by clusters of small, darkly-staining immature neuroepithelial cells forming rosettes. Such aggregates are commonly seen although in some cases the neuroepithelium forms sheets without rosette formation. Note the adjacent immature cartilage and bone (to the lower left) and immature squamous epithelium (to the upper right). H & E × 40

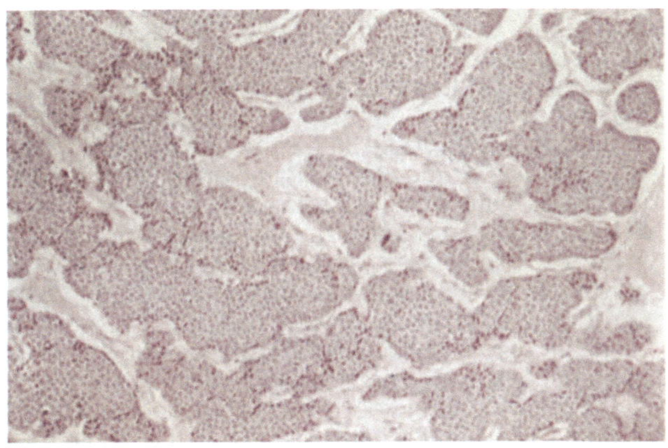

Figure 28.10 Ovary: insular carcinoid. The regular, small oval cells with round central nuclei and clearly defined margins are arranged in islands and nests of rather variable size. The cytoplasm is eosinophilic and contains fine argyrophil granules. The stroma is fibrous. H & E × 100

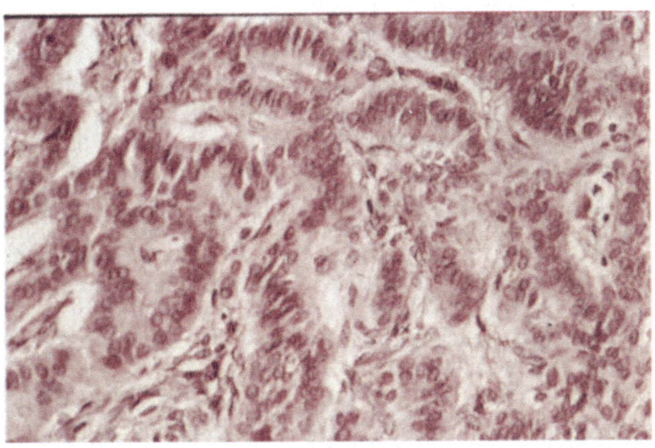

Figure 28.11 Ovary: trabecular carcinoid. The tumour is formed by cells arranged in wavy parallel trabeculae or ribbons set in a fibrous stroma. The cells have round nuclei with stippled chromatin, copious cytoplasm and a somewhat columnar configuration in contrast to the round or polygonal cells of the insular carcinoid. H & E × 250

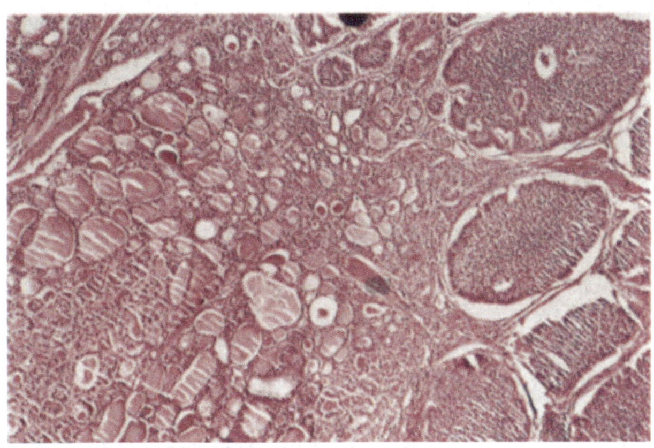

Figure 28.12 Ovary: strumal carcinoid. To the left of the field, there are well-formed thyroid acini, many of which contain colloid, and to the right islands of carcinoid tumour, the latter being formed by regular cells with round or ovoid nuclei, the peripheral layer of which forms a palisade. H & E × 40

Teratomata

The prognosis of any individual teratoma is determined, not by the usual criteria of malignancy, but by the degree of maturity of its constituent tissues. Those in which all the tissue components are fully mature, i.e. resemble adult tissues, run a benign course whilst with increasing degrees and extent of tissue immaturity, i.e. tissues resembling embryonic structures, there is a progressive tendency towards malignant behaviour. Hence teratomata are classed as either mature or immature, the term 'malignant' being reserved for carcinomata, or similar neoplasms, arising in a mature cystic teratoma.

Mature Cystic Teratoma

These neoplasms, the common 'dermoid cysts' of gynaecological practice, are sufficiently well known for little comment to be required as to their usual histological appearances. The classical appearances may, however, be altered by torsion or infection whilst it is not uncommon for their lining of squamous epithelium to be replaced, either wholly or in part, by granulation tissue containing foreign body-type giant cells. Under these circumstances the diagnosis may be dependent on the finding of sieve-like areas in the cyst wall (Figure 28.6): the true nature of these is unknown but they are a characteristic and specific feature of mature cystic teratomata

Rupture of a mature cystic teratoma, which occurs in about 1% of cases, may be sudden but can be chronic with slow leakage of cyst contents into the peritoneal cavity: this includes a chemical peritonitis with 'oily' ascites and multiple peritoneal and omental implants containing sebaceous materal and hair.

Malignant change occurs in between 1 and 2% of mature cystic teratomata, usually in the postmenopausal years. The resulting neoplasm is typically a squamous cell carcinoma, less commonly an adenocarcinoma: a wide range of other neoplasms can, however, arise on occasion, e.g. malignant melanoma, basal cell carcinoma, glioblastoma multiforme.

Mature Solid Teratomata

These rare neoplasms, which occur in childhood and adolescence, differ from their more common cystic counterpart only in being largely or entirely solid. The multiple tissue components, derived from all three germ cell layers, are all fully mature (Figure 28.7) but it must be stressed that these tumours must be very extensively sampled in order to exclude the presence of immature elements.

Mature solid teratomata are benign but some give rise, possibly because of partial capsular rupture, to multiple implants of mature, glial tissue on the peritoneum and omentum (Figure 28.8): this condition of peritoneal gliomatosis is non-progressive.

Immature Teratoma

These rare tumours are usually solid and occur most commonly during the first two decades of life. They usually contain a melange of mature and immature tissue components derived from all three germ cell layers, though the picture is not uncommonly dominated by immature mesenchymal or neuroepithelial tissue (Figure 28.9). These tumours are graded prognostically in terms of the degree and extent of tissue immaturity[1,2] thus:

- Grade 1: minor foci of immature tissue: rare mitotic activity
- Grade 2: moderate quantities of immature tissue: moderate mitotic activity
- Grade 3: large quantities of immature tissue

This grading system is of considerable value, but in recent years attention has also been focused on a quantitative assessment of the content of immature neuroepithelium[3], this adding a further degree of prognostic precision.

Immature teratomata may be confused with a malignant mixed Müllerian tumour but the latter does not contain tissues from all three germ cell layers (neural elements being conspicuously absent), and occurs in a very much older age group. Teratomata containing immature tissue run a malignant course but their prognosis has been transformed for the better in recent years by the introduction of effective chemotherapeutic agents.

Monodermal Teratomata

Teratomata are usually thought of as containing a mixture of tissues but some consist entirely, or predominantly, of one tissue: these may originally have been typical teratomata in which one component has overgrown and obliterated the other tissue elements or may be tumours which have differentiated along only one tissue line.

Thyroid tissue is present in many teratomata but a diagnosis of struma ovarii should be confined to those neoplasms in which thyroid tissue is the sole, or overwhelmingly predominant, component: such tumours are formed of histologically typical thyroid tissue and, although benign, may be complicated by marked ascites. It is debatable if a struma ovarii ever gives rise to 'pelvic hyperthyroidism' whilst malignant change is very rare: the histological diagnosis of malignant change may be relatively straightforward if a typical papillary adenocarcinoma develops, but commonly the only unequivocal evidence of malignancy is the development of metastases. Peritoneal deposits of a malignant struma ovarii may have a deceptively benign appearance though this condition of 'peritoneal strumatosis' is characteristic of an indolently malignant neoplasm and compatible with long survival.

Ovarian carcinoid tumours are uncommon and most occur in association with a mature cystic teratoma or enteric-type mucinous tumour: a minority occur, however, in pure form. The cells in a carcinoid tumour are rather small but have abundant, slightly eosinophilic cytoplasm and clearly defined cell boundaries: their nuclei are round and uniform. These cells may be arranged in an insular pattern (Figure 28.10), cellular islands being set in a variable amount of fibrous stroma: small rounded acini are often present in these islands, particularly at their periphery. The insular carcinoid tumour may be confused with a granulosa cell neoplasm but the presence of argyrophil cells, the rounded nature of the nuclei together with their lack of grooving, the relatively abundant cytoplasm and the well defined cell margins all help to identify a neoplasm as being of a carcinoid, rather than granulosa cell, nature. Another pattern adopted by ovarian carcinoid tumours is a trabecular one (Figure 28.11) in which long, often wavy, parallel, ribbons, one or two cells thick, are set in a fibrous stroma: the distinction between a trabecular carcinoid and a trabecular dysgerminoma or a poorly differentiated Sertoli–Leydig cell tumour does not usually present any great problem, but it may be extremely difficult to distinguish between any type of primary ovarian carcinoid tumour and a metastasis from a gastrointestinal carcinoid tumour: bilaterality and multinodularity suggest a secondary, rather than a primary, tumour.

The strumal carcinoid (Figure 28.12) is a rare neoplasm formed of a combination of a struma ovarii and a carcinoid tumour, usually of trabecular type but sometimes having an insular pattern. The carcinoid component of this neoplasm is thought to be derived from the parafollicular cells of the thyroid tissue and to be, therefore, homologous with the medullary carcinoma of the thyroid gland.

Other rare monodermal teratomata include pure primary malignant melonomata, retinal anlage tumours, primitive neuroectodermal tumours and sebaceous gland tumours. The commonest monodermal teratoma is, however, the enteric type of mucinous cystadenoma.

References

1. Thurlbeck, W. M. and Scully, R. E. (1960). Solid teratoma of the ovary: a clinicopathologic analysis of nine cases. *Cancer*, **13**, 804–813
2. Robboy, S. J. and Scully, R. E. (1970). Ovarian teratoma with glial implants on the peritoneum: an analysis of 12 cases. *Hum. Pathol.*, **1**, 543–653
3. Kurman, R. J. and Norris, H. J. (1977). Malignant germ cell tumors of the ovary. *Hum. Pathol.*, **8**, 551–564

Ovary: Sex Cord Stromal Neoplasms

29

This group of neoplasms includes all those which contain granulosa cells, thecal cells, Sertoli cells or Leydig cells, either singly or in any combination. Both granulosa and Sertoli cells are believed to be derived from the primitive sex cords of the embryonic gonad, and it is thought that in the postnatal ovary undifferentiated cells of sex cord origin retain a bisexual potentiality and can give rise to either granulosa or Sertoli cell neoplasms, these tumours being homologues of each other. Neoplasia of these cells is often accompanied by a stromal reaction which in the case of granulosa cell tumours may add a thecomatous element to the neoplasm, and which in the case of Sertoli cell tumours often shows Leydig cell differentiation. Stromal cells may themselves become neoplastic and can evolve into either thecomata or Leydig cell tumours.

Granulosa Cell Tumours

The cells forming a granulosa cell tumour are small and may be round, ovoid, polygonal or spindle shaped: they have scanty cytoplasm, indistinct cell boundaries and relatively large nuclei which often show a longitudinal groove. These cells are arranged in a variety of patterns and although, in any individual tumour, a particular cellular arrangement may predominate there is usually a mixture of patterns. A follicular pattern is common: microfollicles (Figure 29.1) consist of rosettes of cells arranged around a small central space containing dense eosinophilic material in which scattered shrunken nuclei or nuclear fragments may be seen (the Call–Exner body), whilst macrofollicles represent relatively large areas of liquefaction in islands of granulosa cells: an uncommon type of follicle is that which is large and lined by circumferentially arranged cells. The insular pattern (Figure 29.2) is characterized by islands of polygonal cells arranged, except at the periphery, without polarity and with few microfollicles. In the trabecular pattern (Figure 29.3) anastomosing cords or ribbons of cells are set in a stromal matrix: the ribbons may be one, two or several cells thick, and those cells adjacent to the stroma tend to be regimented at right angles to the axis of the ribbon with their nuclei arranged antipodally. If the ribbons are very thin and the stroma scanty the terms 'watered silk' or 'moire silk' are frequently applied. In the diffuse pattern, often wrongly and misleadingly referred to as a 'sarcomatous' pattern, the cells, usually polygonal or spindle-shaped, are arranged in sheets (Figure 29.4).

A particular variant of the granulosa cell tumour is the 'juvenile granulosa cell tumour' (Figure 29.5) in which there may be either large, thick-walled follicles or a disorderly mixture of granulosa and thecal cells: marked luteinization and nuclear hyperchromatism are common features. Such neoplasms occur, as their name suggests, most commonly in children but they are not confined to this age group[1].

Most granulosa cell tumours exert an oestrogenic effect and all should be considered as malignant[3]: the degree of malignancy is, however, often low and the course pursued by these tumours is frequently extremely indolent with recurrence or metastases appearing many years after removal of the primary neoplasm. The histological pattern of the neoplasm is of no prognostic value, and the only microscopic feature suggestive of a gloomy outlook is the presence of numerous mitotic figures, though even this is by no means a totally reliable criterion.

Thecomata

These neoplasms, which are usually oestrogenic, are particularly prone to develop in ovaries showing cortical stromal hyperplasia and are formed of plump, pale, ovoid or spindle-shaped cells with ill-defined borders, small ovoid nuclei and abundant pale cytoplasm (Figure 29.6): these are arranged in interlacing bundles or anastomosing trabeculae which are intermingled with bands of less cellular fibrous tissue. Reticulin fibres, which surround individual cells, are abundant, plaques of hyalinized collagen are often present and intracellular fat is usually demonstrable: focal or diffuse luteinization may occur.

Thecomata are almost invariably benign: rare instances of a malignant thecoma are, however, encountered[3], the diagnosis in such cases resting upon the presence of cellular pleomorphism and abnormal mitotic figures.

Androblastomata

Androblastomata are tumours composed of Sertoli cells, Leydig cells, or the precursors of either, in pure form or in any combination. These neoplasms were formerly known as 'arrhenoblastomata' but this name gives an impression of invariable accompanying virilization: not all these tumours are, however, androgenic and the term 'androblastomata' is preferred, for this lacks any connotations of endocrinological activity and emphasizes that the histological features of these neoplasms recapitulate morphological phases in the development of the male gonad[4].

Sertoli Cell Tumours

These neoplasms are formed of highly differentiated uniform tubules (Figure 29.7) which are lined by a single layer of radially arranged cells with clear cytoplasm and basal nuclei. The lining cells may have clearly defined lateral and apical borders but it is not uncommon for their apical cytoplasm to trail off towards the tubular lumen to form interlacing fibrils, whilst their lateral boundaries may be sufficiently ill-defined as to impart a syncytial-like appearance. The cells usually contain some cytoplasmic lipid in the form of fine droplets and are occasionally markedly distended and vacuolated by fat.

Pure Sertoli cell tumours are invariably benign and often appear to be oestrogenic.

Leydig Cell Tumours

These may arise either from stromal cells or from pre-existing hilar cells and are formed of regular, ovoid or polygonal, cells arranged in closely packed sheets or solid cords (Figure 29.8). These cells have large nuclei which are often centrally placed, but not uncommonly appear aggregated or 'pooled', and finely granular, markedly eosinophilic cytoplasm in which lipid droplets and granules of lipochrome pigment are frequently present. Reinke's crystals, which are slender rod-shaped, bodies with rounded, tapering or square ends and measure between 10 and 20 μm in length, are present in about 50% of these neoplasms but are irregularly distributed and often only found after extensive sampling: they are best seen in sections stained with Masson's trichrome (in which they appear red) and although their presence is an absolute indication of the Leydig cell nature of a neoplasm their absence does not negate this diagnosis.

A variant of this typical Leydig cell neoplasm is the stromal Leydig cell tumour which is formed largely of spindle-shaped cells but which shows multifocal Leydig cell differentiation.

Leydig cell tumours are usually androgenic though a small minority are oestrogenic. They are nearly always benign but very occasional cases have given rise to metastases: those which have behaved in a malignant fashion have not usually differed histologically from those pursuing a benign course[3].

Sertoli–Leydig Cell Tumours

These neoplasms contain a mixture of Sertoli and Leydig cells but it is possible, indeed probable, that the Leydig cell component is not neoplastic but is due to Leydig cell differentiation in a stromal reaction to a Sertoli cell tumour.

Histologically, well differentiated Sertoli–Leydig cell tumours (Figure 29.9) are formed of clearly defined tubular structures lined by Sertoli-like cells and Leydig cells are present, in variable numbers, between the tubules. In tumours of intermediate differentiation (Figure 29.10) reasonably well defined Sertoli cells are arranged in true tubules, solid tubules, trabeculae or solid cords: the cords may be long and sinuous but are more commonly short and fragmented, being formed of a double layer of cells arranged perpendicular to the axis of the cord. This Sertoli cell component is set in an abundant mesenchymal stroma containing spindle cells and collagen in various proportions: Leydig cells are seen in the stroma, singly, in clusters or as sheets. Poorly differentiated neoplasms (Figure 29.11) are formed largely of sheets of closely packed spindle-shaped cells in which occasional irregular cords or imperfectly formed tubules may be recognized: small groups of Leydig cells are also present and, indeed, if these are not seen the tumour can only be designated as a 'sex cord stromal tumour of indeterminate type'.

A small proportion of Sertoli–Leydig cell tumours also contain heterologous elements such as mucinous epithelium, fat, muscle, bone or cartilage: the presence of these elements has been variously attributed to mesenchymal metaplasia or to a possible teratomatous origin of androblastomata of this type.

Most Sertoli–Leydig cell neoplasms are androgenic but a few, particularly the well differentiated ones, appear to exert an oestrogenic effect. The well differentiated neoplasms appear always to behave in a benign fashion but a small proportion of the less well differentiated tumours, probably less than 5%[5], recur or metastasize: the histological appearances in these tumours offer no guide to prognosis and, in particular, it can not be assumed that a poorly differentiated tumour is more likely to behave in a malignant fashion than is one of our intermediate differentiation.

Gynandroblastoma

These are extremely rare tumours which may be either oestrogenic or androgenic. They should only be diagnosed if undisputable granulosa cell and Sertoli–Leydig cell components are present, and if each forms a significant proportion of the neoplasm.

Sex Cord Tumours with Annular Tubules

These are formed of rounded nests of cells separated by stroma (Figure 29.12). The nests are formed by epithelial-like cells arranged around hyaline bodies to form simple or complex cords: the cells have clear or eosinophilic cytoplasm, indistinct borders and nuclei which are palisaded around the margins of the nests and around the hyaline cores. Many of these cells have a Sertoli-like appearance but there is increasing electron microscopic evidence that they are in fact granulosa cells, a view strengthened by the occasional merging of a tumour of this type with a granulosa cell tumour[6]. Some of these tumours are of only microscopic size and there is a tendency for these small lesions, which are possibly hamartomatous in nature, to be associated with the Peutz–Jeghers syndrome: others are large and more clearly neoplastic, occasional cases having given rise to metastases[7].

References

1. Scully, R. E. (1982). Sex cord-stromal tumors. In Blaustein, A. (ed.) *Pathology of the Female Genital Tract*. 2nd edn. pp. 581–601. (New York, Heidelberg and Berlin: Springer-Verlag)
2. Fox, H., Agrawal, K. and Langley, F. A. (1975). A clinico-pathological study of 92 cases of granulosa cell tumor of the ovary with special reference to the factors influencing prognosis. *Cancer*, **35**, 231–241

3. Fox, H. and Langley, F. A. (1981). Malignant gonadal stromal tumours of the ovary. In Coppleson, M. (ed.) *Gynecologic Oncology*. pp. 697–709. (Edinburgh, London, Melbourne and New York: Churchill Livingstone)

4. Teilum, G. (1958). Classification of testicular and ovarian androblastoma and Sertoli cell tumors. A survey of comparative studies with consideration of histogenesis, endocrinology and embryological theories. *Cancer*, **11**, 769–782

5. Roth, L. M., Anderson, M. C., Govan, A. D. T., Langley, F. A., Gowing, N. F. C. and Woodcock, A. S. (1981). Sertoli–Leydig cell tumors: a clinicopathologic study of 34 cases. *Cancer*, **48**, 187–197

6. Anderson, M. C., Govan, A. D. T., Langley, F. A., Woodcock, A. S. and Tyagi, S. P. (1980). Ovarian sex cord tumours with annular tubules. *Histopathology*, **4**, 137–145

7. Hart, W. R., Kumar, N. and Crissman, J. D. (1980). Ovarian neoplasms resembling sex cord tumours with annular tubules. *Cancer*, **45**, 2352–2363

Figures 29.1–29.2 will be found overleaf.

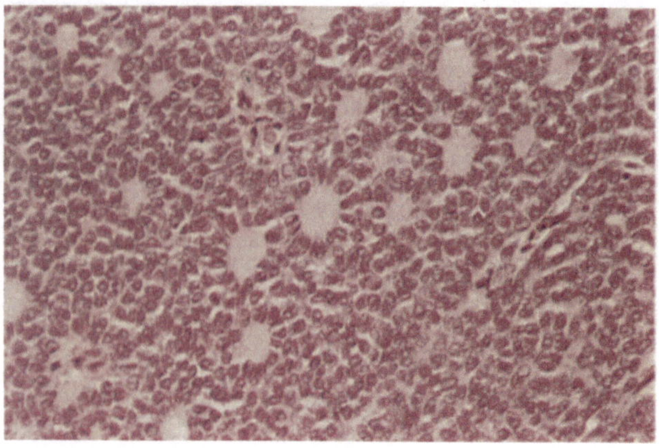

Figure 29.1 Ovary: granulosa cell tumour. In the micro-follicular pattern shown here, the cells are arranged in rosettes around dense eosinophilic material. These are Call–Exner bodies. H & E × 250

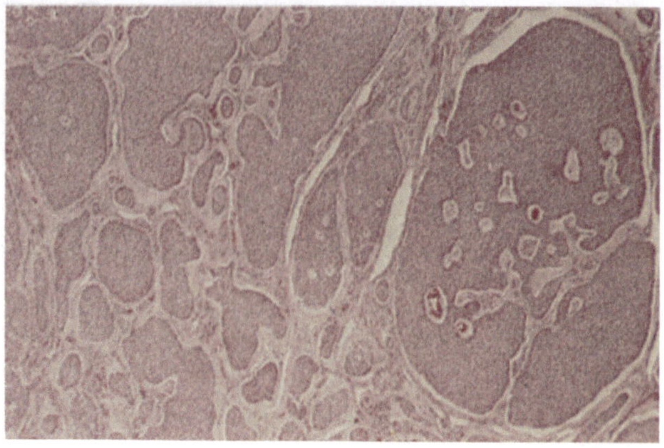

Figure 29.2 Ovary: granulosa cell tumour, insular pattern. The cells are forming islands of varying shapes and sizes, those in the centres of the islands being arranged randomly whilst those at the margin form a definite palisade with their long axes at right angles to the insular margin. Micro-follicles are rare. H & E × 40

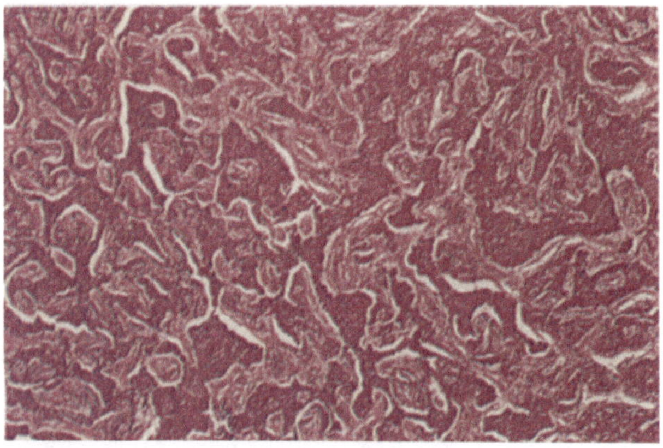

Figure 29.3 Ovary: granulosa cell tumour, trabecular pattern. The granulosa cells are arranged in irregular branching and anastomosing trabeculae which vary in size. Elsewhere the tumour showed both insular and diffuse patterns. H & E × 40

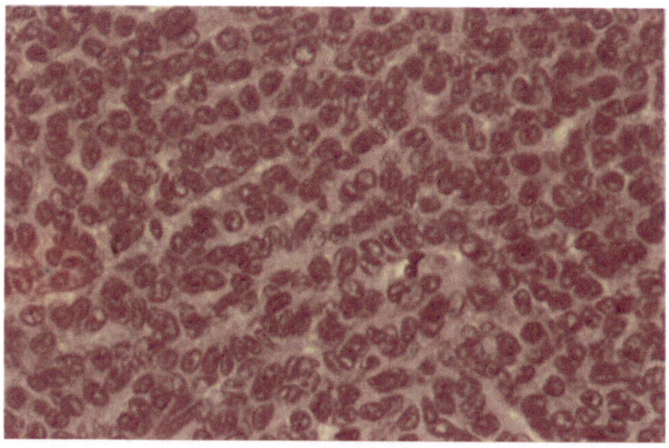

Figure 29.4 Ovary: granulosa cell tumour, diffuse pattern. The neoplasm is composed of diffuse sheets of cells with ill-defined cell boundaries and pale, rather scanty, eosinophilic cytoplasm. The nuclei are predominantly round or ovoid and in many there is a distinct groove. H & E × 400

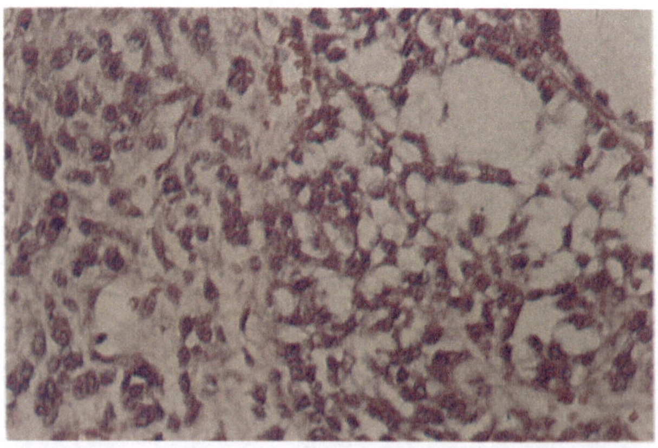

Figure 29.5 Ovary: juvenile granulosa cell tumour. To the right of the field is a follicle-like structure of lipid-containing granulosa cells whilst to the left there are plump, luteinized stromal cells. The nuclei of the granulosa cells are more hyperchromatic than in the common form of the tumour; mitoses are fairly numerous. Elsewhere there was a macrofollicular pattern and in some areas an intermingling of granulosa and thecal cells to form solid sheets. H & E × 25

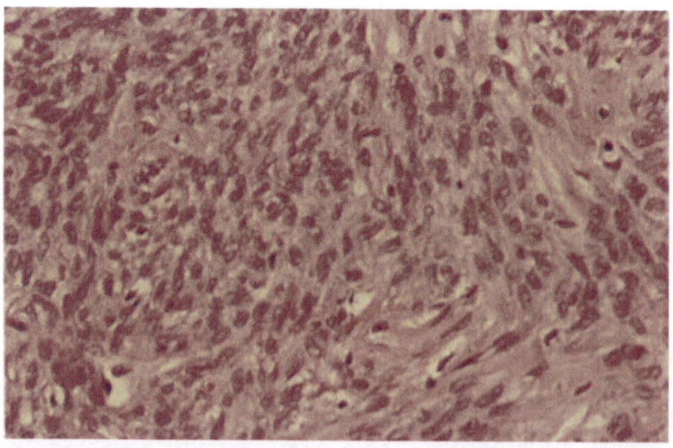

Figure 29.6 Ovary: thecoma. Thecomata vary in appearance, some being very cellular and rich in lipid whilst others show extensive hyalinization. In the left of this field the cells are ovoid or plump spindle-shaped, have pale eosinophilic cytoplasm, vesicular ovoid nuclei and ill-defined cell boundaries. To the right there are bands of hyalinized collagen. H & E × 250

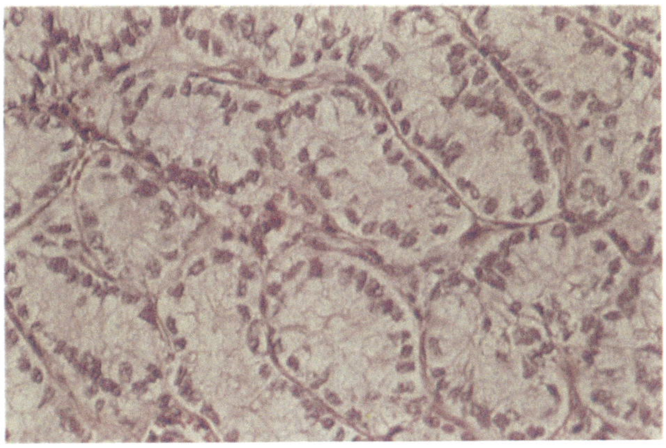

Figure 29.7 Ovary: Sertoli cell tumour. The whole tumour is composed of uniform tubules lined by tall columnar cells with pale faintly granular cytoplasm and round or oval basal nuclei. H & E × 250

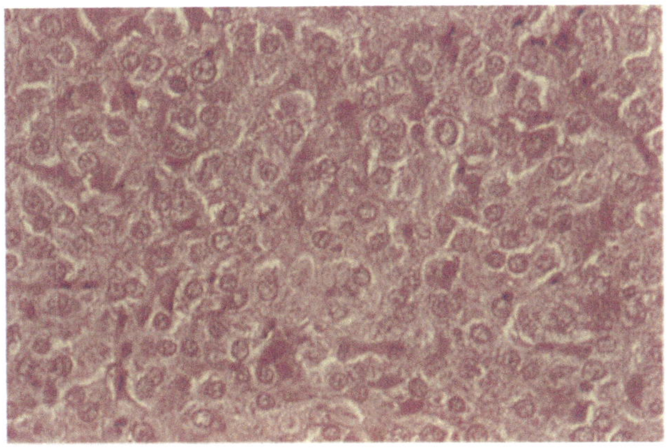

Figure 29.8 Ovary: Leydig cell tumour. The cells are large, ovoid or polygonal, their cytoplasm is copious, granular and eosinophilic. The nuclei are large, round and vesicular. Note that to the lower left foci are seen in which the nuclei appear concentrated or aggregated. H & E × 250

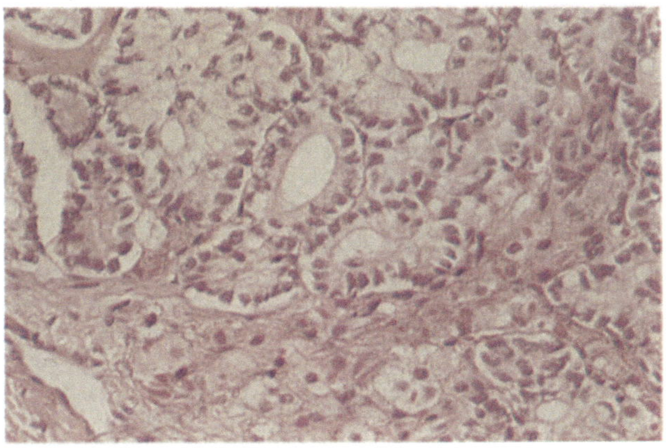

Figure 29.9 Ovary: well-differentiated Sertoli–Leydig cell tumour. The neoplasm is composed of well-defined tubules. They are lined by Sertoli-like cells with ill-defined cellular margins, round basal nuclei and pale granular cytoplasm. Between the tubules and to the lower left of the field there are clusters of Leydig cells which have copious eosinophilic cytoplasm and central, round vesicular nuclei. The cytoplasmic vacuolation is due to the accumulation of lipid. H & E × 250

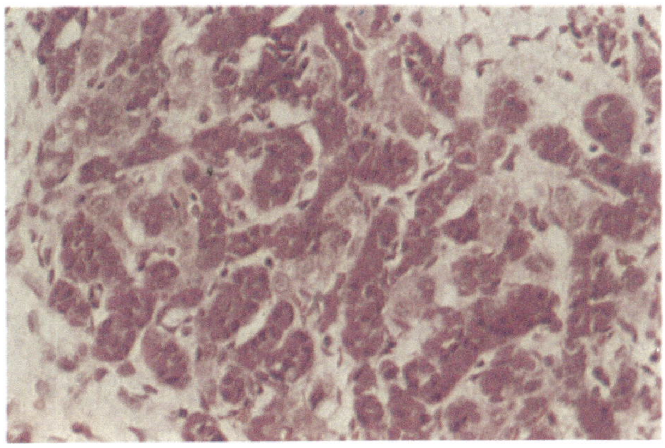

Figure 29.10 Ovary: Sertoli–Leydig cell tumour of intermediate differentiation. Darkly staining immature Sertoli-like cells are arranged in short cords; between the cords there are Leydig cells. This area of intermediate differentiation was present in a tumour showing other, less differentiated areas, a not uncommon occurrence. H & E × 250

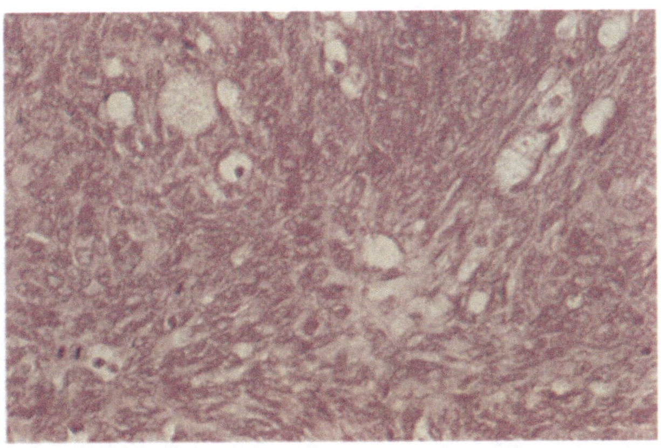

Figure 29.11 Ovary: poorly differentiated Sertoli–Leydig cell tumour. Occasional large vacuolated cells with foamy, eosinophilic cytoplasm lie between interweaving bands of elongated cells resembling fibroblasts. These are Leydig cells and bands of sex cord stromal cells. Note the resemblance to fibrosarcoma and the mitoses (lower left). H & E × 250

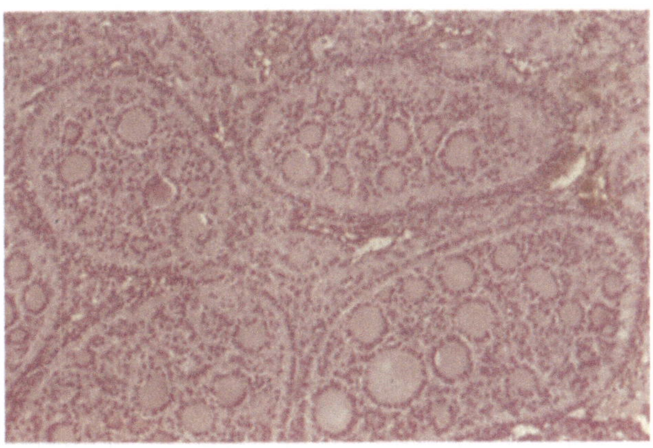

Figure 29.12 Ovary: sex cord tumour with annular tubules. The tumour is composed of round or ovoid nests of cells. Around the margins of the nests there is a palisade of columnar cells with basal nuclei and pale, eosinophilic granular cytoplasm. The centres of the nests are composed of intersecting cords of similar cells. At the points of intersection there are opaque, hyaline eosinophilic cores. The nests and hyaline cords vary in size. H & E × 100

Ovary: Miscellaneous Neoplasms 30

Tumours of Non-specialized Tissues

Tumours can develop from any of the non-specialized ovarian mesenchymal tissues: these may be malignant, and it is not always possible to distinguish such neoplasms from a one-sided development of a mixed Müllerian tumour. The fibroma is the only common tumour in this group and is formed of small, thin, spindle-shaped cells with narrow ovoid nuclei running parallel to their long axis (Figure 30.1): these cells are arranged in interlocking bundles but the appearances may be markedly altered by oedema, hyalinization or myxoid change. Intracellular lipid is absent and this, together with the thinness of the cells, helps to distinguish a fibroma from a thecoma: it is admitted, however, that cases are encountered in which the histological features lie somewhere between those typical of a fibroma and those characteristic of a thecoma, and under such circumstances the rather unsatisfactory diagnosis of 'fibrothecoma' has to be made. Ascites complicate about 15% of ovarian fibromata and fluid may also accumulate in the pleural cavity to give a typical Meig's syndrome: oedema of the legs, vulva and anterior abdominal wall is sometimes seen. Rarely, ovarian fibromata form part of the basal cell naevus or Gardner's syndrome. Ovarian fibrosarcomata are very rare, the diagnosis depending upon the histological evidence of pleomorphism and mitotic activity, both features conspicuously absent from the benign fibroma.

A distinct entity, differing from the fibroma, is the sclerosing stromal tumour (Figure 30.2) which usually develops during the second and third decades, and shows a pseudolobular pattern in which cellular nodules are separated from each other by bands of hyaline or oedematous connective tissue: in the cellular areas there is a mixture of fibroblasts, lipid-containing rounded cells and oval polyhedral cells. This neoplasm is thought to arise from the ovarian stroma, appears to be occasionally oestrogenic and is invariably benign.

A vast range of other non-specific tumours can, on occasion, arise in the ovary, such as leiomyomata, leiomyosarcomata, angiosarcomata, rhabdomyosarcomata, chrondrosarcomata, etc. but their histological features do not differ in any way from those seen in such tumours in extragonadal sites. Only the rare haemangiomata merit comment: these are usually cavernous or capillary–cavernous in type and are formed of thin-walled vessels. Not uncommonly, however, the leash of hilar ovarian vessels is mistaken for a haemangioma, an error that can be avoided if the hilar site and thick-walled nature of the normal ovarian vasculature is borne in mind (Figure 30.3).

Mixed Germ Cell Sex Cord Stromal Tumours

Three forms of mixed tumours of this type are currently recognized, of which the gonadoblastoma is the most common. Gonadoblastomata are small and contain cellular nests surrounded by a collagenous stroma: within the nests there is a mixture of large germ cells and smaller cells which resemble immature Sertoli or granulosa cells (Figure 30.4). The small ovoid cells of sex cord type may be arranged in a microfollicular pattern around blobs of hyaline material, may form an investment around groups of germ cells or surround germ cells in a coronal fashion. The stroma between the cell nests often, but not invariably, contains groups of Leydig or luteinized cells and foci of calcification are extremely common. Gonadoblastomata occur in individuals who, irrespective of phenotype, nearly always have a Y chromosome and who usually have either a pure or a mixed gonadal dysgenesis, and it is possible that they are a hamartomatous malformation rather than a true neoplasm. Nevertheless, a malignant germ cell neoplasm, usually a dysgerminoma but occasionally a choriocarcinoma, yolk sac tumour or immature teratoma, will eventually develop in about 50% of cases.

A very rare form of mixed germ cell–sex cord tumour, distinct from a gonadoblastoma, occurs in young children with a normal karyotype and otherwise normal ovaries[1]; in these tumours, which are usually large, the germ cells and sex cord cells are intimately admixed and arranged in trabeculae, solid tubules or sheets (Figure 30.5). These tumours appear to behave in a benign fashion.

The third type of mixed tumour, a combined sex cord tumour with annular tubules and dysgerminoma (Figure 30.6), is of exceptional rarity.

Lipoid Cell Neoplasms

This term is applied to a group of uncommon neoplasms, usually virilizing, having an endocrine-type architecture and formed of large, oval or polygonal cells which resemble lutein, Leydig or adrenocortical cells (Figure 30.7). It is probable that all are derived from the ovarian stromal cells which may differentiate along a variety of pathways to produce a range of neoplasms of common histogenesis but differing morphology.

The Leydig cell variant of the lipoid cell tumour is, by definition, regarded as a form of androblastoma but some lipoid cell tumours bear a striking morphological resemblance to an adrenocortical adenoma. These adrenal-like tumours are formed of large poly-

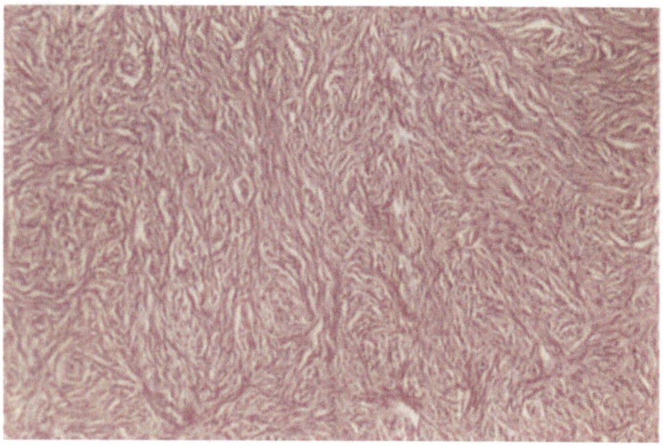

Figure 30.1 Ovary: fibroma. The tumour is composed of interlacing bundles of narrow spindle-shaped cells. The cells which lie parallel to the axes of the bundles have narrow, densely staining tapering nuclei and eosinophilic cytoplasm. H & E × 40

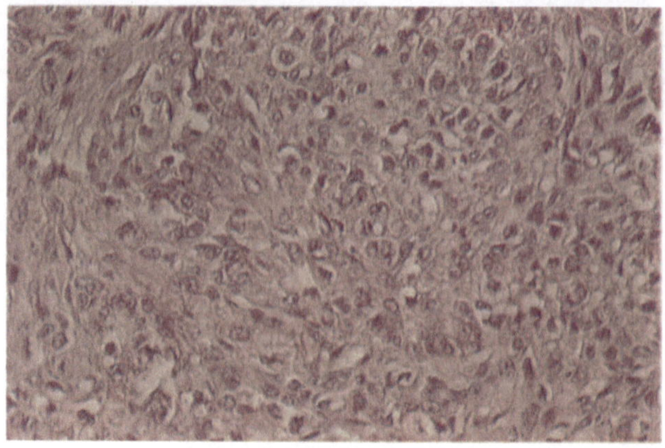

Figure 30.2 Ovary: sclerosing stromal tumour. This field from the centre of one of the cellular pseudolobules contains an intimate mixture of large round cells with clear lipid-laden cytoplasm and spindled fibroblasts. H & E × 250

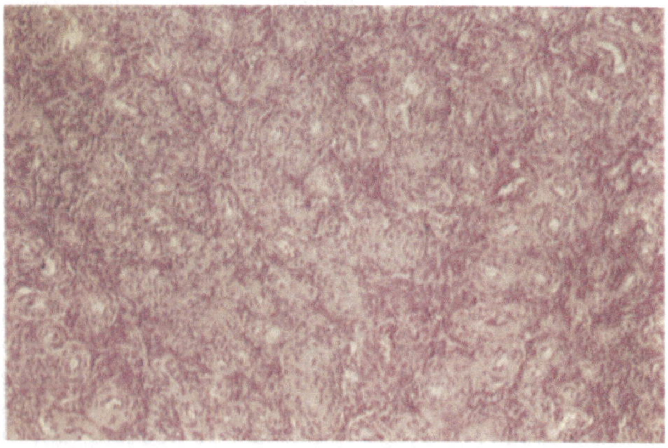

Figure 30.3 Ovary: hilar vasculature. This field gives some idea of the intense vascularity of the ovarian hilum which occurs in some patients. It can be distinguished from a haemangioma by the presence of muscle in the vessel walls and their orderly disposition in the hilum. H & E × 100

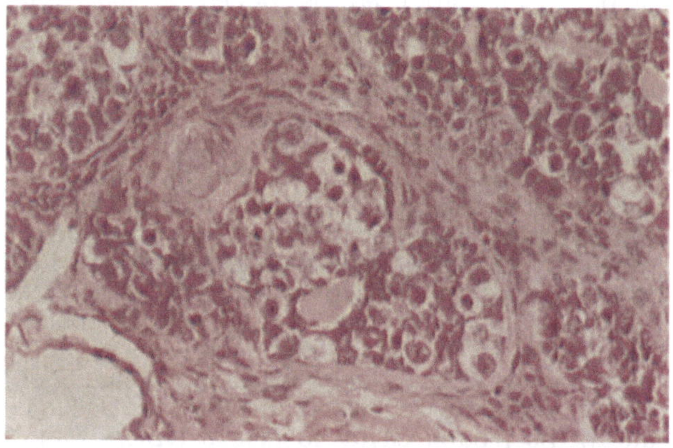

Figure 30.4 Ovary: gonadoblastoma. Several cell nests, set in a fibrous stroma, are present in this field. The nest in the centre contains large germ cells with clear or faintly granular cytoplasm and large round central vesicular nuclei with prominent nucleoli. The germ cells are surrounded by cells of sex cord type and similar cells also surround hyaline material. Focal calcification has occurred in hyaline material to the upper left of the nest and luteinized stromal, or Leydig, cells are seen in the fibrous tissue. H & E × 250

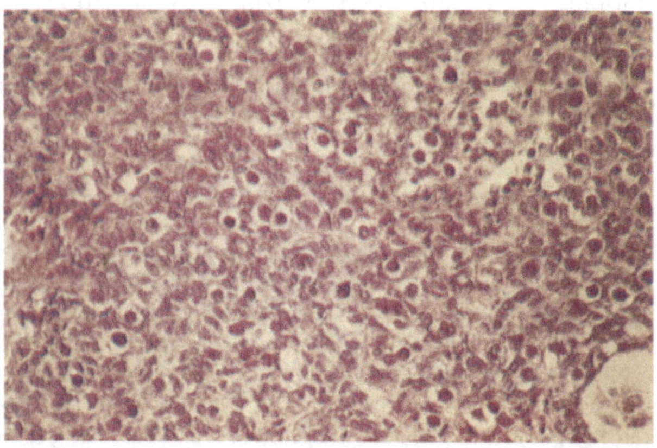

Figure 30.5 Ovary: mixed germ cell–sex cord tumour. The field shows an intimate mixture of round germ cells with large, dense, round, central nuclei and clear cytoplasm and trabeculae and pseudoacini of sex cord cells which are cubo–columnar and have ill-defined cellular margins. H & E × 250

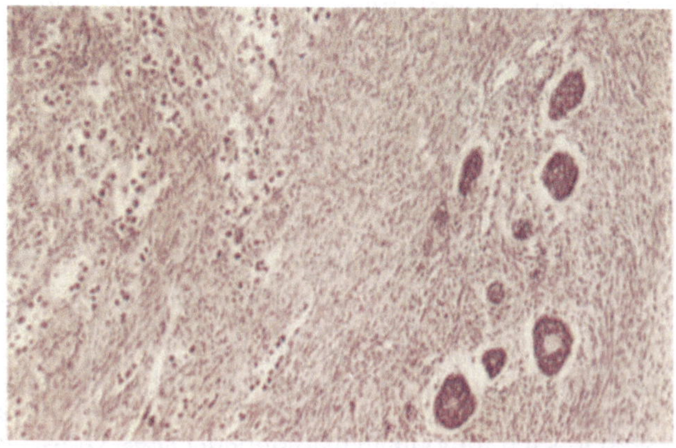

Figure 30.6 Ovary: sex cord tumour with annular tubules and dysgerminoma. To the left of the field is a typical infiltrating dysgerminoma and to the right, nests of sex cord tumour with annular tubules. (For histological details see Figures 28.2 and 29.12.) H & E × 100

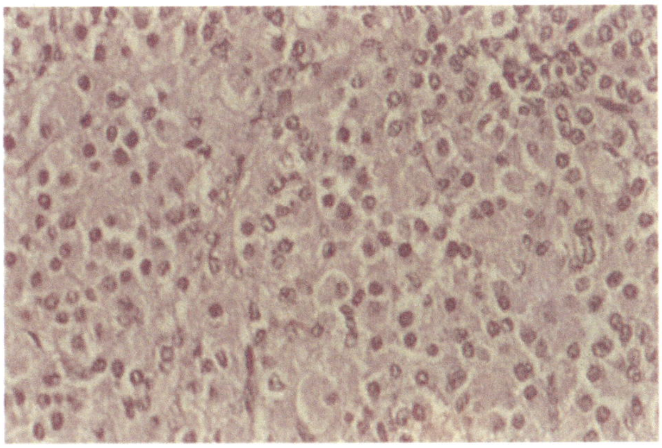

Figure 30.7 Ovary: lipoid cell neoplasm. The tumour is composed of closely packed nests of large round or polygonal cells with copious eosinophilic cytoplasm and round or ovoid vesicular nuclei. H & E × 25

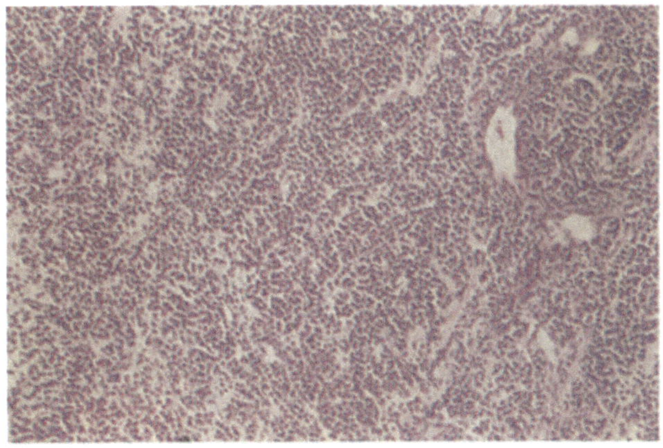

Figure 30.8 Ovary: diffuse lymphoma. The ovarian architecture is obliterated by infiltrating sheets and strands of darkly staining lymphomatous cells. H & E × 100

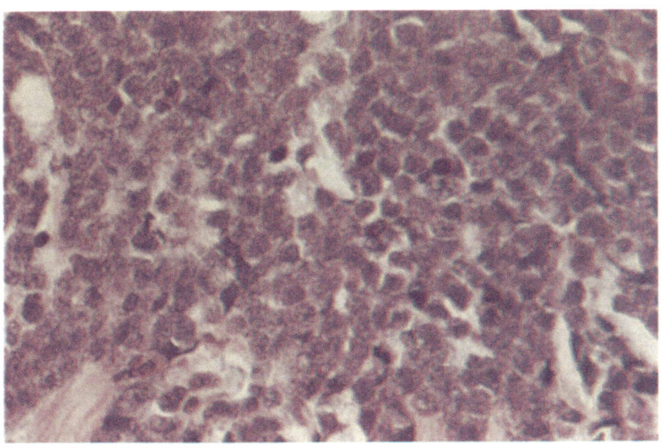

Figure 30.9 Ovary: lymphoma. A detail of the ovary seen in Figure 30.8 showing the sheets of poorly differentiated lymphocytic cells with frequent mitoses. Diffuse granulosa ·cell tumour is sometimes confused with lymphoma because of the superficial similarity in their pattern of growth. H & E × 400

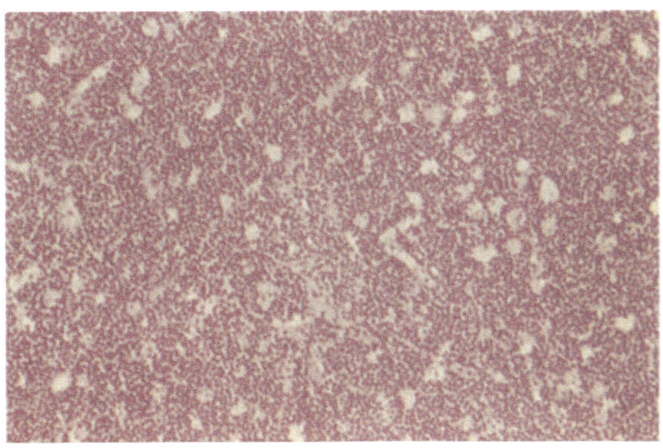

Figure 30.10 Ovary: Burkitt lymphoma. At low magnification the tumour has a 'starry sky' appearance. This is due to the contrast between the pale-staining macrophages and the darkly staining lymphoid cell which constitutes the bulk of the neoplasm. H & E × 100

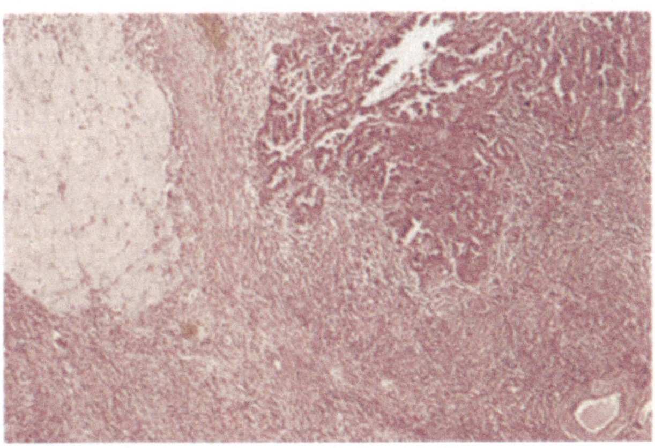

Figure 30.11 Ovary: metastatic adenocarcinoma. This ovary was removed from a patient who had a papillary serous cystadenocarcinoma in the contralateral ovary. The field shows one of several metastatic foci of tumour which were developing in the ovarian cortex. Note the chronic inflammatory cell infiltrate at the advancing margin of the neoplasm. H & E × 4

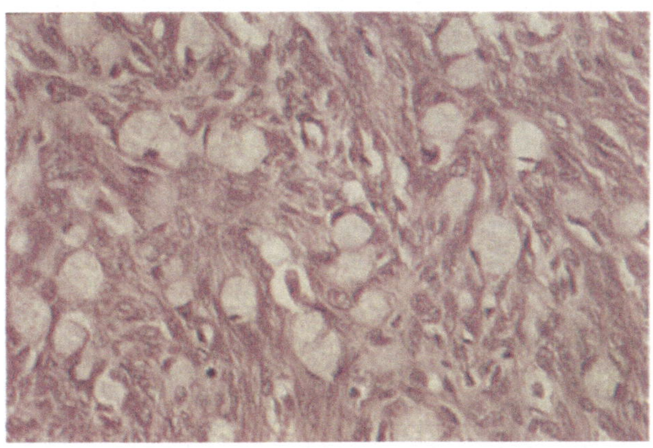

Figure 30.12 Ovary: Krukenberg tumour. Large pale neoplastic epithelial cells with faintly granular, eosinophilic or basophilic cytoplasm and eccentric nuclei lie within dense fibrous stroma. In other examples the stroma may be more oedematous and the tumour cells may form clusters or indistinct acini or tubules. The stroma may present a 'pseudosarcomatous' appearance. H & E × 250

gonal or rounded cells with well defined margins and abundant, usually lipid-containing, cytoplasm which are arranged in nests or columns around a rich capillary network: they are usually virilizing and there is little evidence that they can secrete adrenal corticosteroids. It was originally thought that these neoplasms originated in ovarian adrenal rests but it is extremely doubtful if such rests ever occur in the adult ovary, and a derivation from stromal cells is indicated by the occasional evidence of a peripheral transition between tumour and stromal cells and by the admixture of adrenal-like cells with Leydig cells in some neoplasms. The adrenal-like tumours are usually benign but a few, though lacking the conventional histological characteristics of malignancy, have recurred or metastasized.

Some lipoid cell neoplasms do not show clear cut evidence of either Leydig or adrenal cell differentiation and are often classed as luteomata. It is doubtful, however, if such a neoplasm exists, most tumours bearing this diagnosis have in fact been luteinized Leydig, granulosa or thecal cell neoplasms whilst the luteoma of pregnancy is a non-neoplastic condition. These unclassifiable lipoid cell neoplasms are best called 'lipoid cell tumours of indeterminate type'.

Malignant Lymphoma

The ovary is not uncommonly involved in disseminated malignant lymphoma and occasionally patients with disseminated disease present with a palpable ovarian mass: primary extranodal malignant lymphoma of the ovary can also occur but is distinctly uncommon. The histological appearances are, however, very similar in both these circumstances and it is not possible, simply by studying the ovary, to determine if this is a primary lesion or a secondary involvement.

Malignant lymphomata of the ovary are nearly always of the diffuse non-Hodgkins type, most being either lymphoblastic or poorly differentiated lymphocytic in nature: a minority are histiocytic. The characteristic histological picture (Figure 30.8) is of sheets of uniform cells which totally obliterate all ovarian structures though occasionally ovarian follicles are seen surrounded by tumour cells. The cytological features (Figure 30.9) are those of a lymphoma and need not be discussed fully here. A lymphoma must be differentiated from a metastatic oat cell or breast carcinoma and from a diffuse granulosa cell tumour: the cytological features usually make this distinction relatively easy but in debatable cases the problem is resolved by the application of immunocytochemical stains for B cell markers and histochemical stains for specific histiocytic cell enzymes.

A particular type of ovarian lymphoma is the Burkitt lymphoma (Figure 30.10), usually encountered in the tropics but occasionally seen in temperate zones. The predominant cell is an undifferentiated or primitive stem cell which is arranged in sheets: macrophages are, however, interspersed amongst the tumour cells to give a 'starry sky' appearance.

Metastatic Tumours

The ovary is a common site of metastasis, particularly from primary sites in the breast, gastrointestinal tract and uterus. The proportion of apparently primary malignant ovarian tumours which eventually turn out to be metastatic is probably about 15–20%.

Most metastatic tumours resemble the primary neoplasm from which they are derived (Figure 30.11) and thus do not often present any diagnostic difficulty. It can, however, be extremely difficult to differentiate between a metastasis from a colonic adenocarcinoma and a primary mucinous adenocarcinoma of the ovary: features suggestive of a metastasis rather than a primary tumour include a multifocal tumour pattern and blood vessel invasion, this latter feature being a particular characteristic of metastatic deposits in the ovary.

The subject of metastatic tumours of the ovary has been bedevilled by the loose and inconsistent usage of the term 'Krukenberg tumour': a diagnosis of Krukenberg tumour should be based solely on histological grounds and any mucus-secreting adenocarcinoma, whether it be from a primary site in the stomach, colon, breast or gall bladder, may fall into this category. The true Krukenberg tumour is commonly bilateral and, histologically, consists of plump, rounded epithelial cells set in a dense cellular stroma: the epithelial cells, which may occur singly or in clusters, are frequently mucus-containing and have their nuclei displaced laterally to give a signet-ring appearance (Figure 30.12). The stromal cells are plump, spindle-shaped and show a moderate degree of pleomorphism and mitotic activity, features which have sometimes evoked the incorrect use of the term 'pseudosarcomatous pattern'. Variations on this basic theme are not uncommon, these including the formation of tubules, a trabecular arrangement of mucin-poor cells and the presence of cysts lined by apparently innocuous mucinous epithelium[2]. Focal stromal luteinization is a not uncommon feature of Krukenberg tumours.

The question as to whether a primary Krukenberg tumour of the ovary can occur is a vexed one, but there seems no good reason why a primary mucinous adenocarcinoma of the ovary should not occasionally assume the histological appearances of a Krukenberg tumour. Nevertheless, such a diagnosis should be made with extreme caution for the absence of a primary extra-ovarian tumour can be very difficult to prove, instances of presumed primary Krukenberg tumours of the ovary having been described in which a primary gastric carcinoma did not become apparent until nearly 5 years after removal of the ovarian neoplasm[3]. Indeed, the diagnosis of primary Krukenberg tumour of the ovary should not be entertained until the patient has survived in good health for at least 5 years after removal of the ovarian tumour or has been shown at autopsy to have no extra-ovarian primary tumour.

References

1. Talerman, A. (1982). Germ cell tumors of the ovary. In Blaustein, A. (ed.). *Pathology of the Female Genital Tract*. 2nd edn., pp. 602–664. (New York, Heidelberg, Berlin: Springer-Verlag)
2. Scully, R. E. (1979). Tumors of the Ovary and Maldeveloped Gonads. *Atlas of Tumour Pathology, 2nd Series, Fascicle 16*. (Washington, DC: Armed Forces Institute of Pathology)
3. *Fox, H. and Langley, F. A. (1976). Tumours of the Ovary.* (London: Heinemann)

Endometriosis and Endosalpingiosis 31

Endometriosis

Endometriosis is characterized by the presence of ectopic endometrial tissue in an extra-myometrial site. Attempts have been made to impose a conceptual unity on the two conditions of adenomyosis and endometriosis by referring to the former as 'internal endometriosis' and to the latter as 'external endometriosis': there is, however, no valid justification for this terminology which blurs the fact that adenomyosis and endometriosis, though not uncommonly occurring together in the same patient, are conditions of differing aetiology and pathogenesis.

The pathogenesis of endometriosis is, however, still far from being fully understood though suggested mechanisms are:

(1) Reflux of endometrial tissue through the Fallopian tubes as a result of retrograde menstruation with subsequent implantation on, and growth in, the pelvic peritoneum.
(2) Multifocal endometrial metaplasia of the pelvic peritoneum, either occurring spontaneously or being induced by contact with fragments of regurgitated endometrium which subsequently die and are absorbed.
(3) Haematogenous dissemination of endometrial tissue.
(4) Lymphatic spread of endometrial tissue.

Cogent reasons are forthcoming for supporting each of these theories but it would appear that most instances of endometriosis are due to one or other of the first two suggested mechanisms: not all cases of this disease are, however, explicable on this basis or in terms of any unitary theory and it is almost certain that endometriosis can develop along any of these proposed pathogenetic pathways. Furthermore, genetic and immunological factors probably also play a role[1–3] whilst it has been maintained, with some validity, that many examples of apparent ovarian endometriosis are, in fact, of a benign neoplastic nature[4].

The commonest sites of endometriosis are, in rough descending order of frequency, the ovaries, pouch of Douglas, uterine ligaments, pelvic peritoneum, rectovaginal septum, uterine cervix, appendix, inguinal hernial sacs and large or small bowel; foci of endometriosis are occasionally encountered in surgical scars, in the vulva, at the umbilicus and in the bladder whilst exceptional instances of lesions occurring in lymph nodes, kidney, limbs, pleura and lungs have been described.

The basic pathology of endometriosis is simple as the only criterion for diagnosis of this condition is the finding of histologically recognizable endometrial glands and stroma in an ectopic site (Figure 31.1). The ectopic endometrial tissue may or may not show cyclical changes, more commonly the latter, but any such activity tends to be weakly developed, the glands showing either only a minor degree of proliferative activity or a markedly inadequate secretory transformation. This basic simplicity is, however, often confounded by a number of complicating factors, predominant amongst which is the tendency for haemorrhage to occur in endometriotic foci: bleeding into the lesion itself can cause considerable distortion or damage which may culminate in a 'self-destruction' of the endometrial tissue, whilst leakage of blood into the surrounding tissues releases intensely fibrogenic iron which promotes dense adhesions that may obscure the primary lesion. A second complicating factor is the tendency for some endometriotic lesions, particularly in the ovary, to undergo cystic change with resulting attenuation, or loss, both of the lining epithelium and of the surrounding mantle of stroma.

Ovarian Endometriosis

In the early stages of ovarian endometriosis the lesions are seen as small raised, dimpled or puckered, reddish-blue surface implants: later, tiny cysts appear and these tend to enlarge and grow into the ovarian tissue, commonly attaining a diameter of 2–5 cm and sometimes being as large as 10 cm across. The cysts have a smooth or granular, brownish-yellow lining and, usually, a thick fibrotic wall: their content of old, semi-fluid or inspissated blood commonly has a dark brown or black appearance – hence the term 'chocolate cysts'. Leakage of blood from the endometriotic foci results in the formation of dense adhesions which often bind the ovary down to the posterior surface of the uterus or broad ligament.

The histological diagnosis of ovarian endometriosis is readily made if typical endometrial glands and stroma are present: such foci are usually found on, or just below, the surface epithelium, but may occasionally be seen in the wall of the cyst. In many instances, however, the epithelium lining an endometriotic cyst is reduced to a monolayer of cuboidal cells (Figure 31.2) which may retain, to some extent endometrial characteristics but which is frequently devoid of specific identifying features: recognition of the endometriotic nature of the cyst under the latter circumstances may only be possible if there is still a thin rim of surrounding endometrial stromal tissue but can be presumed if the attenuated epithelium is surrounded by a mantle of large, rounded or polyhedral, haemosiderin-containing macrophages (Figure 31.3). Often, however, the cyst lining is either

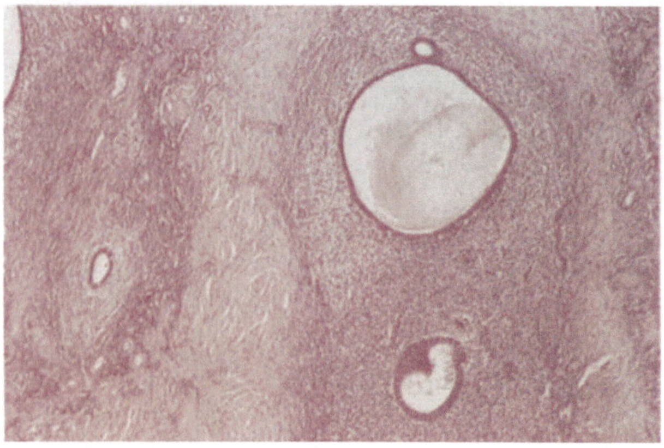

Figure 31.1 Ovary: endometriosis. This ovary shows several typical foci of endometriosis. They contain stroma and non-secretory glands which are cystically dilated. There is no evidence of haemorrhage. H & E × 40

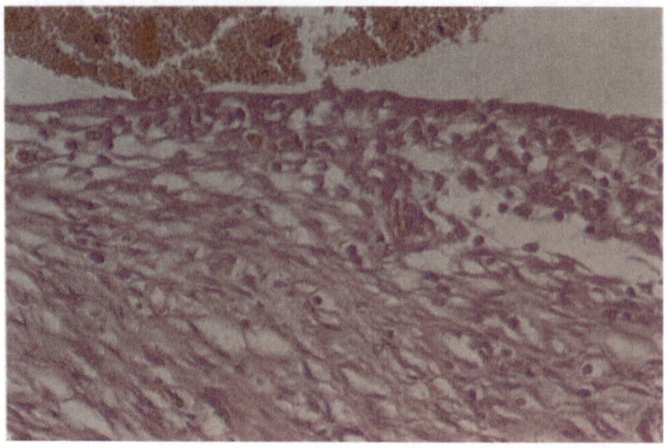

Figure 31.2 Ovary: endometriotic cyst. The cyst is lined by a single layer of flattened cubo–columnar cells beneath which an occasional endometrial stromal cell can be identified. The wall is fibrous and the lumen contains blood which has come from bleeding foci of functional endometrial tissue elsewhere in the cyst. H & E × 250

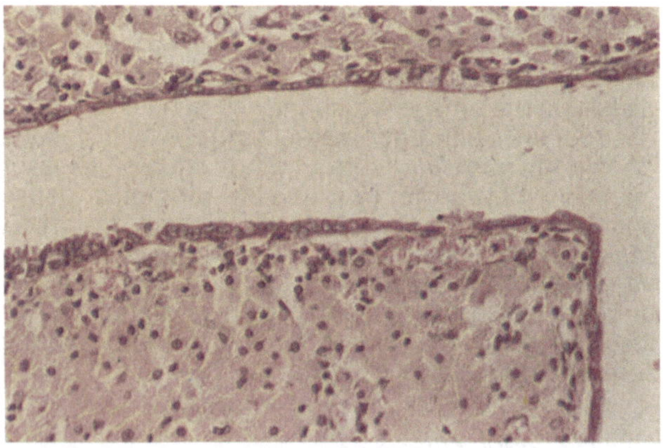

Figure 31.3 Ovary: endometriotic cyst. The cyst is lined by a single layer of cubo–columnar cells similar to those seen in Figure 31.2 but there is no stroma, the underlying tissue is composed chiefly of macrophages. These latter cells are large, round or polyhedral, have round or ovoid central nuclei and their cytoplasm is pale, eosinophilic and granular. There is little haemosiderin in this example. H & E × 250

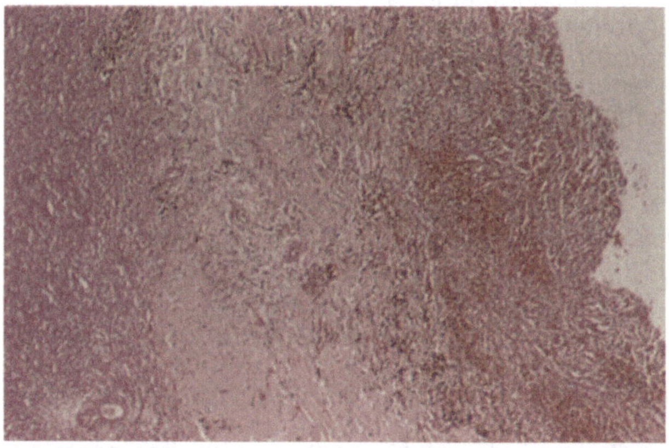

Figure 31.4 Ovary: endometriotic cyst. Endometrial tissue has been completely lost in this example. The cyst is lined (from the right) by successive layers of young granulation tissue showing foci of haemorrhage, more mature granulation tissue and dense fibrous tissue. Haemosiderin-containing macrophages are present in all layers, those in the deeper layers being most heavily pigmented. Ovarian stroma is visible to the left. H & E × 40

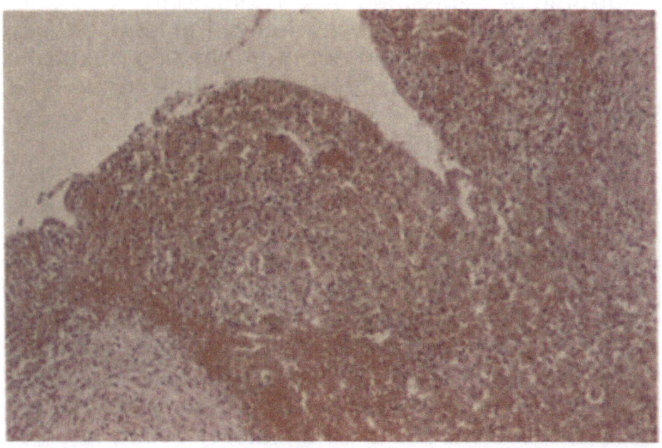

Figure 31.5 Ovary: endometriotic cyst. The cyst is lined predominantly by haemosiderin-containing macrophages and foci of haemorrhage. In cases where characteristic endometriotic tissue is not immediately apparent in a cyst wall a careful examination will often reveal some remnants characteristic of endometrium, areas of which are often well preserved even when there has been extensive destruction and haemorrhage. H & E × 100

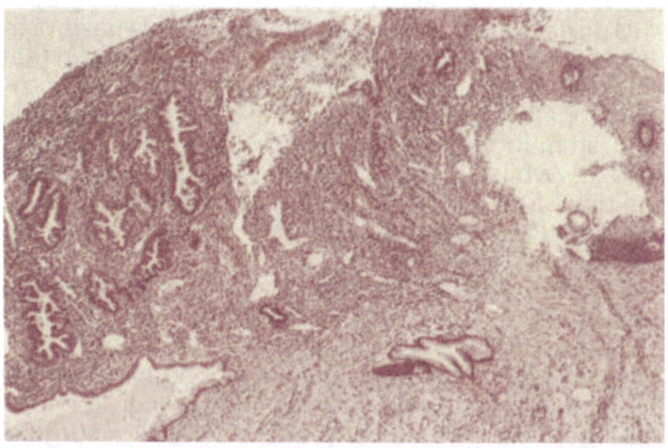

Figure 31.6 Cervix: endometriosis. Endocervical tissue incorporating crypts lined by tall mucus-secreting cells (to the right) is in continuity with secretory endometrium (to the upper left). The endometrium which contains mature secretory glands and copious, partly decidualized stroma undergoes cyclical breakdown and haemorrhage in synchrony with the intrauterine endometrium and may form a visible haemorrhagic focus on the cervix. H & E × 40

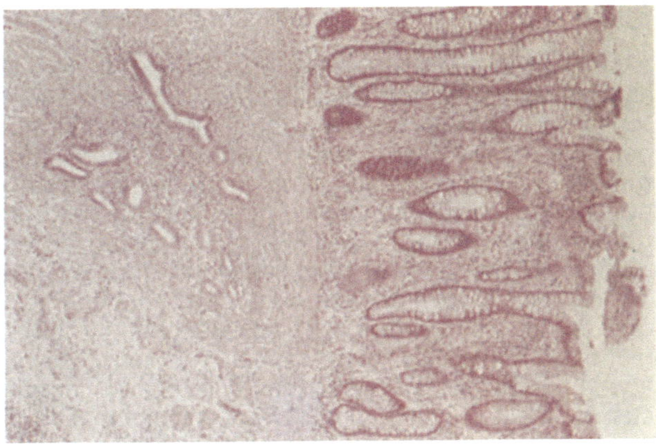

Figure 31.7 Colon: endometriosis. Within the colonic submucosa (to the left) there is a typical focus of endometrial stroma and glands. The mucosa, to the right, is not grossly abnormal in this area but was ulcerated elsewhere, endometrial tissue forming the ulcer base. H & E × 40

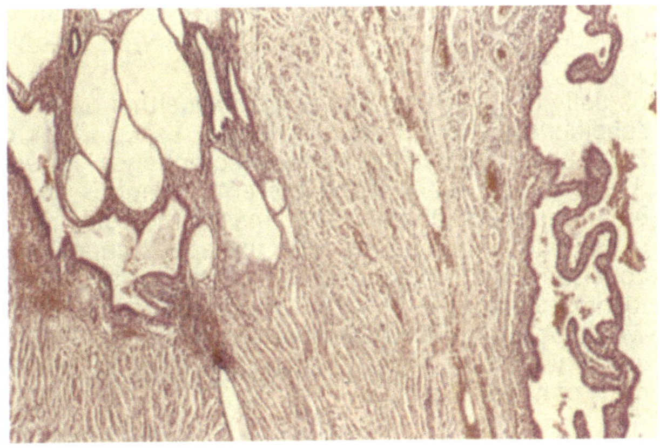

Figure 31.8 Fallopian tube: endometriosis. The tube lumen, which lies to the right is moderately distended and there is a hydrosalpinx. Within the wall (to the left) there is a focus of endometrium comprising basal type glands, some of which are cystically dilated, functional glandular tissue and stroma. H & E × 40

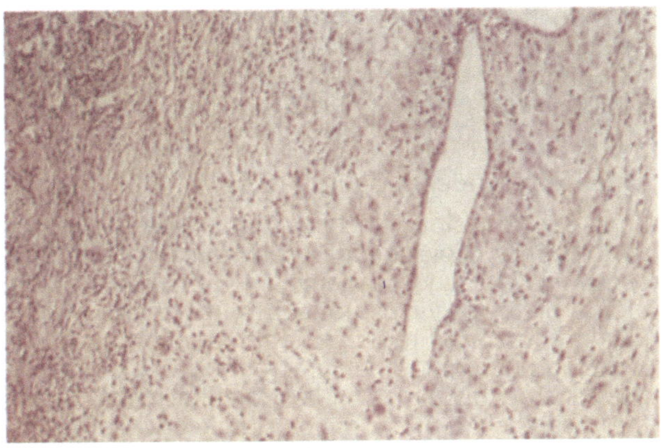

Figure 31.9 Ovary: endometriosis, hormone effect. This example shows the effect of progestagens on endometriosis. The stromal cells are enlarged and have copious eosinophilic cytoplasm: there is an infiltrate of small, dark stromal macrophages (K-cells). The glandular epithelium is flattened and shows neither secretory nor proliferative activity. The biopsy came from a patient who was 14 weeks pregnant. H & E × 100

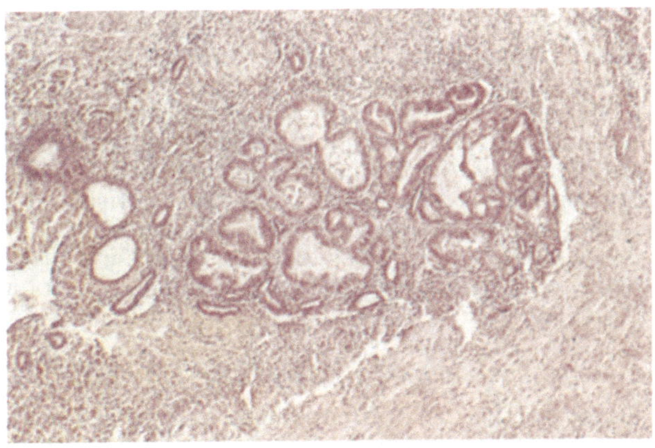

Figure 31.10 Ovary: endometriosis with atypia. This cluster of closely packed endometrial glands in the wall of an endometriotic cyst shows architectural atypia (Figure 14.4). The glands are irregular in outline, show invaginations, outpouching and a mild degree of cellular atypia. The cyst lumen lies to the left and haemosiderin-containing macrophages lie beneath the lining epithelium. H & E × 40

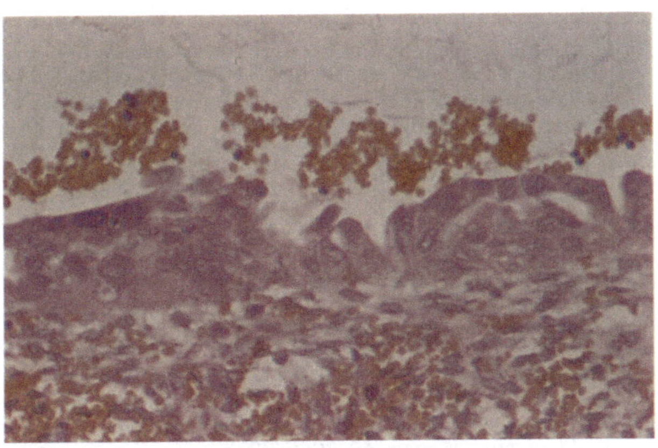

Figure 31.11 Ovary: endometriosis with atypia. The epithelium lining this endometriotic cyst is multilayered; it shows budding, multinucleation and cellular and nuclear pleomorphism; nucleoli are present. Such a picture may be due to intraepithelial neoplasia but a similar appearance may be a reaction to severe inflammation and regeneration. H & E × 250

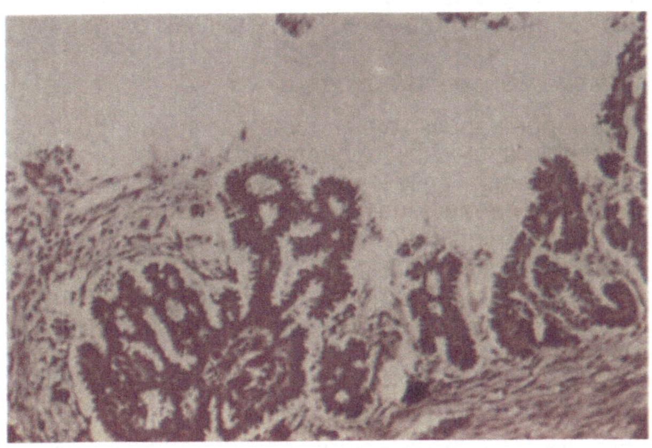

Figure 31.12 Uterine serosa: endosalpingiosis. The peritoneum bears papillary fragments formed by epithelium of tubal type. There is no cytological atypia; small psammoma bodies are present. H & E × 100

partially or totally lost and is replaced either by non-specific granulation tissue, fibrous tissue (Figure 31.4) or aggregated pigmented macrophages (Figure 31.5), these usually being present in various combinations and permutations. In these circumstances it is justifiable to conclude that the appearances 'are consistent with a diagnosis of endometriosis' or even to make a diagnosis of 'probable endometriosis' but it would be imprudent to be more dogmatic than this for virtually identical appearances may be encountered in cysts of luteal origin.

Cervical Endometriosis

Endometriosis at this site (Figure 31.6) needs to be distinguished from atypical endocervical glands and from mesonephric remnants: this distinction is not usually difficult if recognizable endometrial stroma is present, as it usually is, around the glands.

Gastrointestinal Endometriosis

In a typical case endometriosis of the gastrointestinal tract (Figure 31.7) does not give rise to any diagnostic problem. Sometimes, however, endometriosis in the colon forms a nodule or mass which can be mistaken for a primary colonic adenocarcinoma. Such a lesion is usually predominantly fibrous and when cut the firm white fibrous tissue tends to be honeycombed by tiny blood-filled cysts: it is of considerable diagnostic importance to note that the colonic mucosa is usually intact but it has to be borne in mind that a neoplasm may occasionally arise in, and from, colonic endometriosis.

Endometriosis of the Fallopian Tube (Figure 31.8)

Endometriosis can occur on the serosal surface of the tube, usually in typical and easily recognizable form, or can develop within the tubal lumen: in the latter circumstances the endometrial tissue often replaces the tubal epithelium in the proximal portion of the tube, and this may represent an extrusion of uterine endometrium into the tube rather than true endometriosis. In other instances, however, foci of endosalpingeal endometriosis are seen separated from the uterine epithelium by typical tubal epithelium. It has been suggested, not altogether convincingly, that foci of this type may predispose to tubal pregnancy.

Effects of Exogenous Hormones

The appearances of endometriosis can be considerably altered by the administration of progestational agents. These lead to atrophy of the glands and a marked predecidual change in the stroma (Figure 31.9). Administration of oestrogens may have the same effects on endometriotic foci as it does on the normally sited endometrium, and can lead to various patterns of hyperplasia identical in type to those seen in the endometrium.

Atypia and Malignant Change in Endometriosis

There is no doubt that malignant neoplasms can arise from foci of endometriosis, this occurring most commonly in the ovary but having also been noted in many extragonadal sites[5,6]. The resulting tumour is usually an endometrioid adenocarcinoma but mixed Müllerian tumours of both high and low grade malignancy, clear cell adenocarcinoma, carcinosarcomata, squamous cell carcinoma and endometrial stromal sarcoma can all originate in this fashion. Intermediate stages between endometriosis and frank neoplasia have been recognized with increasing frequency in recent years[7]: these include cellular and nuclear atypia in endometriotic glands, cellular atypia, nuclear pleomorphism and irregular budding in the monolayer lining of an endometriotic cyst (Figure 31.10), and an overgrowth of atypical epithelium to give a picture resembling that of an endometrial glandular hyperplasia with cellular and architectural atypia (Figure 31.11). Whether in all these circumstances the lesions should be classed as neoplastic or hyperplastic in type is debatable and whether, if neoplastic, they should be regarded as tumours of borderline malignancy is still a moot point. Nevertheless, it is possible in some cases of endometrioid adenocarcinoma of the ovary to trace a transition between fully benign endometriosis, glands showing irregularity with cellular and nuclear atypia and frank adenocarcinoma. In these circumstances it is clearly justifiable to regard the atypia as a 'pre-malignant' change. It is probable that nuclear and cellular irregularity in the monolayer lining of a cyst should be treated with less suspicion, for in most instances this represents a reaction to the cysts contents rather than a neoplastic change.

Endosalpingiosis (Figure 31.12)

Small cystic lesions lined by tubal-type epithelium and usually containing psammoma bodies are occasionally found scattered on the surface of the uterus, on the pelvic peritoneum and in the omentum. This is considered to be a condition of endosalpingiosis[8] and thought to be homologous to endometriosis: it is probably due to multifocal tubal metaplasia of the mesothelium. The major significance of endosalpingiosis is that the lesions may be misinterpreted as metastases from a serous adenocarcinoma of the ovary, an impression that is usually dispelled by noting the benign nature of the epithelium. In very rare cases foci of endosalpingiosis can, however, undergo malignant change.

References

1. Simpson, J. L., Elias, S., Malinak, L. R. and Buttram, V. C. (1980. Heritable aspects of endometriosis. I. Genetic studies. *Am. J. Obstet. Gynecol.*, **137**, 327–331
2. Malinak, L. R., Buttram, V. C., Elias, S. and Simpson, J. L. (1980). Heritable aspects of endometriosis. II. Clinical characteristics of familial endometriosis. *Am. J. Obstet. Gynecol.*, **137**, 332–337
3. Weed, J. and Arquembourg, P. C. (1980). Endometriosis: can it produce an autoimmune response resulting in infertility? *Clin. Obstet. Gynecol.*, **22**, 169–186
4. Czernobilsky, B. (1982). Primary epithelial tumors of the ovary. In Blaustein, A. (ed.). *Pathology of the Female Genital Tract.* 2nd edn., pp. 511–560. (New York, Heidelberg, Berlin: Springer-Verlag)
5. Brooks, J. J. and Wheeler, J. E. (1977). Malignancy arising in extragonadal endometriosis: a case report and summary of the world literature. *Cancer*, **40**, 3065–3073
6. Mostoufizadeh, M. and Scully, R. E. (1980). Malignant tumors arising in endometriosis. *Clin. Obstet. Gynecol.*, **23**, 951–963
7. Czernobilsky, B. and Morris, W. J. (1979). A histologic study of ovarian endometriosis with emphasis on hyperplastic and atypical changes. *Obstet. Gynecol.*, **53**, 318–323
8. Zinsser, K. R. and Wheeler, J. E. (1982). Endosalpingiosis in the omentum: a study of autopsy and surgical material. *Am. J. Surg. Pathol.*, **6**, 109–117

Pregnancy

32

In this section only those aspects of obstetric pathology which tend to impinge on the practice of the gynaecological pathologist will be considered.

Normal Pregnancy

Implantation of the fertilized ovum normally occurs during the mid-secretory phase of the cycle. After implantation, glandular secretion continues in undiminished fashion and stromal oedema persists despite the stromal cells undergoing a predecidual change. After the 14th day of gestation a fully formed decidua emerges (Figure 32.1), almost all the endometrial stroma being converted into pavement-like sheets of epithelioid-like cells with clearly defined limiting margins and central vesicular nuclei. The stromal vessels are dilated and the glands away from the implantation site tend to show marked scalloping and striking secretory activity. In some cases an Arias-Stella phenomenon will be seen (Figure 32.2): this occurs focally and involves single, or small groups of, glands. The glandular epithelial nuclei are pleomorphic and hyperchromatic whilst the cytoplasm is abundant and usually clear or vacuolated although sometimes deeply eosinophilic. The epithelium lining the glands often shows some degree of stratification and intraluminal tufting is common. The Arias-Stella change is thought to be a hypersecretory phenomenon and can develop when trophoblast, in any form, is present anywhere in the body[1]: it has to be remembered, however, that it can occasionally occur in women given ovulation-inducing drugs or progestagens. The setting of these glands within a secretory, gestational-type endometrium enables a distinction to be drawn between this change and a clear cell adenocarcinoma of the endometrium.

An unsuspected early pregnancy (Figure 32.3) is sometimes encountered in curettings, and it should be noted that as the ovum implants cytotrophoblastic cells stream out from the trophoblast shell to colonize the underlying decidua and immediately adjacent myometrium (Figure 32.4): both mononuclear and multinucleated trophoblastic cells are seen in this 'placental site reaction' which was formerly, and incorrectly, labelled as 'syncytial endometritis'.

During pregnancy, changes also occur elsewhere in the genital tract. Focal decidual-like change may be found in the uterine cervix, uterine serosa, ovarian surface epithelium and in the rugae of the Fallopian tube. Within the cervix the endocervical glands tend to have a hypersecretory appearance and there may also be a degree of microglandular hyperplasia.

Abortion

About 15% of established pregnancies spontaneously abort before the 20th week of gestation, and it is now clear that a majority of first trimester abortions are associated with a fetal chromosomal abnormality. Material from both complete and incomplete abortions are commonly sent for pathological examination and the tissue received may range from a complete embryo and placenta to curetted material which consists mainly of blood clot. If a gestational sac is received it should be opened and the presence or absence of a fetus determined: if a fetus is present an attempt should be made to note any malformations. Most abortion material received by the pathologist is, however, derived from curettage of abortions which are thought to be incomplete. In such cases it is usual to receive a mixture of blood clot, partially necrotic and inflamed decidua and placental villi: it should be noted that a diagnosis of 'products of conception' cannot be made unless placental villi are present, and that inflammatory and necrotic changes in the decidua are a normal phenomenon and not indicative of a septic abortion. In the absence of placental villi the diagnosis of intrauterine pregnancy can be almost fully confirmed if a placental site reaction is seen within the decidual fragments.

The villi in an abortion may show a normal first trimester pattern (Figure 32.5) but very commonly embryonic demise has preceded the abortion by some days or weeks and under such circumstances the villi often show marked stromal fibrosis together with sclerotic occlusion of the fetal villous vessels (Figure 32.6), features which develop after embryonic death as a normal postmortem change. In some instances the villi show hydropic change (Figure 32.7): this term refers to the presence of swollen oedematous villi which, however, are rarely sufficiently distended to form macroscopic vesicles. Fetal vessels may or may not be present but the diagnostic feature of a hydropic abortion, and the finding which distinguishes it from a complete or partial hydatidiform mole, is the complete absence of trophoblastic hyperplasia. A hydropic change of this type is often associated with gross abnormality and early death of the embryo (the so-called 'blighted ovum') but is occasionally seen in placentae from morphologically and chromosomally normal embryos. The term 'hydatidiform change', if used at all, should only be applied to villi showing trophoblastic hyperplasia, such cases being either complete or partial hydatidiform moles (*vide infra*).

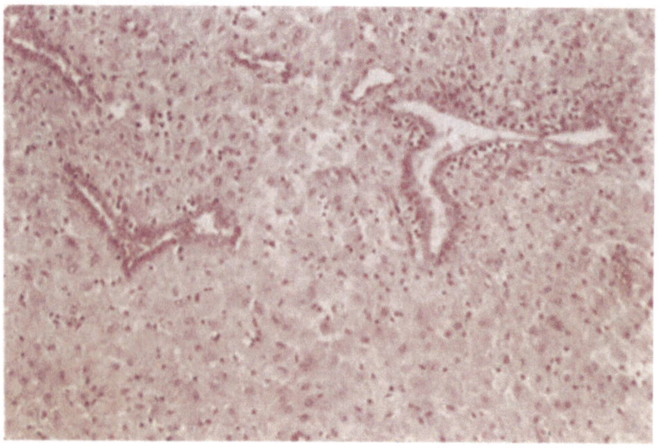

Figure 32.1 Endometrium: decidualization. The endometrial stromal cells are enlarged and have copious eosinophilic cytoplasm. The three glands are cleft-like and their epithelium, which is cuboidal, shows neither secretory nor proliferative activity. The neutrophil polymorphonuclear leukocytes in the stroma around the gland to the right are a reflection of the continuous process of decidual modelling which occurs in pregnancy and are not indicative of infection. H & E × 100

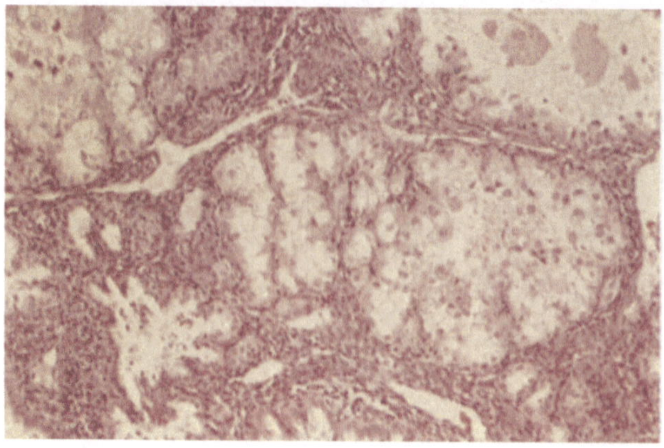

Figure 32.2 Endometrium: Arias Stella change. Arias Stella change is seen as conspicuous foci of pale, enlarged hypersecretory glands. The epithelial cells are enlarged, their nuclei, which may be strikingly hyperchromatic and pleomorphic, have lost their polarity and their cytoplasm is pale, eosinophilic and may be vacuolated. The apparent multilayering of the epithelium and the cytological atypia may give a false impression of neoplasia. H & E × 100

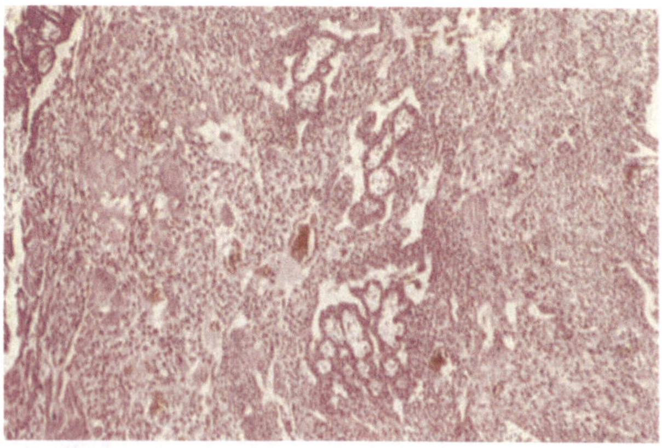

Figure 32.3 Endometrium: early pregnancy. This early implantation site was found unexpectedly in a hysterectomy specimen. It shows villous stems (centrally) surrounded by sheets of cytotrophoblast and syncytiotrophoblast. The presence of an identifiable blastocyst and villous stems distinguish the appearance from choriocarcinoma. If necessary serial sectioning of such a focus should be carried out to identify villi. H & E × 40

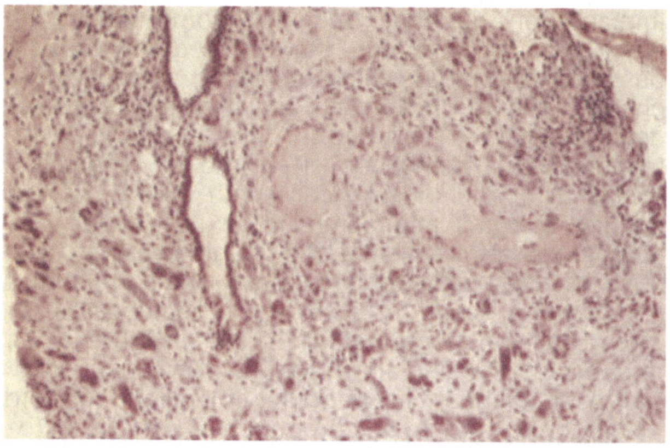

Figure 32.4 Endometrium: placental site reaction. This fragment of decidua is infiltrated by large, darkly-staining, pleomorphic mononuclear and multinucleate trophoblast cells. The walls of the blood vessels to the upper right are infiltrated by similar cells. This is a physiological phenomenon. H & E × 100

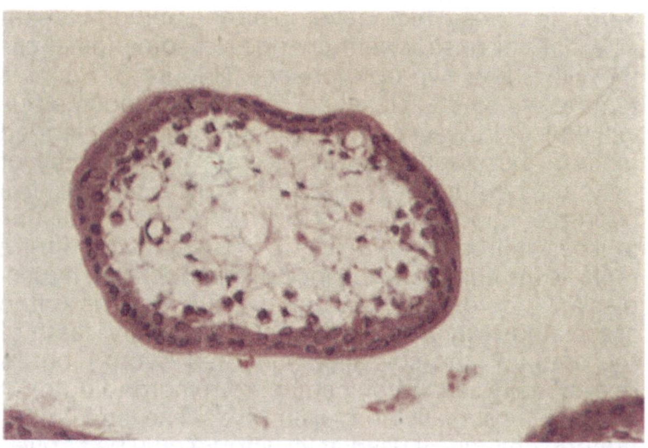

Figure 32.5 Placenta: first trimester villus. The villus has a core of scanty mesenchymal cells in which there is early blood vessel formation. The covering trophoblast forms two distinct, continuous layers, an outer layer of syncytiotrophoblast in which there are nuclear clusters and an inner layer of cytotrophoblast. H & E × 250

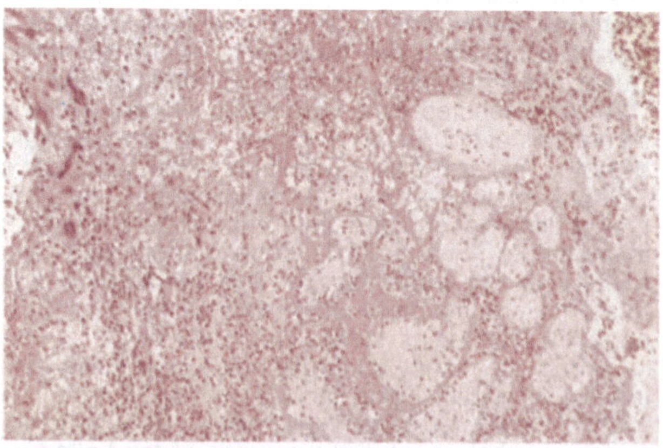

Figure 32.6 Placenta: spontaneous first trimester abortion. The material obtained following spontaneous abortion normally shows changes which have occurred subsequent to fetal death. In this field ghost-like placental villi are seen to the right. Fibrin lies between the villi and at the left, there is decidua in which individual multinucleated trophoblast cells can be seen. The inflammatory cells are a concomitant of tissue breakdown and do not normally indicate infection. H & E × 100

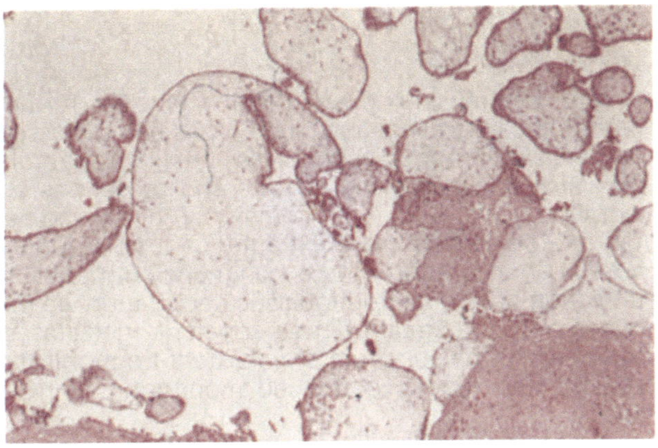

Figure 32.7 Placenta: hydropic abortus. The villi in the centre of the field are enlarged, oedematous and the trophoblast attenuated. There is no evidence of trophoblastic hyperplasia and sclerosed fetal vessels are present in some villi. These changes, which are frequently focal, occur subsequent to fetal death. H & E × 40

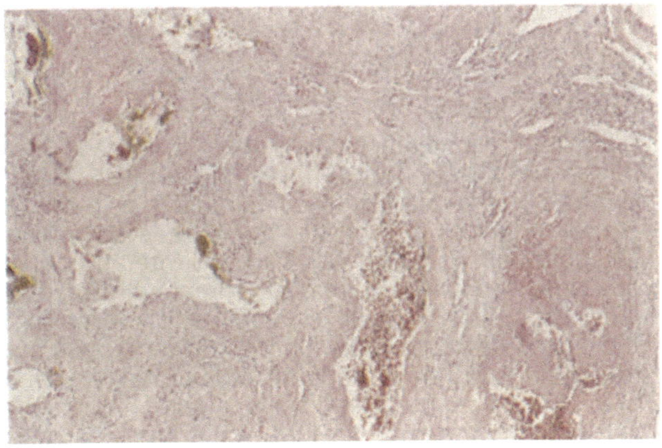

Figure 32.8 Uterus: subinvolution of the placental bed. This uterus was removed from a patient with uncontrollable postpartum haemorrhage. The vessels of the placental bed are patent and their lumena widely open; thrombus has formed in the vessel at the lower right of the field which is only partly occluded. H & E × 4

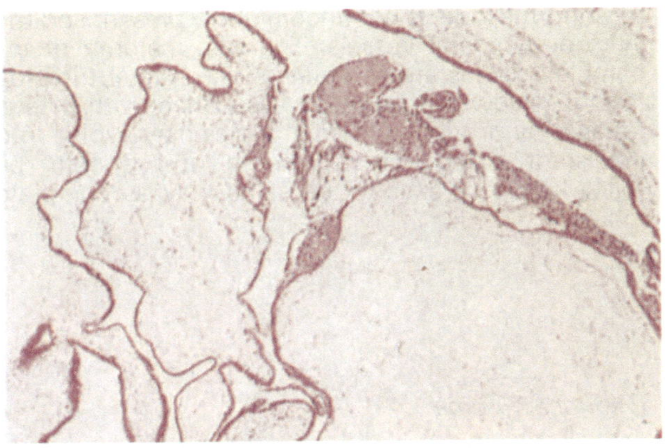

Figure 32.9 Placenta: hydatidiform mole. All the villi in the placenta are enlarged and hydropic; there are no fetal vessels. The trophoblast which is attenuated in many areas shows focal hyperplasia on the two villi in the centre of the field. H & E × 40

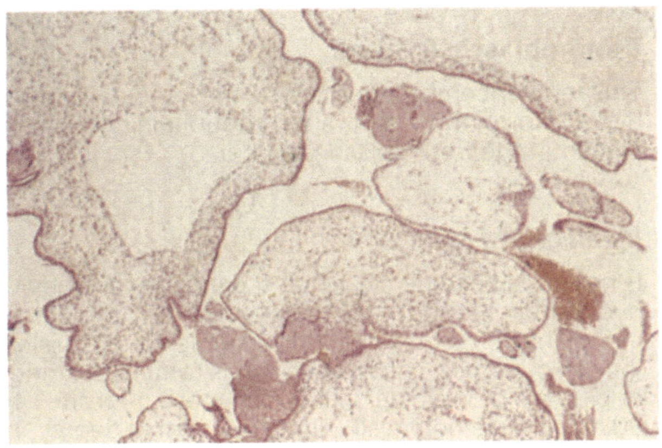

Figure 32.10 Placenta: partial hydatidiform mole. Enlarged, oedematous, vesicular villi and villi of normal size are both present in this placenta from a triploid abortus. The trophoblast is relatively hypoplastic and this particular field shows no evidence of trophoblastic hyperplasia. H & E × 40

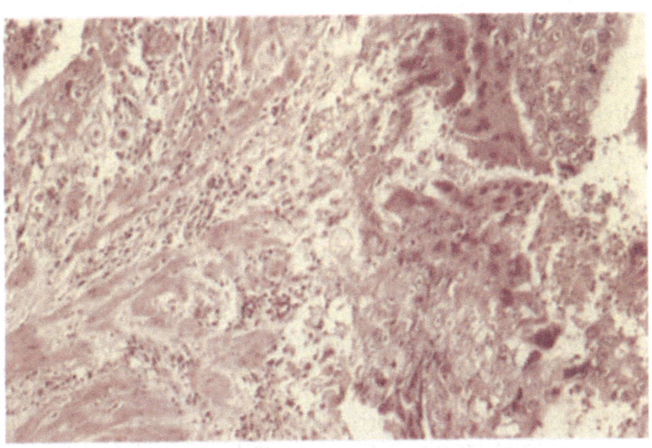

Figure 32.11 Myometrium: choriocarcinoma. To the right of the field there are sheets of syncytiotrophoblast with dense eosinophilic cytoplasm and darkly-staining pyknotic nuclei intermingled with sheets of cytotrophoblast composed of cells with large vesicular nuclei with prominent nucleoli, pale eosinophilic cytoplasm and well-defined cell margins. This neoplastic tissue is infiltrating the myometrium (which lies to the left of the field), where there is a mild chronic non-specific inflammatory cell response. The absence of villi distinguishes the neoplasm from invasive hydatidiform mole. H & E × 100

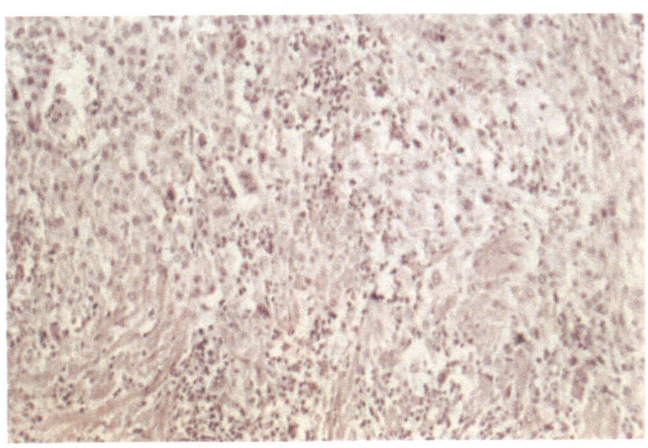

Figure 32.12 Myometrium: placental site trophoblastic tumour. Sheets and columns of cytotrophoblastic cells with small regular round or ovoid central nuclei and pale granular cytoplasm are penetrating deeply into the myometrium. Smooth muscle infiltrated by cytotrophoblast is present in the lower half of the field. The absence of syncytiotrophoblast distinguishes the condition from choriocarcinoma although occasional multinucleate cells may be present. H & E × 100

Puerperium

Curettage is sometimes undertaken because of post-partum bleeding, it often being surmised that a portion of the placenta has been left *in situ*. On occasion pieces of fibrotic, but otherwise normal, placental villous tissue will be encountered in such curettage specimens but more commonly the material received consists largely of blood clot and partially hyalinized decidua: a few fibrotic placental villi may be embedded within the latter. It is probable that in most instances the bleeding is due to inadequate involution of the placental bed, and in some cases the curettings may contain maternal vessels which, instead of being collapsed and occluded by thrombus, are still distended and either thrombus-free or only partially thrombosed[2]. These vascular abnormalities are seen in their fullest expression in uteri removed postpartum for continuing severe bleeding (Figure 32.8).

Trophoblastic Disease

This term encompasses not only the various forms of hydatidiform mole but also choriocarcinoma and placental site trophoblastic tumour.

Hydatidiform Mole

It has now become clear that there are two types of hydatidiform mole, the complete mole and the partial mole. The complete hydatidiform mole has a classical 'bunch of grapes' appearance and is formed of strings or clusters of vesicular villi which measure from 1 to 30 mm in diameter: all villi show some degree of distension and no macroscopically normal placental tissue is present: an empty gestational sac may occasionally be found but a fetus is absent. Histologically, all the villi are abnormal, showing varying degrees of distension and oedema: degenerative changes, often amounting to frank liquefaction, are seen in the villous stroma and fetal vessels are absent. The defining feature of a hydatidiform mole is, however, the presence of a variable degree of trophoblastic hyperplasia (Figure 32.9): this is usually very obvious in complete hydatidiform moles but is occasionally rather focal in distribution. It is necessary to distinguish between trophoblastic hyperplasia and the normal actively growing trophoblast of the first trimester placenta but true hyperplasia is usually circumferential around a villus whilst normal, but actively growing, trophoblast is commonly polar. It should be noted that the degree of trophoblastic hyperplasia is of no prognostic importance in terms of the possibility of subsequent development of a choriocarcinoma. The pathogenesis of a complete hydatidiform mole is still uncertain but it is now known that they invariably have an XX chromosomal constitution, both X chromosomes being of paternal origin.

Some complete moles are invasive and penetrate deeply into the myometrium: the histological diagnosis is dependent upon finding vesicular villi within the uterine wall and such cases may terminate in death because of haemorrhage or uterine perforation. The diagnosis of invasive mole is, however, now largely obsolete for continuing high hCG titres in a woman from whom a mole has been evacuated are usually treated with chemotherapy without further pathological investigation, such cases being classed as 'persistent trophoblastic disease'. An invasive mole may also apparently metastasize and present as an extrauterine nodule, most commonly in the vagina. Villi are present in these extrauterine lesions which are not an indication of true malignancy but rather a reflection of normal trophoblastic deportation via the maternal blood stream. These apparent 'metastases' form part of the spectrum of persistent trophoblastic disease and require continued monitoring of hCG levels.

The partial hydatidiform mole differs from the complete mole in that only a proportion of the villi show vesicular change, the mole commonly appearing as an identifiable, largely normal, placenta in which there are scattered vesicles. Histologically, markedly vesicular villi are scattered amongst a villous population of normal diameter (Figure 32.10): the trophoblastic mantle of the vesicular villi, though tending to be thin and hypoplastic, shows occasional foci of trophoblastic hyperplasia. A fetus, albeit often an abnormal one, is not uncommonly present and the villi contain fetal vessels. The vast majority of incomplete moles are associated with a fetal triploidy though a few are probably associated with a fetal tetraploidy or trisomy. Partial moles may evolve into persistent trophoblastic disease and should be followed up in exactly the same way as complete moles.

Choriocarcinoma

This malignant tumour of trophoblast follows a hydatidiform mole in 60% of cases, an abortion in 30% and a normal pregnancy in 20%, the time interval between the preceding pregnancy and the development of a choriocarcinoma varying between a few months and 15 years. A choriocarcinoma forms single or multiple haemorrhagic nodules within the uterus which histologically show central necrosis with a surrounding core of viable tumour tissue. The neoplastic tissue shows a basic bimorphic pattern which usually recapitulates that of the early implanting blastocyst (Figure 32.11), central cores of cytotrophoblast being surrounded by a peripheral rim of syncytiotrophoblast: the cytological features commonly do not differ significantly from those of proliferating normal trophoblast. It should be emphasized that villi are not present in a choriocarcinoma and that the presence of villous structures refutes this diagnosis. The diagnosis of choriocarcinoma is relatively easy in a hysterectomy specimen but may be more difficult in curettings. In such samples, the presence of villous tissue negates a diagnosis of choriocarcinoma, this diagnosis being only valid if non-villous, invasive trophoblastic tissue showing an orderly arrangement of cyto- and syncytiotrophoblast is present. Often the non-villous trophoblast in curettings lack the typical features of a choriocarcinoma: if the preceding pregnancy was a hydatidiform mole a diagnosis of persistent trophoblastic disease should be made under these circumstances, whilst if the gestation was either an abortion or a normal pregnancy the presence of non-villous trophoblast is an almost certain indication of a choriocarcinoma[3].

Placental Site Trophoblastic Tumour

This uncommon lesion, which has also been called trophoblastic pseudotumour and atypical choriocarcinoma, usually presents months or years after a normal pregnancy and is characterized by a massive cytotrophoblastic cell infiltration of the myometrium (Figure 32.12): no true syncytiotrophoblast is present though occasional multinucleated cells are seen. The cytotrophoblastic cells infiltrate between the muscle fibres, show only minimal vascular invasion and cause little or no haemorrhage or necrosis. Many cases of this condition run an apparently benign course but some have metastasized and caused death[4]: it has been suggested that only those lesions which have a mitotic count of more than 4 per 10 high power fields are likely to behave in a malignant fashion[5].

References

1. Arias-Stella, J. (1972). Atypical endometrial changes produced by chorionic tissue. *Hum. Pathol.*, **3**, 450–455
2. Robertson, W. B. (1981) *The Endometrium*, (London and Boston: Butterworths)
3. Elston, C. W. (1981). Gestational tumours of trophoblast. In Anthony, P. P. and MacSween, R. N. M. (eds.). *Recent Advances in Histopathology II*. pp. 149–161, (Edinburgh, London, Melbourne and New York: Churchill–Livingstone)
4. Eckstein, R. P., Paradinas, F. J. and Bagshawe, K. D. (1982). Placental site trophoblastic tumour (trophoblastic pseudotumour): a study of four cases requiring hysterectomy including one fatal case. *Histopathology*, **6**, 211–226
5. Scully, R. E. and Young, R. H. (1981). Trophoblastic pseudotumor: a reappraisal. *Am. J. Surg. Pathol.*, **5**, 75–76

Hormone-Induced Changes in the Female Genital Tract

33

Steroid hormones administered to a woman may induce changes in many tissues but it is their effects on the endometrium which most frequently pose a problem to the pathologist, and it is to these that this section is particularly directed. The use of exogenous hormones, either for contraceptive purposes, as therapy for disease states or as replacement for a diminished or absent production of endogenous hormones, is now so widespread that a pathologist called upon to interpret endometrial histology must insist upon a detailed history of the possible exposure of the patient to hormones: furthermore, a full knowledge of the administration of non-hormonal drugs is also mandatory for some of these may, as a side-effect, influence pituitary or ovarian function and hence alter endometrial morphology, e.g. the hyperprolactinaemia resulting from the use of dopamine antagonists in the treatment of psychiatric disorders.

Progestagens

Synthetic progestagens are more potent than progesterone and are derived either from 17α-hydroxyprogesterone or from 19-nortestosterone[1]. Progestagens act only on an endometrium in which progesterone receptors have been induced by prior exposure to oestrogen but nevertheless exert an anti-oestrogenic effect, partly by blocking oestrogen receptors and partly by inducing the enzyme 17β-dehydrogenase which converts oestriol into the less potent oestrone. Progestagens derived from 17α-hydroxyprogesterone are partially converted to oestrogens and hence are more markedly anti-oestrogenic than are those derived from 19-nortestosterone which do not undergo any conversion to oestrogens.

Effects on Normal Endometrium

In women receiving high dosage progestagens, e.g. for the treatment of endometriosis, derivatives of 17α-hydroxyprogesterone tend, during the earlier stages of administration, to exert a progestational effect which partially overshadows their anti-oestrogenic activity. Thus, although the endometrial stroma shows a florid predecidual change and is heavily infiltrated by K cells the glands are small, straight, poorly developed and are either inactive or show only weak activity (Figures 33.1 and 33.2) whilst spiral artery development is either absent or poor, the endometrial vasculature tending to consist mainly of thin-walled dilated vessels. With continuing use of progestagens the anti-oestrogenic effect becomes predominant and the endometrium will become atrophic with sparse inactive glands set in a fibrous, but patchily decidualized, stroma. Progestagens derived from 19-nortestosterone will, when used in high dosage, tend to produce endometrial atrophy from the onset of therapy.

In women taking small doses of progestagens for contraceptive purposes, a situation now rather uncommon, it is unusual to find the florid stromal predecidual change that is encountered in patients receiving progestagens in therapeutic dosage. Long term low-dose usage results in a variable endometrial appearance (Figures 33.3 and 33.4) but the picture encountered most commonly is of small glands showing a minor, or moderate, degree of secretory activity set in a mildly, and often irregularly, decidualized stroma which is infiltrated by K cells and contains thin-walled, poorly developed vascular channels: in many instances the appearances resemble those found in spontaneously occurring luteal phase insufficiency. Even with low dosage progestagens, their continued usage will eventually lead to endometrial atrophy.

Effects on Abnormal Endometrium

Administration of progestagens to patients with endometrial hyperplasia creates a picture of secretory change (Figure 33.5) superimposed on an arrested hyperplastic endometrium: the secretory change may be uniform or irregular, and often the resulting complex pattern cannot be distinguished from that seen after spontaneous ovulation has occurred in a woman with endometrial hyperplasia resulting from previous anovulatory cycles.

Oestrogens

Oestrogen therapy is given to patients with absent gonadal function, e.g. gonadal dysgenesis, to women with severe menopausal symptoms and to cases of carcinoma of the breast. In recent years postmenopausal oestrogen replacement therapy has been quite widely used, particularly for the prevention of osteoporosis.

Effects on the Endometrium

The morphological changes in the endometrium of women receiving oestrogens vary with the duration of administration and with the potency and dosage of the hormone, but, in general, oestrogens will stimulate endometrial growth, induce glandular and stromal proliferation and cause development of immature vessels[2]. The appearances in the endometrium after short term oestrogen therapy in pre- or perimenopausal women resemble those encountered in patients with a persistent follicle, breakdown and bleeding occurring in a thick endometrium showing only proliferative changes. In postmenopausal women given cyclic, low-dosage oestrogens there may be either a normal or a weakly proliferative pattern in the endometrium: not uncommonly the endometrium is relatively shallow with rather widely spaced glands showing cystic dilatation or non-complex budding, this being referred to as 'the disordered proliferative endometrium' (Figure 33.6).

In many women, long-continued, unopposed oestrogen administration will lead to the development of a cystic glandular hyperplasia of the endometrium, whilst a pure glandular hyperplasia, often only with architectural atypia but sometimes with cellular atypia, will be found in a significant proportion of cases. There is now little doubt that long term unopposed usage of oestrogens is, whether given continuously or cyclically, also associated with an increased risk of endometrial adenocarcinoma[3, 4]: hence endometrial biopsy must always be undertaken if bleeding occurs in women on this form of treatment, such specimens meriting careful study.

Combinations of Oestrogen and a Progestagen

Administration of both oestrogen and a progestagen is widely used for contraceptive purposes, and it is also becoming increasingly common to combine post postmenopausal oestrogen replacement therapy with a progestagen. The hormones may be given consecutively (sequential regime) or concurrently (combined regime).

Effects on the Endometrium of Sequential Regime

Sequential hormones were widely used for contraceptive purposes, the regime usually consisting of 14 days of oestrogens followed by 5 or 7 days of oestrogen together with a progestagen and then a 7 day hormone-free interval. With such a regime the exogenous oestrogen produces a normal proliferative pattern in the endometrium but inhibits pituitary gonadotrophin release and thus prevents ovulation. The subsequent addition of a progestagen produces, in the absence of a corpus luteum, an abortive delayed secretory phase with inadequate secretory transformation of the glands, poor development of the spiral arteries and suboptimal decidualization of the stroma. Prolonged sequential contraception can, rarely, lead to endometrial atrophy but generally the progestagen is unable to nullify the stimulatory effect of the oestrogen, and the emergence of an increased risk of both endometrial hyperplasia and adenocarcinoma with this form of contraception has led to its being discontinued.

Paradoxically, sequential hormonal therapy is being reintroduced in postmenopausal women on oestrogen replacement therapy, progestagens being administered for 7 days in each calendar month of continuous oestrogen therapy in the hope of diminishing the risk of endometrial adenocarcinoma whilst retaining the beneficial effects of oestrogen. The endometrial morphology in women receiving this form of therapy have not yet been fully described though the incidence of endometrial hyperplasia is undoubtedly diminished.

Effects on the Endometrium of Combined Regime

This is the most widely used form of steroid contraception, a combination of oestrogen and a progestagen being taken for 21 days after which there is a hormone-free interval of 7 days. The currently used low dosage contraceptive regimes rarely produce the rather bizarre histological changes, such as a pseudosarcomatous reaction in the endometrial stroma, which were seen in association with earlier high dosage regimes, and which figure prominently in earlier accounts of endometrial morphology in contraceptive users. The endometrial appearances with low dosage pills vary with differing combinations but, in general, endometrial proliferation occurs during the first 8–10 days of administration, the degree of proliferative change being, however, restrained by the anti-oestrogenic effect of the progestagen: hence, the endometrium tends to be rather shallow whilst the glands are straight, poorly developed and show only sparse mitotic activity. Subnuclear vacuoles develop prematurely (Figure 33.7), on about day 9 or 10, in an irregular fashion in only a small proportion of the glands and this is followed by a premature, inadequate secretory phase (Figure 33.8), the progestagen being unable to exert its full effect because of insufficient priming of the endometrium by the oestrogen. The exogenous oestrogen does, however, prevent ovulation and because of the absence of a corpus luteum the secretory phase is short and poorly sustained, lasting only until about day 15: a variable degree of stromal oedema is seen transitorily, stromal predecidual change only occurs focally and the spiral vessels are poorly developed, thin-walled vascular channels predominating in the endometrium. After day 15 or 16 the glands undergo involution and are set in a weakly decidualized stroma. With continuing usage of the combined contraceptive regime the anti-oestrogenic effect of the progestagen usually becomes dominant and the endometrium undergoes atrophy, small inactive glands being set in a mildly oedematous and rather fibrous stroma showing focal, weak predecidual change (Figures 33.9 and 33.10). Severe atrophy is, however, seen much less commonly since the introduction of the low dosage regime (Figure 33.11)

Combination hormonal contraception is not associated with any increased risk of endometrial hyperplasia or neoplasia; indeed such regimes appear to confer some degree of protection against the development of an endometrial adenocarcinoma.

Effects of Exogenous Hormones on Other Female Genital Tract Tissues

Myometrium

Myometrial hypertrophy is sometimes encountered in women taking high dose progestagens whilst both with this form of therapy and, to a lesser extent in patients using combined oestrogen/progestagen preparations, any leiomyomata present may become enlarged, oedematous and focally necrotic. Leiomyomata may also undergo an increase in cellularity, and these regimes occasionally result in bizarre cellular atypia, a change seen, however, much less frequently since the introduction of low dosage combination contraceptives.

Cervix

Combined steroid regimes not infrequently lead to cervical ectopy, hypersecretion of mucus, stromal oedema and focal decidua-like change: many women using a contraceptive regime of this type will also develop microglandular hyperplasia, usually only apparent on histological examination but sometimes sufficiently marked to form a visible polypoidal mass (Figure 33.12).

Women using a combined steroid contraceptive regime have an increased incidence of cervical intra-epithelial neoplasia and of cervical invasive carcinoma[5]. There is no evidence, however, of a causal relationship between the administration of exogenous hormones and cervical neoplasia, the association reflecting a multitude of factors associated with the use of a highly effective non-barrier form of contraception.

Ovary

Steroidal contraceptives inhibit ovulation, and after several successive cycles there is a substantial reduction in the size and number of developing follicles and an absence of corpora lutea: after several years of use there is atrophy of the cortex and reduced ovarian size. There is reasonably good evidence that the prolonged inhibition of ovulation associated with steroid contraception provides a degree of protection against the development of ovarian epithelial neoplasms.

Figures 33.1–33.12 will be found overleaf.

Fallopian Tube

After several years of combined steroid contraception there is often quite marked atrophy of the tubal epithelium. By contrast, administration only of oestrogens may result in proliferative changes in the tubal epithelium with multilayering and epithelial budding.

References

1. Henzl, M. R. (1978). Natural and synthetic female sex hormones. In Yen, S. C. and Jaffe, R. B. (eds.). *Reproductive Endocrinology.* (Philadelphia, London, Toronto: W. B. Saunders)
2. Hendrickson, M. R. and Kempson, R. L. (1980). *Surgical Pathology of the Uterine Corpus.* (Philadelphia, London, Toronto: W. B. Saunders)
3. Cramer, D. W. and Knapp, R. C. (1979). Review of epidemiologic studies of endometrial cancer and exogenous estrogen. *Epidemiol. Rev.*, **54**, 521–526
4. Shapiro, S., Kaufman, D. W., Slone, D., Rosenberg, L., Miettinen, O. S., Stolley, P. D., Rosenheim, N. B., Watring, W. G., Leavitt, T., and Knapp, R. C. (1980). Recent and past use of conjugated estrogens in relation to adenocarcinoma of the endometrium. *N. Engl. J. Med.*, **303**, 485–489
5. Schaude, H., Dallenbach-Hellweg, G., and Schlaefer, K. (1980). Histologic changes of the cervix uteri following contraceptive use. In Dallenbach-Hellweg, G. (ed.). *Functional Morphologic Changes in Female Sex Organs Induced by Exogenous Hormones.* (Berlin, Heidelberg and New York: Springer-Verlag)

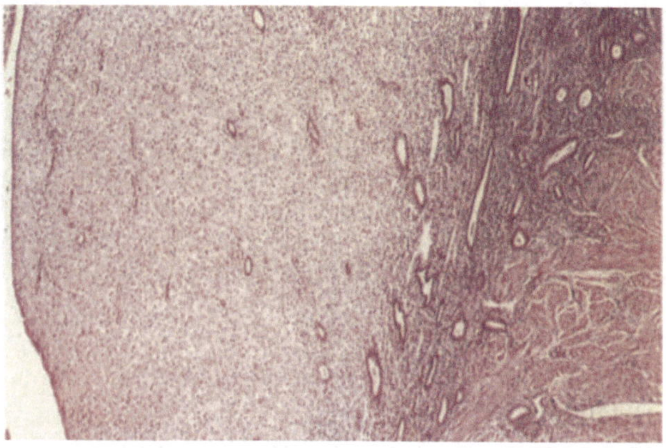

Figure 33.1 Endometrium: progestagen effect. The endometrium, from a patient who had received norethisterone, shows marked stromal pseudo-decidualization and glandular atrophy. Note that this change is very sharply limited to the functional layer, the basal endometrium, to the right, being unresponsive to the exogenous hormone. H & E × 40

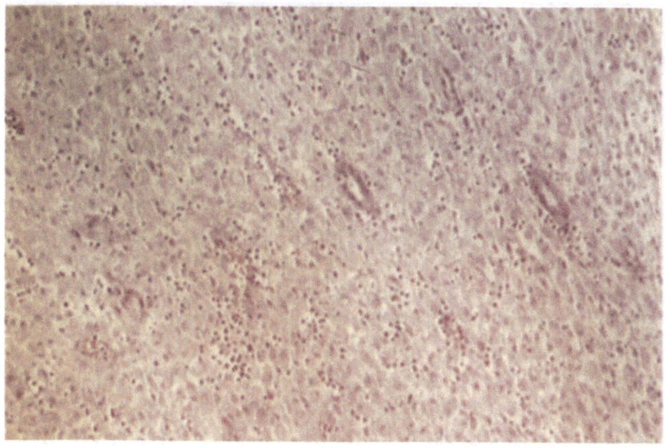

Figure 33.2 Endometrium: progestagen effect. A detail from Figure 33.1 showing narrow, tubular glands which are exhibiting neither secretory nor proliferative activity. There is pronounced stromal decidualization, the individual cells being enlarged and their cytoplasm copious and eosinophilic. The tissue is infiltrated by small, darkly-staining stromal macrophages (K-cells). H & E × 100

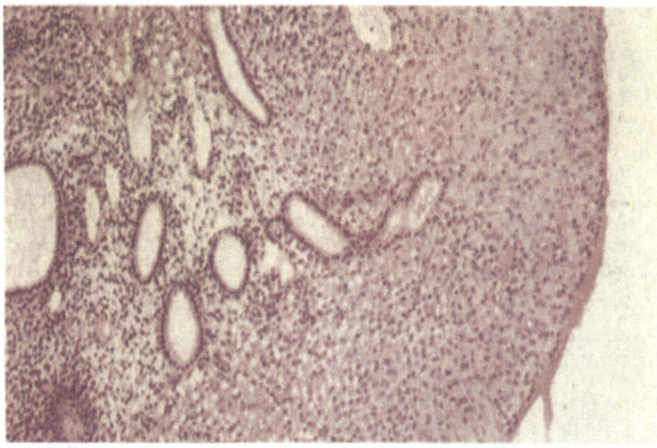

Figure 33.3 Endometrium: progestagen contraceptive. The glands are small, tubular, are lined by cuboidal epithelium and show no secretory activity. The superficial stroma shows a moderate degree of decidualization and the spiral arteries are poorly developed. The progestational effects are much less marked than those seen with high dose progestagen therapy. H & E × 100

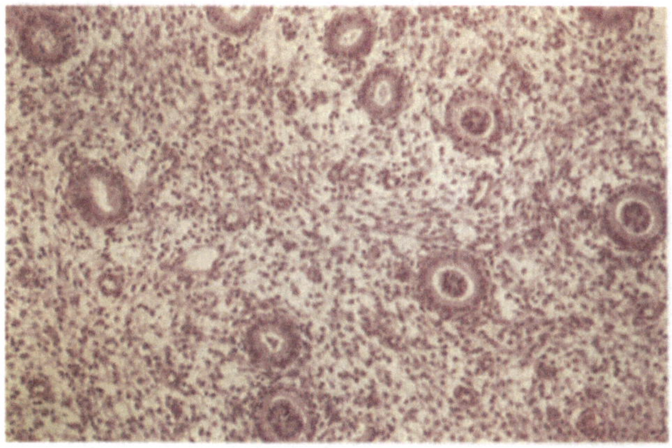

Figure 33.4 Endometrium: progestagen contraceptive. The glands are small, tubular and show minimal secretory transformation. Spiral artery growth is absent and there is little stromal decidualization. The appearances are similar to those seen in luteal phase insufficiency (Figure 11.2). H & E × 100

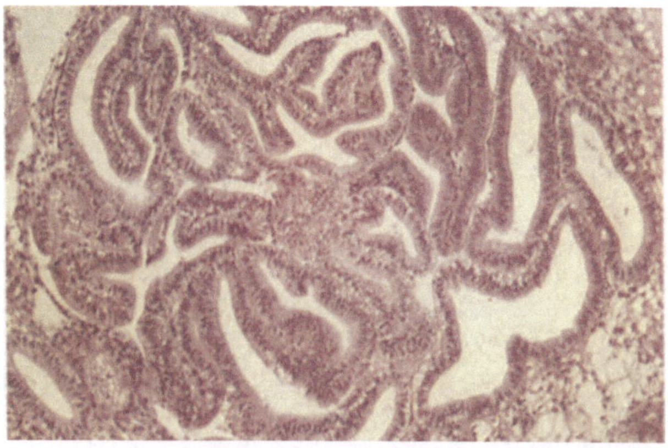

Figure 33.5 Endometrium: the effect of progestagens on hyperplastic endometrium. The field shows a cluster of closely packed glands showing moderately severe architectural atypia. The patient had been given norethisterone for 5 days prior to operation and there is well developed subnuclear vacuolation of the glandular epithelium. A similar appearance would have been seen had the patient ovulated. H & E × 100

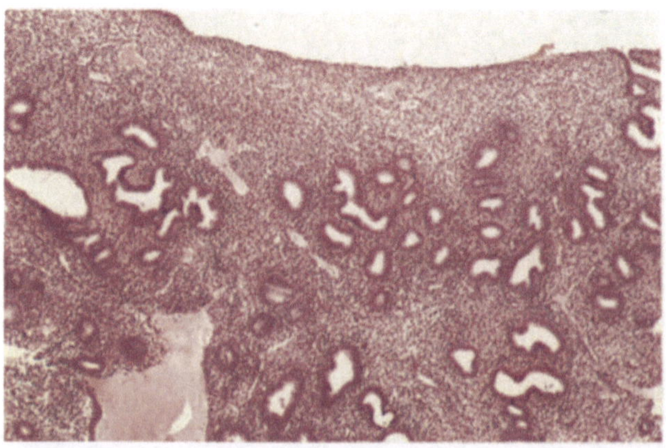

Figure 33.6 Endometrium: disordered proliferative endometrium. This biopsy was from a woman of 51 years who was receiving oestrogens for menopausal symptoms. The endometrium is shallow, the glands, which are a little crowded, show a mild degree of budding and their epithelium is multilayered; an occasional glandular epithelial mitosis was seen. There is no cytological atypia. H & E × 40

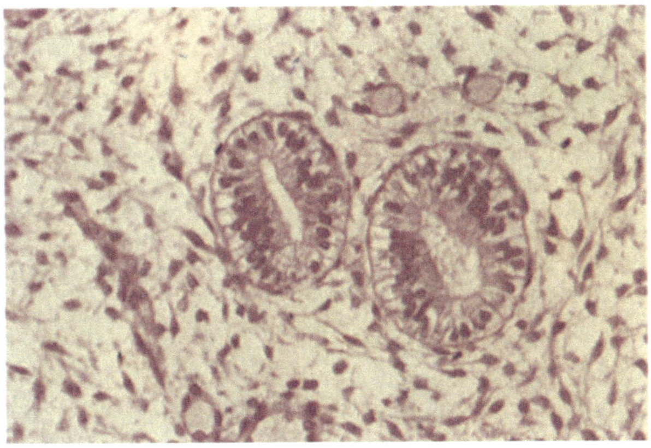

Figure 33.7 Endometrium: combined steroid contraceptive. A biopsy taken on the 9th day after the onset of withdrawal bleeding from a woman taking a combination of 0.25 mg levonorgestrel and 0.03 mg ethinyloestradiol. The glands are straight and tubular and there are subnuclear vacuoles in the glandular epithelium; the stroma is immature and spindled. H & E × 250

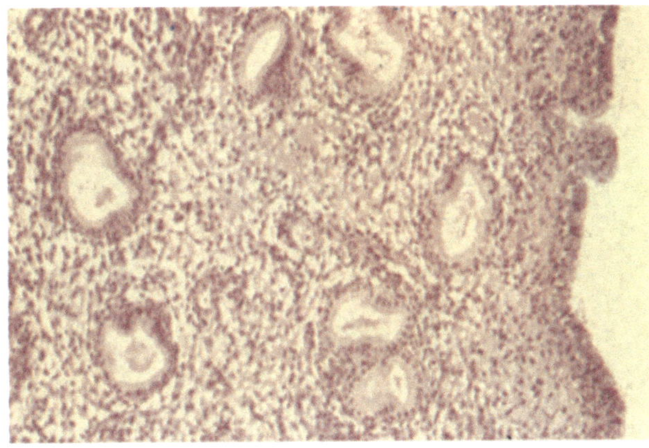

Figure 33.8 Endometrium: combined steroid contraceptive. A premature, abortive secretory endometrium biopsied on the 13th day after the onset of withdrawal bleeding. The glands are small, lined by tall columnar cells with pale cytoplasm and the lumena contain a little secretion. The stroma is minimally oedematous, the spiral arteries are poorly developed and there is no pseudodecidual change. H & E × 100

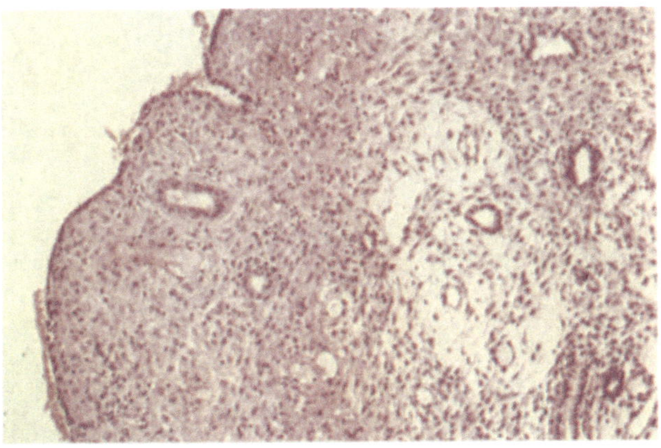

Figure 33.9 Endometrium: combined steroid contraceptive. The appearance of the endometrium on the 26th day following withdrawal bleeding in a woman taking a combination of 0.25 mg levonorgestrel and 0.05 mg ethinyloestradiol. The glands are small, narrow tubes showing neither secretory nor proliferative activity whilst the stroma shows a marked pseudodecidualized compacta. There is no spiral artery maturation. H & E × 100

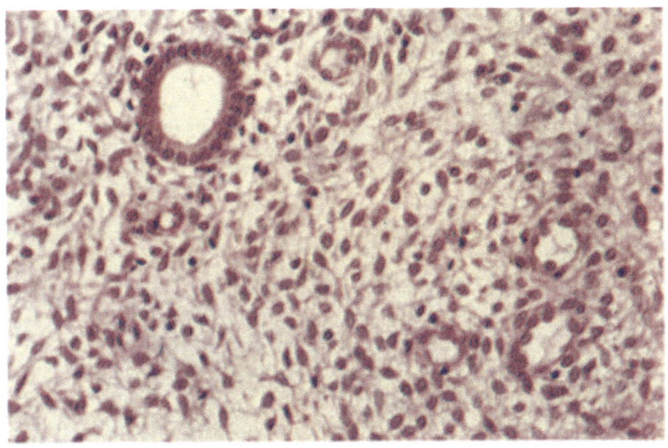

Figure 33.10 Endometrium: combined steroid contraceptive. This sample of endometrium like that in Figure 33.9 was taken on the 26th day after withdrawal bleeding in a woman using a combination of 0.25 mg levonorgestrel and 0.03 mg ethinyloestradiol. The gland is similarly inactive and the spiral arteries (to the right) poorly matured but the stroma remains spindle-celled showing virtually no pseudodecidual change. H & E × 250

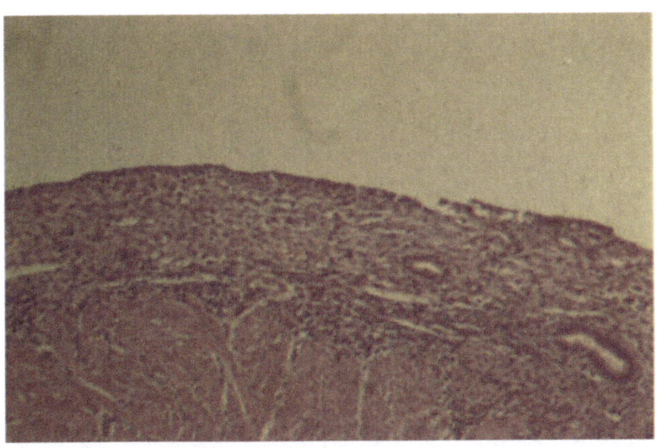

Figure 33.11 Endometrium: combined steroid contraceptive. Severe endometrial atrophy follows the prolonged use of a variety of combined steroid contraceptives. The endometrium is shallow, the stroma compact and the glands, which are narrow, show neither secretory nor proliferative activity. The specimen comes from a sterilizing hysterectomy. H & E × 100

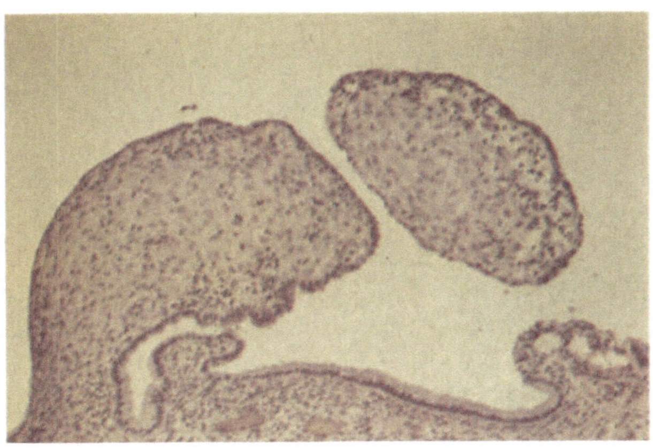

Figure 33.12 Cervix: combined steroid contraceptive. The stroma of the endocervix shows focal pseudodecidual change; the stromal cells are enlarged and have small central nuclei and copious eosinophilic cytoplasm. At the lower right corner there is a focus of microglandular hyperplasia (Figure 7.10). H & E × 100

Mechanical Contraception

34

Intrauterine contraceptive devices (IUCDs) fall into three main categories, inert, chemically active and hormonally active. Uterine perforation, usually occurring at the time of insertion, occurs in approximately 1 in 1000 patients. The perforation may be virtually asymptomatic and the device, particularly if copper coated, may, if left in the abdominal cavity, lead to peritoneal adhesions and intestinal obstruction: very rarely a device has been removed from the bladder or bowel.

Effects on the Endometrium

In most cases the effects of an IUCD on the endometrium are attributable to its acting as a foreign body. There is a generalized mild or moderate increase in stromal lymphocytes and a number of minor focal abnormalities at, or adjacent to, the site of contact with the device[1–3]. These latter changes include alterations in the surface epithelium, such as papillary changes (Figure 34.1), epithelial atypia (Figure 34.2), focal ulceration (Figure 34.3) and, occasionally, squamous metaplasia, whilst there is commonly a focal inflammatory reaction (Figures 34.4 and 34.5) characterized by the presence of neutrophil polymorphonuclear cells within glandular lumens (Figure 34.6) and of stromal plasma cells, macrophages and, occasionally, foreign body type giant cells within the stroma or glands (Figure 34.7). Microthrombi may be seen within stromal vessels adjacent to the contact site and there may be focal atrophy or stromal scarring. Focal pseudodecidual change is often present at the contact site at an inappropriate stage of the cycle (Figure 34.8): cyclical changes within the endometrium generally occur normally, but it is not uncommon to find localized irregular ripening or inadequate secretory transformation in those glands which are immediately adjacent to the contact site. These focal changes are usually most severe in women using a copper device. When the device is progestagen impregnated the endometrium will show changes similar to those seen after administration of oral progesterone, though even in these circumstances the glandular atrophy and stromal predecidual change are often clearly localized to the contact site.

In a proportion of cases a true infective endometritis complicates the use of an IUCD and this results in a diffuse inflammation of the endometrium with widespread exudation of polymorphonuclear leukocytes into the glandular lumens and a diffuse lymphoplasmacytic infiltration of the stroma (Figure 34.9). True infection, though not rare in users of copper devices, is most commonly found in women using an inert IUCD: the infection is an ascending one and is usually polymicrobiol in nature, the infecting organisms including anaerobic and microaerophilic *Streptococci*, *Bacteroides* and *Chlamydiae*. In rare instances *Actinomyces* are found[4] but their presence in curettings or in a cervical smear does not necessarily indicate an active infection, such a diagnosis requiring the identification of tissue responses to the organism (Figure 34.10). *Actinomyces* should not be confused with pseudosulphur granules which are partly calcified collections of cellular debris and fibrin, shed from the surface of the device (Figure 34.11).

Uterine Cervix

A minor degree of microglandular hyperplasia, together with reserve cell hyperplasia and immature squamous metaplasia, are commonly seen in women with IUCDs (Figure 34.12): these changes are usually focal and may be due to local mechanical irritation from the string of the device. There is commonly also a quite well marked non-specific chronic inflammatory cell infiltration in the cervix and this may be accompanied by reactive cellular atypia in the endocervical epithelium and, to a lesser extent, in metaplastic squamous epithelium.

Adnexae

An incidence of endosalpingitis, this including all degrees of severity, of up to 35% has been recorded in IUCD wearers, the frequency of this complication being greatest in young nulliparous women who frequently change their sexual partner. In many cases the endosalpingitis is mild and asymptomatic but acute symptomatic endosalpingitis still occurs three times more frequently in IUCD users than in non-users. Severe pelvic inflammatory disease (PID) is found in up to 8% of a IUCD-using population, the exact incidence varying with the nature of the population studied and the type of device used: the risk is greatest with the inert device. The various pelvic inflammatory complications encountered include tubo-ovarian abscess, intraovarian abscess, severe chronic salpingitis, peri-oophoritis, pelvic cellulitis and pelvic peritonitis: rather surprisingly, tubo-ovarian or intraovarian abscesses in IUCD users tend to be unilateral[5]. The patient is at greatest risk of developing PID in the months immediately after insertion, or re-insertion, of the device and the degree of risk is not related to the duration of use. After removal of the device ex-users have a higher inci-

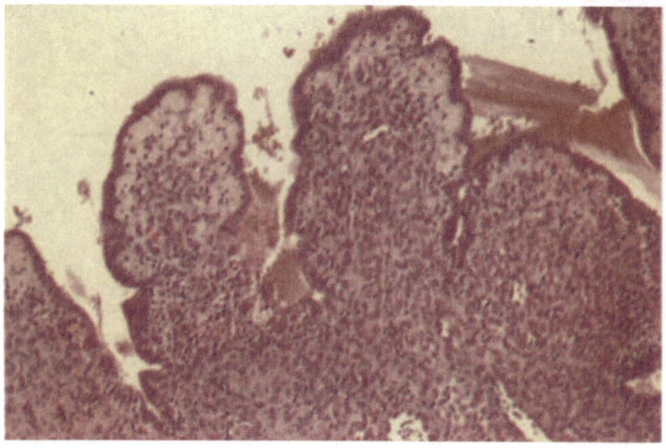

Figure 34.1 Endometrium: IUCD-associated papillary change. The biopsy was taken on the 24th day of the cycle (10th post-ovulatory day). The papillary contour of the surface corresponds to the copper wire on the stem of the device and there is focal acute non-specific inflammation. H & E × 100

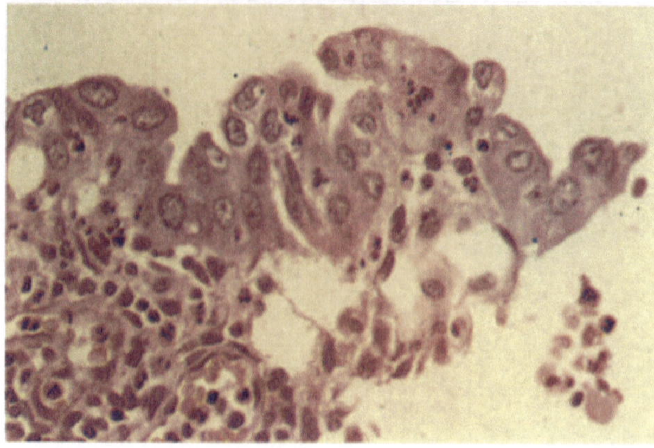

Figure 34.2 Endometrium: IUCD-associated cellular atypia. This fragment of endometrial surface epithelium shows cellular and nuclear pleomorphism. The nuclei contain irregularly dispersed chromatin and there is irregular cytoplasmic vacuolation. Similar atypia occurs in the endocervix and is usually associated with inflammation. In its extreme form, the detection of such cells in a cervical smear may suggest the presence of an adenocarcinoma. H & E × 400

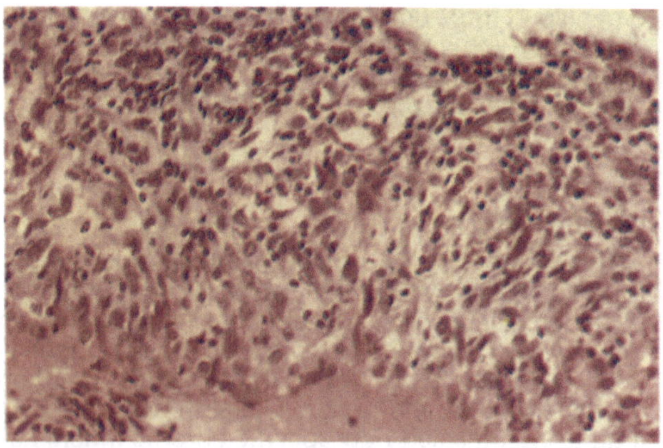

Figure 34.3 Endometrium: IUCD-associated ulceration. This fragment of non-specific granulation tissue was obtained in curettings from a woman wearing an IUCD. The surface epithelium is lost and the underlying stroma which is infiltrated by polymorphonuclear leukocytes and lymphocytes shows a pseudodecidual change and partial replacement by fibroblasts. H & E × 250

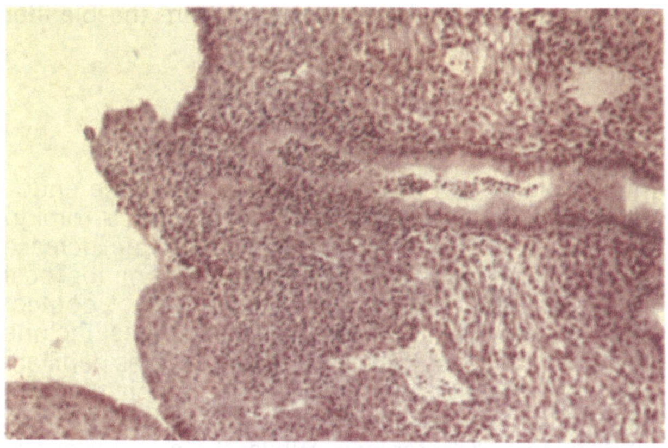

Figure 34.4 Endometrium: IUCD-associated inflammation. The inflammation in this biopsy was limited to one, sharply defined, superficial inflamed wedge (to the left). The inflammatory infiltrate consists of polymorphonuclear leukocytes, plasma cells and occasional lymphocytes. A focal inflammatory response such as this is usually the consequence of irritation rather than of infection. H & E × 100

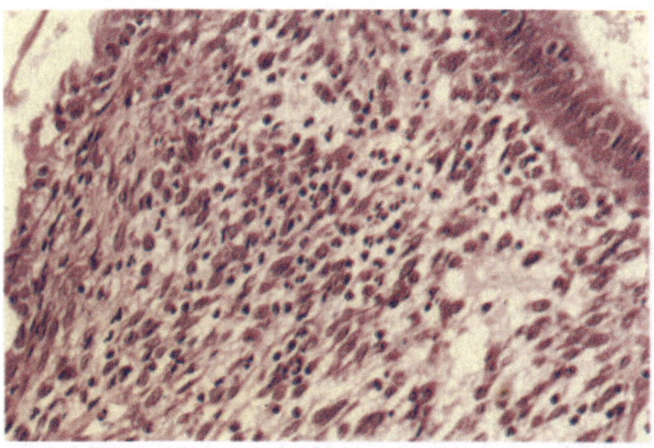

Figure 34.5 Endometrium: IUCD-associated inflammation. This biopsy from the 12th day of the cycle shows stroma focally infiltrated by a mixture of polymorphonuclear leukocytes and occasional plasma cells. The surface epithelium (to the left) shows a minor degree of reactive atypia. This appearance is very characteristic of that seen in the IUCD wearer who has inflammation limited to the contact site. H & E × 250

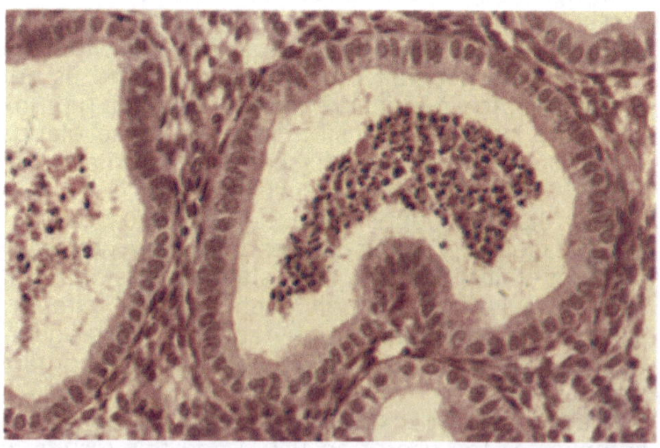

Figure 34.6 Endometrium: IUCD-associated inflammation. The glands in this secretory endometrium contain polymorphonuclear leukocytes but there is little or no interference with glandular maturation and no stromal inflammation. This biopsy which was obtained on the 22nd day of the cycle (8th post-ovulatory day) is extremely similar to the non-specific inflammatory changes seen at this stage of the menstrual cycle in some cases of endometrial tuberculosis. H & E × 250

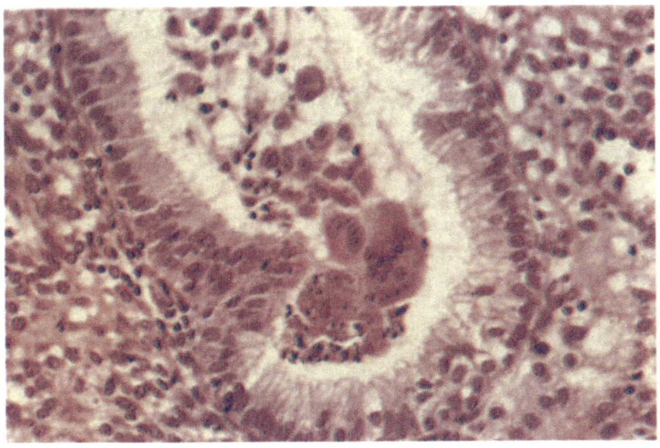

Figure 34.7 Endometrium: IUCD-associated inflammation. A biopsy taken on the 24th day of the cycle (10th post-ovulatory day) contains a gland in which there is a collection of macrophages, including macrophage giant cells. Again, the similarity to tuberculosis and the need to distinguish the two conditions is emphasized. H & E × 250

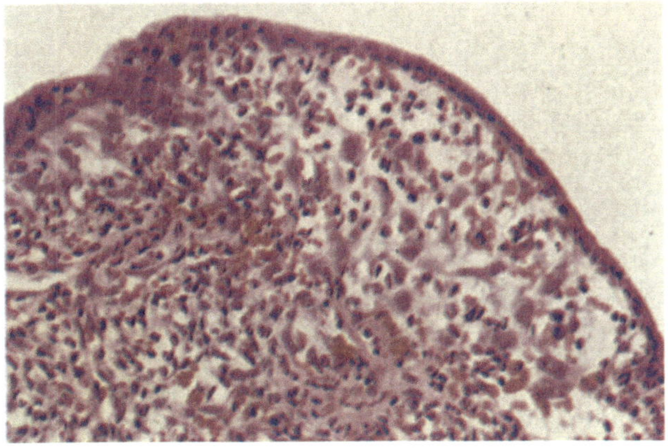

Figure 34.8 Endometrium: IUCD-associated pseudodecidual change. This biopsy from an IUCD contact site presents a very typical appearance. The surface epithelium shows a mild to moderate reactive atypia and the underlying stroma shows a poorly developed pseudodecidual change characterized by cytoplasmic eosinophilia. H & E × 250

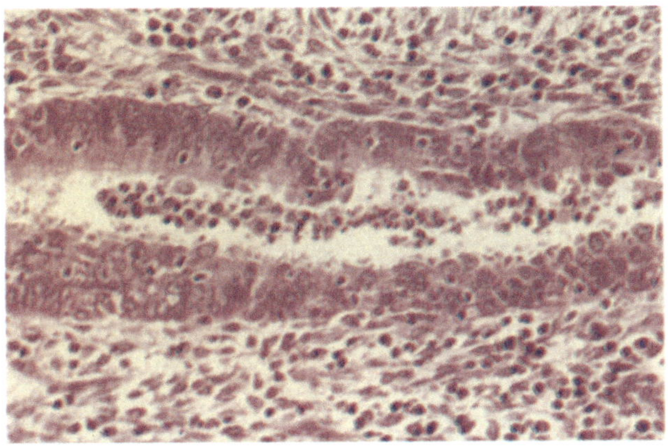

Figure 34.9 Endometrium: IUCD-associated inflammation. The endometrial gland traversing the field contains polymorphonuclear leukocytes and the stroma is heavily infiltrated by plasma cells which are most numerous in the stroma immediately adjacent to the gland. This is the appearance encountered when there is endometrial sepsis. Note that there is a failure of normal glandular maturation: this is probably due to inflammatory interference with normal receptor development. H & E × 250

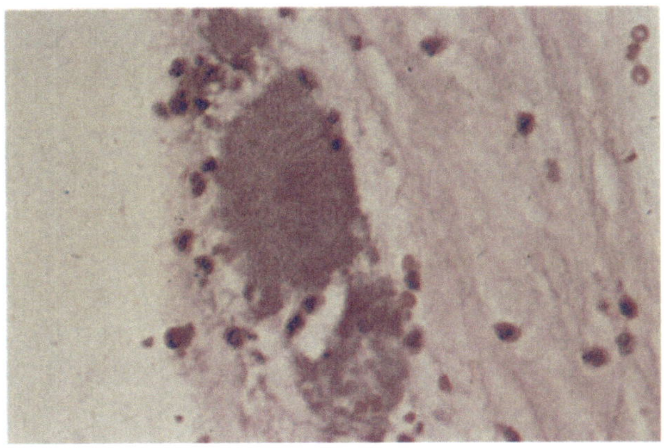

Figure 34.10 Endometrium: *Actinomyces*. In haematoxylin and eosin stained tissue sections, 'sulphur granules', colonies of *Actinomyces*, appear as clusters of eosinophilic, radiating filaments. Gram stains distinguish them from pseudo-sulphur granules (Figure 34.11) but careful microbiological cultures are required for a definite diagnosis. H & E × 400

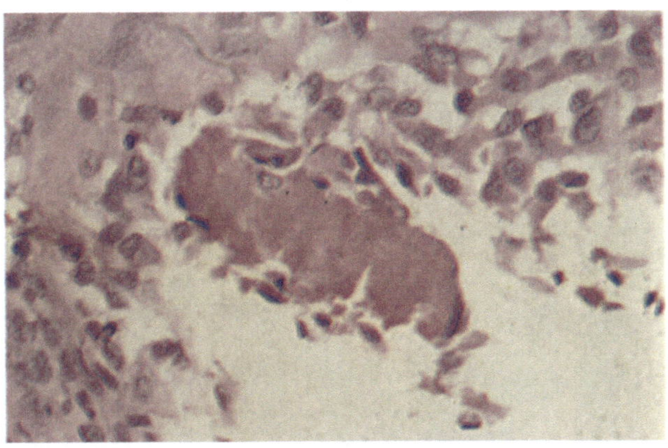

Figure 34.11 Endometrium: 'pseudo-sulphur granule'. In haematoxylin and eosin stained sections there is a strikingly close similarity between these structures which consist of cellular debris and fibrin shed from the surface of the IUCD and colonies of *Actinomyces*. Gram stains demonstrate the absence of filaments. H & E × 400

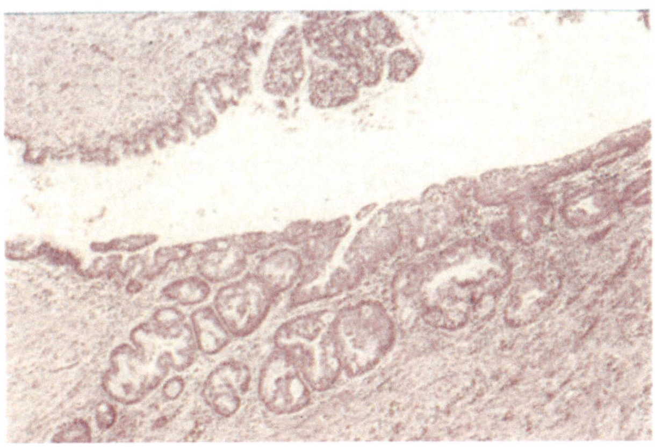

Figure 34.12 Cervix: IUCD-associated change. There is extensive immature squamous metaplasia extending into the endocervical crypt. There is no evidence of cytological atypia. H & E × 40

dence of PID than do 'never users'[6] and the risk of developing PID persists for several months[7].

In patients who have salpingeal disease there is an increased incidence of tubal ectopic gestation[8] whilst IUCD use is also associated with an increased incidence of ovarian ectopic gestation. This is not because an IUCD *causes* ectopic implantation but because although the IUCD does not prevent fertilization it does prevent uterine implantation and, to a lesser extent, inhibits tubal nidation: users have a greatly increased rate of conception, and within this context the incidence of ectopic ovarian implantation is not significantly raised.

References

1. Moyer, D. L. and Mishell, D. R. Jr. (1971). Reactions of human endometrium to the intrauterine foreign body. II. Long term effects on the endometrial histology and cytology. *Am. J. Obstet. Gynecol.*, **111**, 66–80
2. Craig, J. M. (1975). The pathology of birth control. *Arch. Pathol.*, **99**, 233–236
3. Ragni, N., Rugiati, S., Rossato, P., Venturini, P. L., Foglia, G. and Capitanio, G. L. (1977). Histological and ultrastructural changes of the endometrium in women using inert and copper-coiled IUDs. *Acta Eur. Fertil.*, **18**, 193–210
4. Bhagavan, B. S. and Gupta, P. K. (1978). Genital Actinomycosis and intrauterine contraceptive devices. *Hum. Pathol.*, **9**, 567–578
5. Ober, W. B. (1977). Effects of oral and intrauterine administration of contraceptives on the uterus. *Hum. Pathol.*, **8**, 513–527
6. Vessey, M. P., Yeates, D., Flavel, R. and McPherson, K. (1981). Pelvic inflammatory disease and the intrauterine device: findings in a large cohort study. *Br. Med. J.*, **282**, 855–857
7. Burkman, R. T. and The Women's Health Study (1981). Association between intrauterine device and pelvic inflammatory disease. *Obstet. Gynecol.*, **57**, 269–276
8. Weström, L., Bengtsson, L. Ph., and Mårdh, P-A. (1981). Incidence, trends and risks of ectopic pregnancy in a population of women. *Br. Med. J.*, **282**, 15–18

Index

(*Italics refer to figures*)

abortion
  spontaneous, incidence 147
  villi appearance 147, *32.6*
abscesses
  eosinophilic 11
  intraovarian 111, *24.3, 24.4*
acantholytic squames *1.5*
actinomycosis
  and IUCD 159, *34.11*
  ovarian abscesses 111, *24.4*
  tubal 98
adenocarcinoma
  differences with hyperplasia 70, *14.9–14.12*
  infiltration 70, *14.11*
  mitotic figures 70, *14.12*
  stromal role 70, *14.9, 14.10*
adenocarcinoma of the cervix
  clear cell 50
  endocervical, incidence and histology 47, *9.6, 9.7*
  endometrioid 47, *9.8*
  intestinal type 50
  mesonephric type 50, *9.9*
  serous 47
adenocarcinoma, endometrioid 71, *15.1–15.3*
  anaplastic cells 71, *15.3*
  clear cell 71, 74, *15.6, 15.7*
  mucinous 74, *15.8*
  poor therapy effects 74, 75, *15.12*
  secretory 74
  with squamous metaplasia 71, *15.4*
adenocarcinoma of Fallopian tube
  histology 99, *21.4*
  incidence 99
  solid growth 99, *21.5*
  staging 99
  survival rate 102
  and tuberculosis 99, *21.6*
adenocarcinoma, intraendometrial 67, 70, *14.8–14.12*
adenocarcinoma, ovary
  endometrioid 123, 126, *27.5, 27.7*
  mesonephroid 126, *27.9–27.11*
  metastatic 142, *30.11*
  mucinous 123, *27.3, 27.4*
  serous 123, *27.1, 27.2*
  undifferentiated 126, *27.11*
  vacuolated cells 124, *27.7*
adenocarcinoma, papillary of endometrium 71, *15.5*
adenocarcinoma of vagina
  clear cell 38, 50
  histological features and patterns 38, *6.7–6.9*
  increase in frequency 35
  and prenatal diethylstilboestrol 35, 38
adenoid cystic carcinoma, cervical 50, *9.12*
adenomata malignum 47, *9.7*
adenomatoid tumours
  canalicular 86, *17.6*
  cystic 86, *17.7*
  myometrium 83, 86, *17.5–17.7*
  tubular 86, *17.5*
adenomyosis
  foci 83, *17.2*
  myometrium 83, *17.1*
  pregnancy 83, *17.3*
adenosis, vaginal
  atypical changes 34, *5.9*
  epithelial metaplasia 34, *5.8*
  glandular structures 34, *5.7*
  oestrogen exposure 34
adenosquamous carcinoma
  cervix 50
  endometrium 74, *15.9, 15.10*
adnexal 159
  and IUCD 159, 162
androblastoma cell composition 133, 134
androgen insensitivity syndrome
  genotype 114
  gonad appearance 114, *24.11*
angiokeratoma, vulval in children 26, *4.9*
anovulation, forms and functional disorders 58, *11.8, 11.9*
argyrophil cells 50
Arias-Stella change 42, 147, *32.2*
Asherman's syndrome
  endometrial adhesions 62
  hyalinized endometrial stroma 62, *12.10*

Bartholin duct
  cyst 14, *1.9*
  dilated and infection 18, *2.7*
Bartholin's gland
  adenoma and age 27, *4.12*
  carcinomata types 27
  organisms infecting 18
basal cell carcinoma, vulval arrangement 26, *4.6*
basal cell papilloma, features and age 25, *4.1*
basaloid carcinoma, histology of cervical 47, *9.5*
Behçet's syndrome, vulval ulcers 18, *2.11*
benign mucosal pemphigoid 14, *1.7*
  differentiation 14
  tense bullae 14
bowenoid atypia 22
Bowen's disease 22
Brenner tumours, ovary 118
  borderline malignancy 122, *26.10*
  cystic 118, *25.9*
  fibrous 118, *25.7*
  grooved 118, *25.8*
  malignant types 126, *27.8*
broad ligament
  adnexal tumour 102, *21.8–21.10*
  adrenal cortical rest 94, *19.11*
  cysts 94, *19.12*
  embryonic remnants 94, *19.10*
  neoplasms 102
Burkitt lymphoma 142, *30.10*

Call–Exner body 133
Calymmatobacterium granulomatis 15
Canal of Nuck cysts 14
Candida albicans, features of vaginitis 31, 32
carcinoid tumours of cervix 50
carcinoma *see also individual carcinomata*
  cervix 50
  vulva, *in situ* 22, *3.7, 3.8*
carcinomata, mixed of cervix 50
caruncle, urethral 18, *2.8, 2.9*
cellular atypia 19, 22 *see also* vulval intraepithelial neoplasia
  development 22
cervical ectopy
  factors affecting 39
  metaplastic epithelium 42, *7.6*
  villous pattern 39, 42, *7.4, 7.5*
cervical epithelium at menopause 43, 46, *8.6*
cervical intraepithelial neoplasia (CIN)
  CIN I feature 43, *8.1*
  CIN II features 43, *8.2*
  CIN III features and variants 43, *8.3, 8.4*
  CIN differential diagnosis 43, 46
  definition 43
  large cell keratinizing 43
cervicitis, follicular 39, *7.1*
cervix
  carcinoid tumours 50
  epithelial abnormalities 43–6
  factors affecting bulk 39
  inflammatory disease 39–42
  microinvasive carcinomata 46, *8.9–8.11*
  mixed carcinomata 50
  neoplasms 47–50
  non-specific infection 39
  steroid effects 155, *33.2*
Chlamydia sp. cervical 39
choriocarcinoma 150, *32.11*
  fallopian tube 102
  hydatidiform mole 150
  ovarian 127
  vulval metastasis 27, *4.11*
cicatrical pemphigoid *see* benign mucosal

ciliated cell metaplasia 63
condyloma acuminatum
  vaginal 35, *6.1*
  vulval, features 25, *4.2*
  vulval, origins and virus 22, 25, *3.9*, *4.2*
condylomata of cervix, flat 46, *8.7*, *8.8*
corps ronds 14
corpus luteum
  cyst 107, *23.4*
  cyst of pregnancy 107, *23.6*
  normal in pregnancy 103, 106, *22.9*
Crohn's disease
  Fallopian tube 98, *20.11*
  ovary 111, *24.5*
  vulval, features 18, *2.10*
curettage 150
cysts
  Canal of Nuck 14
  Gartner's duct 14, 31, *1.12*, *5.3*
cysts, ovarian *see also* corpus luteum
  corpus albicans 107, *23.5*
  endometriotic 143, 144, *31.2–31.5*
  follicular 107, *23.1*, *23.2*
  germinal inclusion 110, *23.8*
  giant luteinized and pregnancy 107, *23.7*
  luteinized follicular 107, *23.3*
  theca-luteal 107, 110
cysts, paraovarian 94, *19.12*
cysts, vaginal; mesonephric 31, *5.3*
cysts, vulval 14, *1.8–1.12*
  Bartholin duct 14, *1.9*
  epidermoid and surgery 14, *1.11*
  granulomatous reaction 14
  infection 14
  mucinous, wall, 14, *1.10*
  sebaceous (pilar) 14, *1.8*

Darier's disease 11
  histological features 14
  inheritance 11
Donovan bodies 15
dysgerminomata
  anaplasm 127
  cell arrangements 127, *28.1*, *28.2*
dystrophies, vulval 19–23

ectopic pregnancy
  calcifications 94, *19.8*
  incidence 94
  IUCD role 162
  tubal site 94, *19.9*
embryonal carcinomata 127
  clefts 127, *28.3*
emphysematous cysts, popping of vagina 34, *5.5*
endodermal sinus tumours, vagina and age 38
endometrial hyperplasia 67, *14.1*, *14.7*
  adenomatoid 67, *14.3*
  cystic glandular 67, *14.1*, *14.2*
  glandular 67
  glandular and cellular atypia 67, *14.5–14.7*
endometrial stromal sarcoma
  high grade 77, *16.5*
  low grade 77, *16.2–16.4*
endometrial stromal tumours 77, *16.1*
  sex cord pattern 77, 78, *16.6*
endometrioid tumours, borderline malignancy 122, *26.9*
endometriosis 143–6
  atypia 146, *31.10*
  cervical 146, *31.6*
  Fallopian tube 146, *31.8*
  foci 47
  gastrointestinal 146, *31.7*
  hormone effects 146, *31.9*
  malignancy 146, *31.11*
  pathogenic mechanisms 143
  pathology 143, *31.1*
  sites 143
endometriosis, ovarian
  cyst 143, 146, *31.2–31.5*
endometritis
  epithelial neoplasms 71–5
  granulomatous 59, 62, *12.6*
  histiocytic 59, *12.2*
  infective features 59, *12.3–12.5*
  and malakoplakia 59
  non-infective 59, *12.1*
  non-tuberculous 62
  polymorph infiltrate 59, *12.1*
endometrium
  basal layer 51, *10.1*
  cyclical changes 51–4
  disordered proliferative 154, *33.6*
  glycogen secretion 55
  hormonal effects 153–7
  inflammatory disease 59–62
  isthmus 51, *10.2*
  menopause 54, *10.11*
  menstruation 54, *10.9*, *10.10*
  metaplasia 63–6
  ovarian function 51, *10.1*, *10.2*
  pregnancy 147, *32.1–32.4*
  proliferative phase 51, *10.3*
  secretory phases 51, 54, *10.4–10.8*
  senile cystic 54, *10.12*
  spiral artery development 54, 55
endometrium, functional disturbances
  delayed shedding 58, *11.7*
  follicular phase length 55
  irregular ripening 55, *11.4*
  luteal phase deficiency 55, *11.1–11.3*
  oestrogen persistence 55, 58, *11.5*
  short luteal phase 58, *11.6*
  spiral artery 55
endosalpingiosis 146, *31.12*
endosalpingitis
  causes 95
  exudate 95, *20.1*
  reactive cellular atypia 95, *20.2*
eosinophilic metaplasia, endometrium 63, *13.4*
epidermoid cysts of vagina 34, *5.4*
erythroplasia of Queyrat 82 *see also* carcinoma, vulval

Fallopian tube
  cyclic and hormonal effects 91, *19.2*, *19.3*
  embryonic remnants 94, *19.10*
  epithelial metaplasia 91, *19.5*
  inflammatory conditions 95–8
  normal appearance 91, *19.1*
  oestrogenic stimulation 91, *19.4*
  prolapse and metastasis 34, *5.6*
  sterilization effects 91, 94, *19.6*, *19.7*
  steroid effects 155
Fallopian tube neoplasias 99–102
  adenofibroma 99, *21.2*
  benign 99, *21.1*
  intraepithelial 99, *21.3*
  malignant 99–102
familial benign pemphigus (Hailey–Hailey disease) 14, *1.5*
  brick wall appearance *1.6*
  inheritance 14
  Malphigian layer 14
α-fetoprotein 127
fibroma, ovary 139, *30.1*

Gardnerella vaginalis, infection features 31
Gartner's duct
  cysts 14, 42, *1.12*, *7.12*
  description 42
glassy cell carcinoma, features of cervical 50
gonad
  abnormal differentiation 114
  streak 114, *24.10*
gonadoblastoma, ovary 109, *30.4*
granular cell tumour, vulval 26, 27, *4.10*
granuloma inguinale
  lesions 15, *2.3*, *2.4*
  vulva features 15
granulosa cell tumours of ovary 133
  diffuse 133, *29.4*
  insular pattern 133, *29.2*
  juvenile 133, *29.5*
  microfollicules 133, *29.1*
  oestrogenic 133
  trabecular pattern 133, *29.3*
gynandroblastomas 134

haemangiopericytoma
  myometrial diagnosis 86
  reticulum fibres 86, *17.12*
  undifferentiated mesenchyme 86, *17.10*
  vascular pattern 86, *17.11*
Hailey-Hailey disease *see* familial benign pemphigus
herpes infections of cervix
  features 39
  histology, ground glass 39, *7.2*
herpes simplex
  symptoms of infection 15
  vaginitis 31
  vulva infections 15
hob-nail metaplasia, endometrium 66, 74
hydatidiform mole 147
  partial 150, *32.10*
  trophoblastic hyperplasia 150, *32.9*
  types 150
  XX paternal 150
hydropic degeneration 11
hydrosalpinx 95, 98
  histology 98, *20.7*
hydrosalpinx follicularis, features 95, *20.6*
hyperplasia and neoplasia in endometrium 70
hyperplastic dystrophy, vulva
  condtions classed 19
  histology 19, *3.1*
  incidence 19

infections 15–18
intrauterine contraceptive devices (IUCD) 98
  adnexal effects 159, 162
  cellular atypia 159, *34.2*

intrauterine contraceptive devices – *continued*
cervix effects 159, *34.12*
ectopic pregnancy 162
endometrial effects 159, *34.1–34.11*
infection 159, *34.10, 34.11*
inflammation 159, *34.4–34.9*
myometritis 83, *17.4*
organisms infecting 159, *34.4*
papillary change 159, *34.1*
pseudodecidual change 159, *34.8*
and tuberculosis 59
types 159
ulceration 159, *34.3*
IUCD *see* intrauterine contraceptive device

keratoacanthoma appearance 25
keratosis follicularis *see* Darier's disease
Krukenberg tumours, ovary 142, *30.12*

leiomyomata
cellular variant 87, *18.4*
clear cell 87, *18.5*
cystic degeneration 87, *18.3*
epithelioid 87
histology 87, *18.1*
hyaline degeneration 87, *18.2*
nuclear palisading 90, *18.9*
plexiform 87, *18.6*
symplastic, giant cells 87, *18.7*
unusual growth 90, *18.9*
leiomyomatosis peritonealis, dissemination 90, *18.10*
leiomyosarcoma
myometrial 90, *18.11, 18.12*
uterine, survival rate 90
vaginal 38
Leydig cell tumours 134, *29.8*
androgenic 134
lichen nitidus 11, *1.3*
intradermal lymphocyte foci 11, *1.3*
lichen planus 11, *1.2*
histological features in vulva 11, *1.2*
lichen sclerosis of vulva 19
bullae 19, *3.3*
histology of vulval lesion 19, *3.2*
hyperplastic dystrophy 19, *3.4*
lipoid cell neoplasms of ovary 139, 140, *30.7*
lymphangiocystic fibroma 86, *17.9*
lymphogranuloma venereum
Chlamydia sp. cause 15
symptoms 15

malakoplakia
causes 62
histology 62, *12.9*
malignant lymphoma of the ovary 142
Burkitt 142, *30.10*
cytological features 142, *30.9*
histology 142, *30.8*
malignant melanoma
cervix 50
growth patterns 26, *4.5*
incidence in vulva 26
staging 26
vaginal 38
malignant mesothelioma 86, *17.8*
menopause
cervical epithelium 43, *8.6*
endometrium 54, *10.12*
ovary 106
premature 114
menstrual cycle and endometrium 51
mesonephroid tumours, borderline malignancy 122, *26.12*
mesothelioma 118, *25.11*
Michaelis–Gutman bodies 59
microglandular hyperplasia
cell infiltration 42, *7.10*
cervix, histology 42, *7.10*, 7.11
microinvasive lesions of cervix
definition 46
early stromal 46, *8.9, 8.10*
microcarcinoma 46, *8.11*
molluscum contagiosum
virus shedding 15
vulva lesions 15, *2.1, 2.2*
Monroe abscesses 11, *1.1*
mucinous metaplasia, endometrium 63, *13.5*
mucinous tumours of ovary
borderline malignancy 119, *26.4–26.8*
glandular epithelium 119, *26.5*
pseudomyxoma peritonii 122, *26.7*
pseudosarcoma 122, *26.8*
serrated 122, *26.6*
muco-epidermoid carcinomata, cervix 50, *9.10, 9.11*
Müllerian tumours, endometrium mixed
benign mixed 78, *16.7*
carcinosarcoma 78, *16.9*
high grade malignancy 78, *16.9–16.12*
low grade, malignancy 78, *16.8*
mixed mesenchyme sarcoma 78, *16.10*
rhabdomyoblasts 78

myometrial hypertrophy, uterine weight 83
myometritis 83, *17.4*
myometrium, hypertrophy and hormones 154
myometrium tumours 83–6 *see also* smooth muscle neoplasms

Neisseria gonorrhoeae 18
vaginal, features 31
neurolemmoma 87, 90

oestrogen–progestagen combination
combined effects 154
endometrial atrophy 154, *33.11*
endometrial effects 154
gland appearance 154, *33.9, 33.10*
secretory phase 154, *33.8*
sequential effects 154
subnuclear vacuoles 154, *33.7*
oestrogens
endometrial effects 153, 154, *33.6*
prenatal exposure 35, 38
oophoritis, acute 111, *24.2*
oral contraception *see* oestrogens, progestogens
ovarian tumours, prognostic criteria 119
ovary *see also* corpus luteum
borderline malignant tumours 119–22
disorders 111–14
epithelium 103, *22.1, 22.2*
epithelium origin 115
follicular atresia 106, *22.10*
germ cell neoplasms 127–31
gonadotrophin resistance 114, *24.9*
hilar cells 106, *22.11, 22.12*
hilar vasculature 139, *30.3*
infertile 111
luteoma of pregnancy 110, *23.10*
malignant epithelial neoplasia 123–6
metastatic tumours 142, *30.11, 30.12*
non-specialized tissue tumours 139
normal 103–6
oedema 110, *23.9*
polycystic 110
post menopause 106
postovulatory follicle 103, *22.6–22.8*
preovulatory follicle 103, *22.3–22.5*
steroid effects 155
stromal hyperplasia 110, *23.12*
ovary, benign neoplasm 115–19
endometrioid 118, *25.6*
histiogenesis concept 115
incidence 115
mesonephroid 118, *25.10*
mucinous 115, 118, *25.3–25.5*
serous 115, *25.1, 25.2*
stromal luteinization 118, *25.12*
ovotestis 114, *24.12*

Paget's disease
dermis invasion 22, 23
neoplasia associated 22
vulval 22, *3.12*
Paneth cells 118, *25.5*
papillary hidradenoma, vulval benign neoplasm 26, *4.7*
papillary metaplasia of endometrium 63, *13.6, 13.7*
pelvic inflammatory disease 159
pemphigus vegitans 11
pemphigus vulgaris 11, *1.4*
bullae in vagina 11, *1.4*
epithelial antibodies 11, *1.4*
peri-oophoritis 111
fibrous tissue 111, *24.1*
Peutz–Jeghers syndrome 134
placenta
in abortion 147, *32.6, 32.7*
endometrial site 147, *32.4*
placental site trophoblastic tumour 151, *32.12*
polycystic ovary 110, 111
atretic follicles 111, *24.6–24.8*
thickened capsule 111, *24.7*
polyps, cervical
and age 42
fibroblast enlargement 42, *7.9*
hyperplastic epithelium 42, *7.8*
polyps, endometrial 66, *13.9, 13.10*
adenomyomatous 66, *13.11*
polyps, vaginal
fibroepithelial, stroma 34, *5.10, 5.11*
pregnancy *see also* ectopic, placenta
early 147, *32.3*
normal, endometrial changes 147, *32.1–32.4*
trophoblastic disease 150, 151 *see also* hydatidiform mole, choriocarcinoma
progesterone *see also* oestrogen
and endometriosis 146
levels and ovulation 55
progestagens
abnormal endometrium 153, *33.5*
endometrial effects 153, *33.1–33.4*
low dose contraceptives and endometrium 153, *33.3, 33.4*
stromal pseudodecidualization 153, *33.1, 33.2*

psammoma bodies 123
pseudosulphur granules 159, *34.11*
psoriasis 11, *1.1*
histological features 11, *1.1*
inheritance 11
puerperium, vascular abnormalities 150, *32.8*
pyosalpinx 95, *20.5*

Reinke's crystals 134
rhabdomyomata features 35, *6.2*

salpingitis
interstitial 95, *20.3, 20.4*
microabscesses 95, *20.4*
salpingitis, granulomatous
calcifications 98, *20.9*
hyperplasia 98, *20.10*
infective, forms 98
Schaumann bodies 98, *20.8*
tuberculous incidence 98
salpingitis isthmica nodosa 98, *20.12*
sarcoma
cervix 50
incidence of vulval 27
sarcoma botyroides
and age 38
histological features 38, *6.10, 6.11*
Schiller–Duval bodies 127
Schistosoma haematobium 18
schistosomiasis, vulva involvement 18, *2.5, 2.6*
serous tumours, ovary
borderline malignancy 119, *26.1–26.3*
fibrous 119, *26.1*
layered epithelium 119, *26.2*
Sertoli cell tumours 134, *29.7*
Sertoli–Leydig cell tumours
cell composition 134, *29.9, 29.10*
poorly differentiated tumours 134, *29.11*
sex cord stromal neoplasms of ovary 133–7
annular tubules 134, *29.12*
mixed germ cell 139, *30.4–30.6*
smooth muscle neoplasms
and malignancy 90
myometrium 87–90
squamous cell carcinoma, cervix
histology 47, *9.1–9.4*
incidence 47
large cell keratinizing 47, *9.1*
large cell non-keratinizing 47, *9.2*
single cell non-keratinizing 47, *9.3*
spindle cell form 47, *9.4*
squamous cell carcinoma, endometrium 74, *15.11*
squamous cell carcinoma, vaginal
and age 35
histological features 35, *6.6*
incidence 35
survival rate 35
squamous cell carcinoma, vulval
frequency 25
grading 25
histology 25, *4.3*
labia origin 25
microinvasive, features 22, *3.11*
rete ridge *3.11*
squamous metaplasia
cervix 46
endometrium 63, 71, *13.1–13.3, 15.4*
IUCD 63
keratinizing 63, *13.1, 13.2*
morules 63, *13.3*
Staphylococcus spp., Bartholin's gland 18
Stein–Leventhal syndrome *see* polycystic ovary
stromal metaplasia 66, *13.8*
stromal tumour, sclerosing of ovary 139, *30.2*
sweat gland tumours and Paget's disease 26, *4.8*
syphilis
chancre 18
vulva features and development 18

teratomata of ovary 130, 131
immature grading 130, *28.9*
insular carcinoid 130, *28.10*
mature cystic 130, *28.6*
mature solid 130, *28.7, 28.8*
monodermal 130, 131, *28.10–28.12*
stromal carcinoid 131, *28.12*
trabecular carcinoid 130, *28.11*
thecomata of ovary, features 133, *29.6*
therapy, poor and endometrial carcinoma 74, 75, *15.12*
Treponema pallidum 18
Trichomonas vaginalis
cervix infection 39, *7.3*
features in vagina 31, *5.2*
tuberculosis
and granulomatous endometritis 59, 62, *12.6, 12.7*
IUCD 59
menopause 62, *12.8*
salpingitis 98
tubal 59
tumours *see also* individual tumours
benign epithelial 25
endometrial 77–81
malignant epithelial 25, 26
metastatic of vagina 38, *6.12*
metastatic vulval 127, *4.11*
mixed of vagina 35, *6.3*
ovary 115–42
Turner's mosaic 114
Turner's syndrome 114, *24.10*

urethra
caruncle 18, *2.8, 2.9*
tumours 26
uterus prolapse, cervical inflammation 42, *7.7*

vagina
cysts 31, 34, *5.3–5.5*
inflammation 5
neoplasms 35–8
non neoplastic conditions 31–4
prolapse 31, *5.1*
ulceration and tampons 31
vaginal intraepithelial neoplasia (VAIN)
grading criteria 35, *6.4, 6.5*
progression 35
vaginitis
atrophic and oestrogen levels 31
infective, causes 31
non-infective, causes 31, *5.1*
verrucous carcinoma
cervix 47
diagnostic features, vulval 26, *4.4*
virilization 110
vulva
cysts 14
dermatological disorders 11-14
epithelial abnormalities 19–23
inflammatory disease 15–18
neoplasms 25–7
skin appendage tumours 26
vulval intraperitoneal neoplasia 19, 22
epithelial pearls 22, *3.10*
invasive carcinoma 19
mild atypia 22, *3.5*
moderate atypia 22, *3.6*
recognition 22
severe atypia 22, *3.7*

Wickham's striae 11, *1.2*

yolk sac tumours 127, *28.4*
polyvesicular vitelline 127, *28.5*

Zollinger-Ellison syndrome 118

GPSR Compliance

The European Union's (EU) General Product Safety Regulation (GPSR) is a set of rules that requires consumer products to be safe and our obligations to ensure this.

If you have any concerns about our products, you can contact us on ProductSafety@springernature.com

In case Publisher is established outside the EU, the EU authorized representative is:

Springer Nature Customer Service Center GmbH
Europaplatz 3
69115 Heidelberg, Germany

Batch number: 10585057

Printed by Printforce, the Netherlands